Pharmaceutics

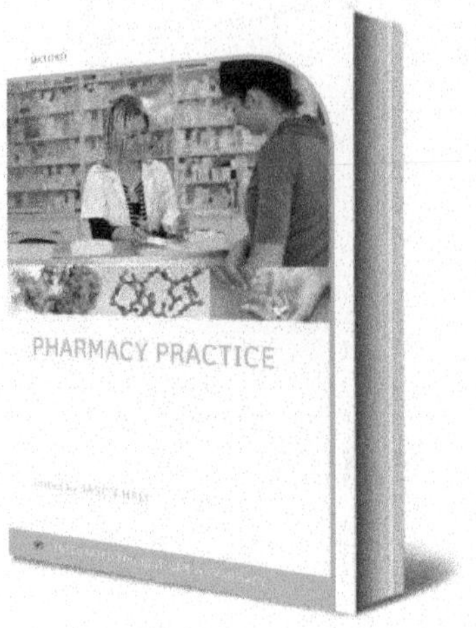

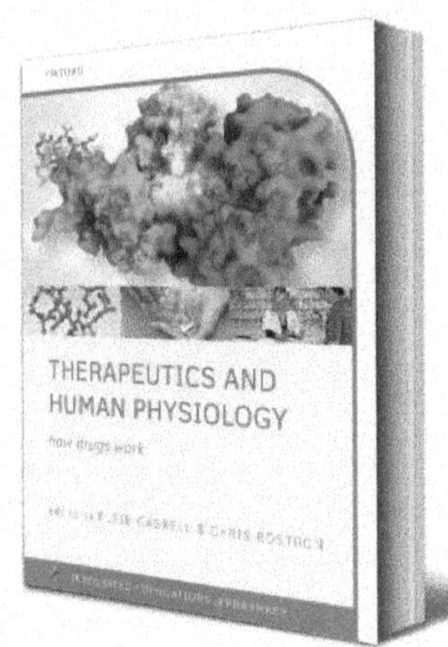

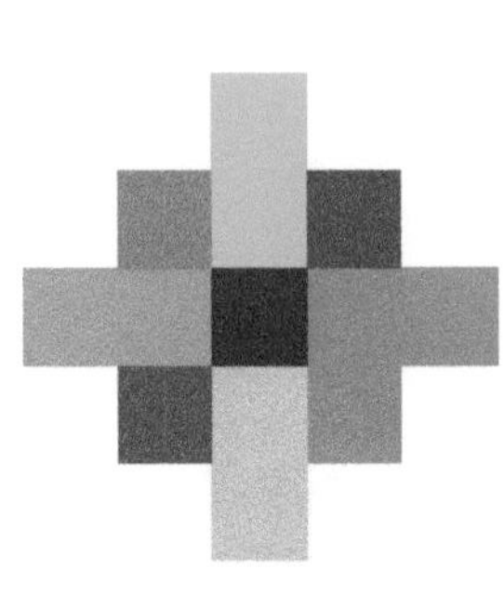

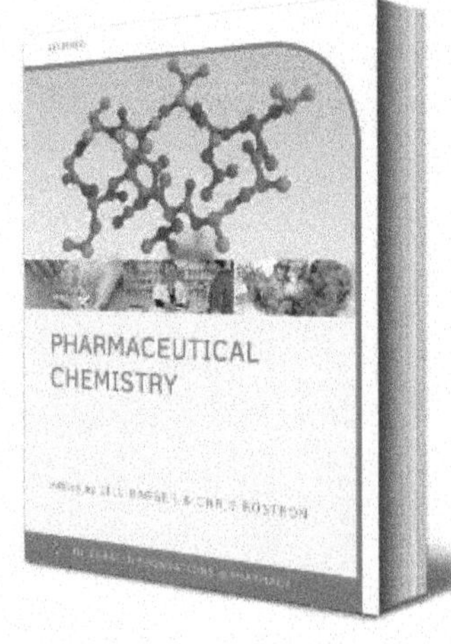

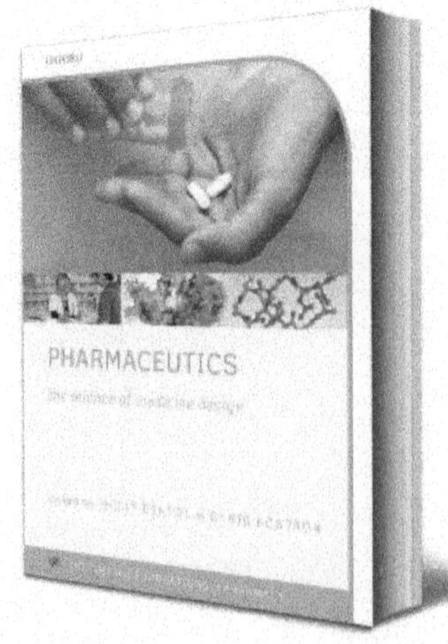

INTEGRATED FOUNDATIONS *of* PHARMACY

Pharmaceutics

The Science of Medicine Design

Edited by Philip Denton and Chris Rostron

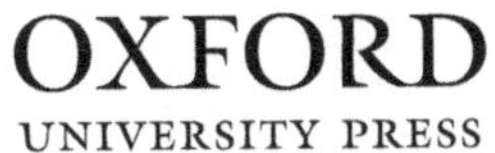

OXFORD
UNIVERSITY PRESS

INTEGRATED FOUNDATIONS *of* PHARMACY

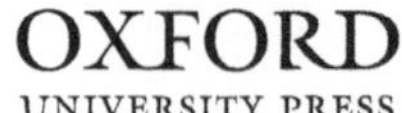

Great Clarendon Street, Oxford, OX2 6DP,
United Kingdom

Oxford University Press is a department of the University of Oxford. It furthers the University's objective of excellence in research, scholarship, and education by publishing worldwide. Oxford is a registered trade mark of Oxford University Press in the UK and in certain other countries

Impression: 10

British Library Cataloguing in Publication Data
Data available

ISBN 978–0–19–965531–1

Printed in Great Britain by
Ashford Colour Press Ltd, Gosport, Hampshire

Preface

As a result of significant changes taking place within the profession of pharmacy, there is an increasing trend for universities to adopt an integrated approach to pharmacy education. There is now an overwhelming view that pharmaceutical science must be combined with the more practice-oriented aspects of pharmacy. This assists students to see the impact of, and relationships between, those subjects which make up the essential knowledge base for a practising pharmacist.

This series supports integrated pharmacy education, so that from day one of the course students can take a professionally relevant approach to their learning. This is achieved through the organization of content and the use of key learning features. Cross-references highlight related topics of importance, directing the reader to further information; Integration Boxes flag relevant topics in a different strand of pharmacy; and Case Studies explore the ways in which pharmaceutical science and practice impacts upon patients' lives, allowing material to be addressed in a patient-centred context.

There are four books in the series, covering each main strand: *Pharmaceutical Chemistry*, *Pharmaceutics: The Science of Medicine Design*, *Pharmacy Practice*, and *Therapeutics and Human Physiology: How Drugs Work*. Each book is edited by a subject expert, with contributors from across pharmacy education. They have been carefully written to ensure an appropriate breadth and depth of knowledge for the first year student. Each book concludes with an overview of the subject and application to pharmacy, building on students' understanding of the concepts and bringing it all together. It applies the material to pharmacy practice in a variety of ways and places it in the context of all four pharmacy strands.

Pharmaceutics: The Science of Medicine Design

Put simply, pharmaceutics is the scientific study of converting a pharmacologically active compound (drug) into a commercially available pharmaceutical product (medicine). Pharmaceutics is therefore not concerned with the chemical synthesis of the drug and this topic is covered within the *Pharmaceutical Chemistry* book in this series. The physicochemical properties of a drug are of importance within pharmaceutics, however, as these will influence the selection of dosage form. The study of the body's response to an administered dosage form is considered within *Therapeutics and Human Physiology: How Drugs Work*. By comparison, pharmaceutics includes the study of the design of dosage forms. This might involve, for example, formulating a drug in the form of an oral sustained release (SR) tablet so that it may be administered less frequently.

Each of the chapters in this book is written by a subject expert and together they cover the main inter-related themes of dosage form design and the physicochemical properties of drugs. Medicine manufacturing techniques, including the control of microorganisms, represent another branch of pharmaceutics and these are introduced at various points throughout the book. Although not strictly a topic within pharmaceutics, the packaging of medicines is considered within this volume as it directly impacts on the quality of the dosage form that is presented to the patient. Chapter 1 provides further information on where specific topics are covered. It is recommended that you read this chapter first if you are new to this subject as it also defines some technical terms that are used throughout this book.

Philip Denton and Chris Rostron, January 2013

Acknowledgements

The editors wish to acknowledge the support of all the contributing authors who have spent a considerable amount of time writing and reviewing their chapters. We would also like to extend our thanks to the staff at Oxford University Press, especially Holly Edmundson and Alice Mumford (Publishing Editors) for their continued support, encouragement, and guidance. In addition we are grateful to Jonathan Crowe and Philippa Hendry for their assistance with preparing the manuscripts.

The supportive feedback from the reviewers: Dr Paul Carter, Dr Colin Melia, Dr Bridgeen Callan, and an anonymous reviewer was greatly appreciated.

Finally we would like to thank out past, present, and future students who have motivated the production of this book.

Contents

An introduction to the *Integrated Foundations of Pharmacy* series

The path to becoming a qualified pharmacist is incredibly rewarding, but it requires diligence. Not only will you need to assimilate knowledge from a range of disciplines, but you must also understand—and demonstrate—how to apply this knowledge in a practical, hands-on environment. This series is written to support you as you encounter the challenges of pharmacy education today.

There are a range of features used in the series, each carefully designed to help you master the material and to encourage to you to see the connections between the different strands of the discipline.

Mastering the material

Boxes

Additional material that adds interest or depth to concepts covered in the main text is provided in the Boxes.

> BOX 2.1
>
> **Bacteria versus archaea**
>
> Archaea are often found living in some of the most extreme environments found on Earth, in conditions where humans would not be able to survive. These

Key points

The important 'take home messages' that you must have a good grasp of are highlighted in the Key points. You may find these form a helpful basis for your revision.

> KEY POINT
>
> All our cells contain identical genetic information; however the cells differentiate to make up the various types of tissues, organs, and body systems that we are made of.

Self-check questions

Questions are provided throughout the chapters in order for you to test your understanding of the material. Take the time to complete these, as they will allow you to evaluate how you are getting on, and they will undoubtedly aid your learning. Answers are provided at the back of each volume.

> SELF CHECK 1.2
>
> Why may it be important for health care professionals to establish the family medical history?

Further reading

In this section, we direct you to additional resources that we encourage you to seek out, in your library or online. They will help you to gain a deeper understanding of the material presented in the text.

> FURTHER READING
>
> Boarder, M., Newby, D., and Navti, P. *Pharmacology for Pharmacy and the Health Sciences: A Patient-Centred Approach.* Oxford University Press, 2010.

Glossary

You will need to master a huge amount of new terminology as you study pharmacy. The glossaries in each volume should help you with this. Glossary terms are shown in pink.

> **ACE inhibitor** Drug that inhibits angiotensin-converting enzyme.
>
> **Acetylcholine (Ach)** The neurotransmitter at preganglionic autonomic neurons and postganglionic parasympathetic neurons and at the neuromuscular junction. It acts on nicotinic and muscarinic receptors. Unusually, acetylcholine is also released from sympathetic nerves that

Online resources

Visit the Online Resource Centre for related materials, including 10 multiple choice questions for each chapter, with answers and feedback.

Go to: **www.oxfordtextbooks.co.uk/orc/ifp**

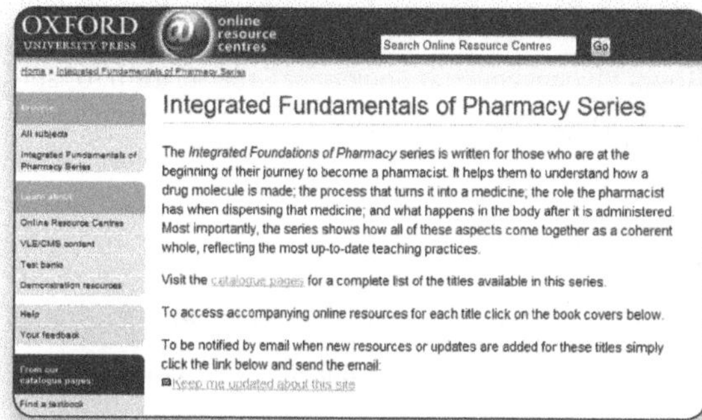

Seeing the connections

Case studies

Case studies show how the science you learn at university will impact on how you might advise a patient. Reflection questions and sample answers encourage you to think critically about the points raised in the case study.

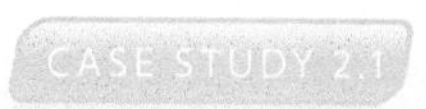

Angela has told Ravi she is pregnant and they are both thrilled at the prospect of being parents. However, Angela had an older brother who had cystic fibrosis (CF)

Cross references

Linking related sections across all four volumes in the series (as well as other sections within this volume), cross references will give you a good idea of just how integrated the subject is. Importantly, it will allow you to easily access material on the same subject, as viewed from the perspectives of the different strands of the discipline.

The study of dosage forms is covered in the **Pharmaceutics** book within this series.

Lecturer support materials

For registered adopters of the volumes in this series, the Online Resource Centre also features figures in electronic format, available to download, for use in lecture presentations and other educational resources.

To register as an adopter, visit www.oxfordtextbooks.co.uk/orc/ifp, select the volume you are interested in, and follow the on-screen instructions.

Any comments?

We welcome comments and feedback about any aspect of the series. Just visit www.oxfordtextbooks.co.uk/orc/feedback and share your views.

About the editors

Editor, Dr Phillip Denton, completed both his first and higher degrees at the University of East Anglia, Norwich. After completing a Postgraduate Certificate in Education (PGCE) at the University of Manchester, he taught 'A' level Chemistry in the Further Education Sector for 3 years. In 1998 he was appointed as a Lecturer in Physical Chemistry at Liverpool John Moores University. He is a Fellow of the Higher Education Academy (FHEA) and holds a Postgraduate Certificate (PGCert) in Learning and Teaching in Higher Education. His research work has investigated the relationship between molecular structure and (bio)chemical reactivity. More recently, he has developed computer systems to support lecturers as part of his role as Learning Development Manager within the Faculty of Science at Liverpool John Moores University.

Series Editor, Dr Chris Rostron, graduated in Pharmacy from Manchester University and completed a PhD in Medicinal Chemistry at Aston University. He gained Chartered Chemist status in 1975. After a period of post-doctoral research he was appointed as a lecturer in Medicinal Chemistry at Liverpool Polytechnic. He is now an Honorary Research Fellow in the School of Pharmacy and Biomolecular Sciences at Liverpool John Moores University. Prior to this he was an Academic Manager, and then a Reader in Medicinal Chemistry at the school. He was a member of the Academic Pharmacy Group Committee of the Royal Pharmaceutical Society of Great Britain and chairman for the past 5 years. He is currently chairman of the Academic Pharmacy Forum and deputy chair of the Education Expert Advisory Panel of the Royal Pharmaceutical Society. He is a past and present external examiner in Medicinal Chemistry at a number of Schools of Pharmacy both in the UK and abroad. In 2008 he was awarded honorary membership of the Royal Pharmaceutical Society of Great Britain for services to Pharmacy education.

Contributors

Professor Barbara Conway, Division of Pharmacy and Pharmaceutical Sciences, University of Huddersfield, UK

Dr Matthew Roberts, School of Pharmacy and Biomolecular Sciences, Liverpool John Moores, UK

Dr Ben Forbes, Institute of Pharmaceutical Science, King's College London, UK

Dr Linda Seton, School of Pharmacy and Biomolecular Sciences, Liverpool John Moores, UK

Dr Judith Madden, School of Pharmacy and Biomolecular Sciences, Liverpool John Moores, UK

Dr Steve Enoch, School of Pharmacy and Biomolecular Sciences, Liverpool John Moores, UK

Dr William McAuley, School of Pharmacy, University of Hertfordshire, UK

Dr Imran Saleem, School of Pharmacy and Biomolecular Sciences, Liverpool John Moores, UK

Ali Al-Khattawi, Aston Pharmacy School, Aston University, UK

Professor Jayne Lawrence, Institute of Pharmaceutical Science, King's College London, UK

Dr Gary Moss, School of Pharmacy, Keele University, UK

Craig A. Russell, Aston Pharmacy School, Aston University, UK

Dr Afzal R. Mohammed, Aston Pharmacy School, Aston University, UK

Abbreviations

ADME(T)	Absorption, distribution, metabolism, and excretion (and toxicology)
API	Active pharmaceutical ingredient
BBB	Blood–brain barrier
CMC	Critical micelle concentration
CNS	Central nervous system
CSF	Cerebrospinal fluid
DMSO	Dimethyl sulphoxide
DPI	Dry powder inhaler
DSC	Differential scanning calorimetry
DTO	Deodorized tincture of opium
EMA	European Medical Agency
FBLD	Fragment-based lead discovery
FDA	United States Food and Drug Administration
GIT	Gastrointestinal tract
HLB	Hydrophile–lypophile balance
HPLC	High pressure/precision liquid chromatography
HTS	High-throughput screening
IA	Intra-arterial
IC	Intracardiac
IC50	Half maximal inhibitory concentration
ID	Intradermal
IM	Intramuscular
IT	Intrathecal
IV	Intravenous
LE	Ligand efficiency
LiPE	Lipophilicity
MAD	Multiple ascending dose
MDI	Metered dose inhaler
MTD	Maximum tolerated dose
NCE	New chemical entity
o/w	Oil in water
o/w/o	Oil in water in oil
ODT	Orally disintegrating or orodispersible tablet
OROS™	Osmotic-controlled release oral delivery system
OTC	Over-the-counter
PAMPA	Parallel artificial membrane permeability assay
QSAR	Quantitative structure–activity relationship
SAD	Single ascending dose
SAR	Structure–activity relationship
SC	Subcutaneous
SDS	Sodium dodecyl sulphate
SLS	Sodium lauryl sulphate
STP	Standard temperature and pressure
TLC	Thin layer chromatography
TPN	Total parenteral nutrition
UV	Ultraviolet
vHTS	Virtual high-throughput screening
w/o	Water in oil
w/o/w	Water in oil in water
WFI	Water for injection

1

Introduction to pharmaceutics

PHILIP DENTON

Think about the last time that you were inside a high street pharmacy (Figure 1.1). Behind the sales counter, you would have seen a range of over-the-counter (OTC) medications in various packages. You may have glimpsed the area where the prescription-only medicines are stored. All these pharmaceutical products are designed to prevent, alleviate, or treat a medical condition, from coughs and colds to mental disorders. Perhaps you have wondered how these products came to be there.

All pharmaceutical products start their life as a **drug**, a chemical compound that interacts with a target in the body and exhibits desirable **pharmacology**. Subject to satisfying regulatory requirements, it would be made available commercially as a medicine. Consider the last two sentences and notice how the description of the pharmaceutical product changes from 'drug' to 'medicine'. This transition is called **formulation** and pharmaceutics is the science of converting a drug into a form that is suitable for presenting to the patient as a medicinal dose. More succinctly, pharmaceutics is the study of **dosage form** design.

FIGURE 1.1 A typical high street pharmacy
Source: Copyright iStockphoto/georgeclerk

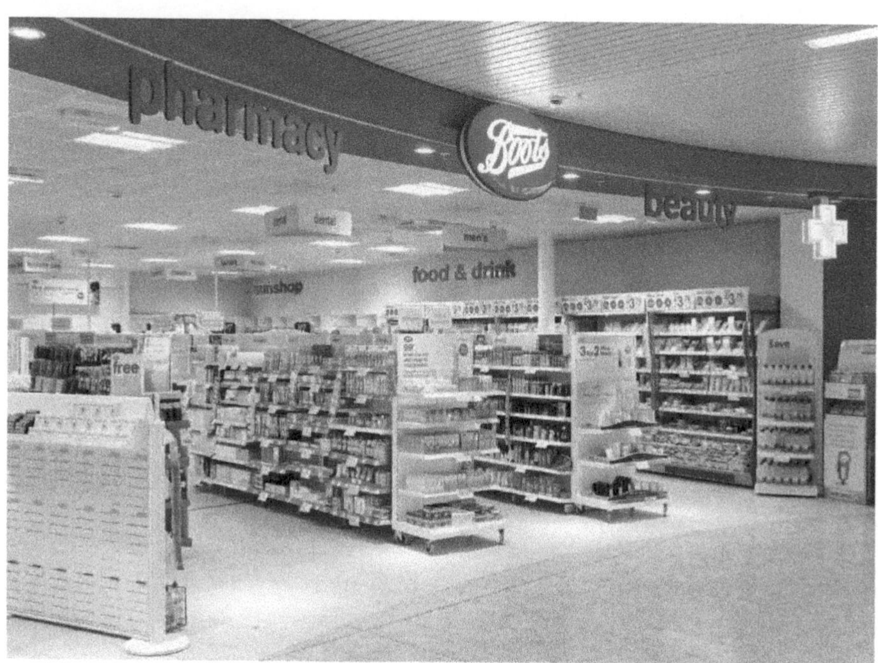

This introductory chapter aims to outline some key concepts in pharmaceutics to help you understand the material presented in subsequent chapters. Examples are given to illustrate important concepts, and some will be familiar to you from your everyday experience. Where appropriate, reference will be made to subsequent chapters where more detail is provided. Although you will encounter a large number of specialized words throughout this book, it is worth emphasizing that pharmaceutics has its foundations in chemistry. You will be familiar with some of the theories that can be used to understand the **physicochemical** properties of compounds contained in beakers and test tubes, such as why table salt is soluble in water. These same principles can be used to comprehend:

- the behaviour of dosage forms prior to their administration and *in vitro*,
- the fate of dosage forms *in vivo* as they make their way to the biological target.

Ultimately, the aim of pharmaceutics is to use these principles to design and manufacture effective and stable pharmaceutical products that are both safe and convenient to use. This includes techniques to eliminate micro-organisms and to inhibit their growth.

Learning objectives

Having read this chapter you are expected to be able to:

- Define pharmaceutics and state its main aims.
- Recognize that a dosage form consists of an Active Pharmaceutical Ingredient (API) and excipients.
- Understand that the design of a dosage form will depend on the chosen route of administration.
- Recall the definition of some key terms relating to the administration of medicines and delivery of drugs.
- Appreciate that human factors will influence the selection of the most appropriate dosage form.
- Give some examples of how the physicochemical properties of an API can impact on the design of a dosage form.
- Appreciate why pharmacists require an understanding of pharmaceutics.
- Understand that a measured pharmaceutical quantity has no meaning if its units are not stated.

1.1 Dosage forms

You will know from experience that medicines encompass a wide range of dosage forms, including solid tablets, liquid syrups, and inhalers that use a carrier gas to deliver the drug to the patient (Figure 1.2). Chapters 2, 3, and 4 of this book will cover the three main phases of matter, solids, liquids, and gases, and describe the range of medicines with formulations that rely on these three states.

For more information on solid dosage forms, please refer to Chapter 2.

For more information on liquid dosage forms, please refer to Chapter 3.

For more information on gaseous dosage forms, please refer to Chapter 4.

FIGURE 1.2 The contents of this typical bathroom cabinet include various dosage forms; solid tablets to be swallowed; liquid drops to be placed in the eye; and an inhaler for drawing medicine into the lungs
Source: Carolyn A. Mckeone/Science Photo Library

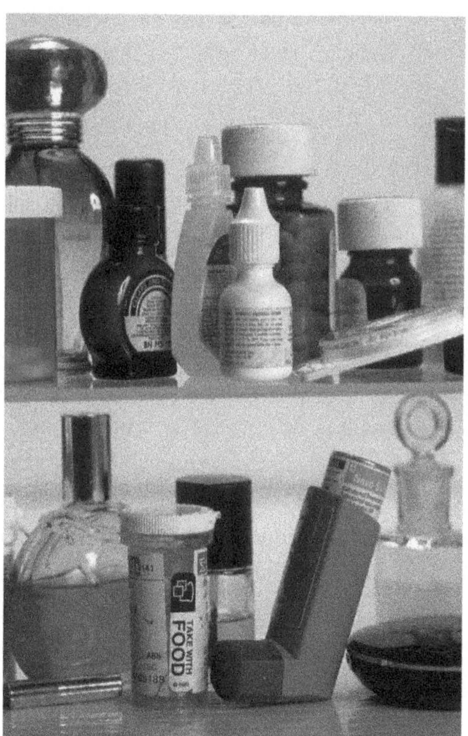

Regardless of their physical state, all medicines are composed of an **active pharmaceutical ingredient (API)**, mixed with one or more **excipients**. Any component of a medicine, other than the API, is an excipient and these are usually added during formulation for a specific purpose. Although categorized as pharmacologically inactive, we will see excipients can have a significant impact on pharmaceutical performance of a medication.

There are many reasons why we cannot normally use medicines that are simply a pure form of the API. For example, the API could be unstable and decompose before it is administered. Pharmaceutics includes the study of kinetics, as these principles can be used to understand and retard the rate of degradation reactions. Alternatively, the API might have acidic or basic properties that could irritate the body. The majority of APIs are either acids or bases and this has a number of implications for dosage form design.

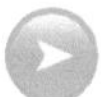
For more information on reaction rates and degradation reactions, please refer to Chapter 12.

For more information acidic and basic behaviour, please refer to Chapter 6.

In many cases, the high potency of an API requires that it is diluted in some way before it can be administered safely. For example, paracetamol for children is typically supplied as a flavoured liquid with a concentration of 120 mg of API per 5 mL. This may be conveniently delivered using a medicinal spoon. If the amount of excipient were less then the concentration of API might be, say, 10 times greater. In this case, only 0.5 mL of syrup would be required and this smaller volume would be much harder to measure accurately. This a particular issue for any drug with a small **therapeutic index (TI)** where overdosing can lead to serious health issues.

KEY POINT

Medicines may be formulated as a range of dosage forms, including tablets, eye drops, and inhalers. All medicines are composed of an active pharmaceutical ingredient (API), mixed with one or more excipients. Excipients are pharmacologically inactive but can have a significant impact on the performance of a medication.

SELF CHECK 1.1

Give three reasons why an API might not be administered to a patient in its pure form.

SELF CHECK 1.2

Why are APIs with high therapeutic indices always preferred to those with low therapeutic indices?

1.2 Drug delivery

The **route of administration** of a medicine is the path by which it is taken into the body. Thus, a liquid for **intravenous (IV)** delivery would be injected directly into a vein, while tablets are designed for oral delivery. We will encounter other routes of administration throughout this book. Regardless of the path through which a commercially available medicine enters the body, the API will have gone through a common series of stages before reaching the marketplace. These commence with the use of specialized techniques to discover new drugs, and continue with the development of the dosage form that will be used to deliver the drug.

For more information on the various routes of administration and details of drug discovery and development, please refer to Chapter 13.

Before an API can exert any pharmacological effect, the API must first dissolve in a physiological fluid; the nature of this fluid depends on the route of administration. A tablet that is swallowed, for example, will ultimately dissolve in the liquid of the gastrointestinal tract (GIT), an example of **dissolution**. Alternatively, a liquid medicine directly injected into a vein will enter the blood plasma. After administration, the API is delivered to the biological target in a process that is generally referred to as drug delivery.

Phase transitions, including dissolution, are of general importance in drug delivery. In order for a tablet to dissolve, it is important that the exterior of the solid is effectively exposed to the surrounding fluid. A specialized coating may be used and this requires an understanding of surface phenomena. Dissolution is an example of a change of state and is subject to thermodynamic laws. The enthalpy change accompanying dissolution can be **exothermic** or **endothermic**. While exothermic processes, such as combustion, are generally more common, dissolution occurs naturally due to the associated increase in disorder, regardless of the enthalpy change. Thus, as with chemical systems, the principles of thermodynamics can be used to ascertain if a process will spontaneously happen.

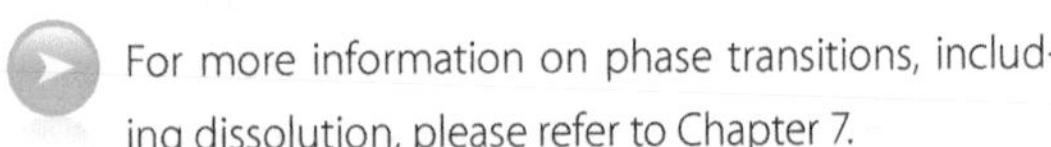
For more information on phase transitions, including dissolution, please refer to Chapter 7.

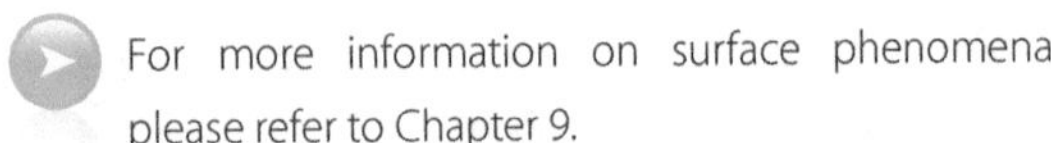
For more information on surface phenomena, please refer to Chapter 9.

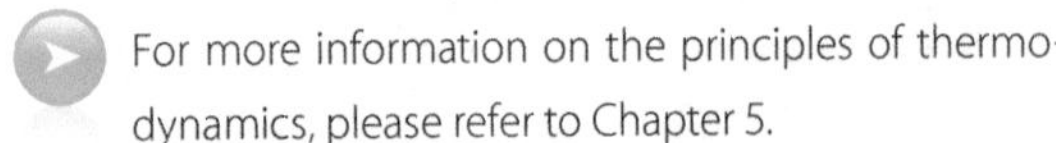
For more information on the principles of thermodynamics, please refer to Chapter 5.

Any API will ultimately interact with the biological target that plays a role in a medical condition, and this is normally a **receptor**. The drug propofol, for example, is used in clinical settings to induce general anaesthesia through IV infusion (Figure 1.3). It binds to receptors located throughout the central nervous system (CNS). Generally, receptors may be present on the surface of cells, such as those in the stomach, or within physiological fluids. The outcome of the interaction between receptors and APIs, or drug action, is not the direct concern of pharmaceutics.

For more information on drug action please refer to Chapter 4 'An introduction to drug action' of the ***Therapeutics and Human Physiology*** book within this series.

FIGURE 1.3 **(A) The structure of propofol, an API that induces general anaesthesia through IV delivery. (B) A fluid bag for an IV infusion**

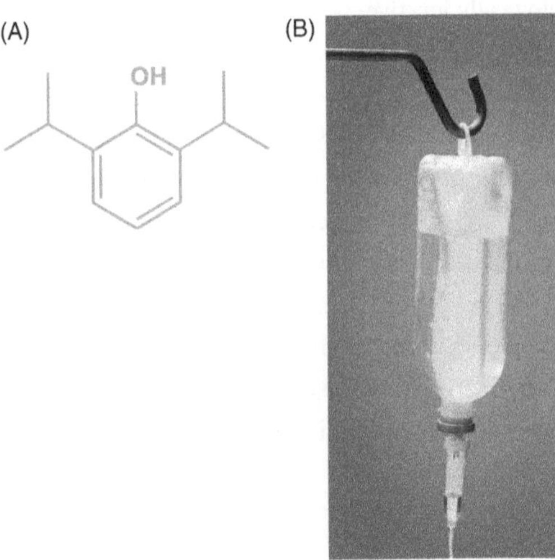

> **KEY POINT**
>
> The route of administration of a medicine is the path by which it is taken into the body. Before an API can exert any pharmacological effect, it must dissolve in a physiological fluid. It can then interact with the biological target that plays a role in the medical condition.

The manner in which the API reaches the target receptor is dependent on the site of administration. For example, intravenously administered profofol is transported to the CNS *via* the patient's circulatory system. This is referred to as **systemic delivery** and it increases the possibility that the drug might bind to an unintended site. An ideal API is a 'magic bullet', a term originally coined by Ehrlich (Figure 1.4) to describe a drug that targets a specific receptor without adverse side-effects. Occasionally, however, unintended side-effects can have desirable outcomes, e.g. minoxidil (see Integration Box 1.1).

FIGURE 1.4 Paul Ehrlich, winner of the 1908 Nobel Prize for Medicine and one of the first proponents of receptor theory
Source: Published in 1909 in *Les Prix Nobel*. Reproduced under Commons Copyright

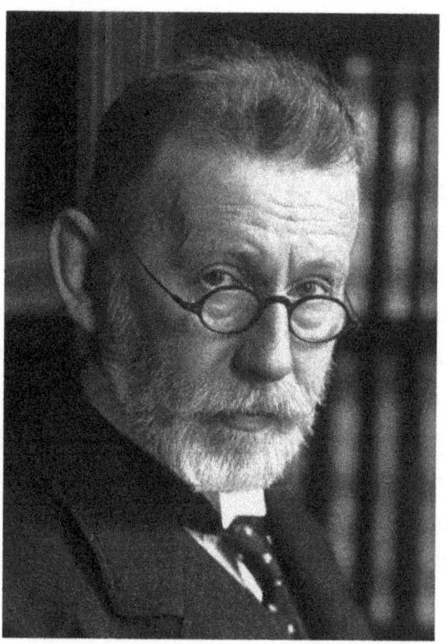

> **INTEGRATION BOX 1.1**
>
> ## Minoxidil
>
> The drug minoxidil is prescribed to patients with high blood pressure and its molecular structure is shown in Figure 1.5A. It was originally available in tablet form and, as a vasodilator, it treats hypertension by widening blood vessels. Patients using minoxidil reported a thickening and darkening of body hair as a side-effect. Consequently, the drug has been available as a foam for direct application to the scalp, marketed under the name Rogaine™. It is thought that the API interacts with receptors on the scalp, improving blood flow to this region and stimulating hair growth.
>
> Within pharmaceutics, it is not uncommon for the same API to be formulated in different dosage forms, such as tablets (Figure 1.5B) and foams (Figure 1.5C). In the case of minoxidil, the different dosage forms give rise to different therapeutic outcomes. In addition to minoxidil, there are other examples where an accidental discovery has ultimately led to a new pharmaceutical product.

FIGURE 1.5 **(A) The structure of the API minoxidil. (B) A blister pack of tablets for oral delivery. (C) A foam for external application**

(A)

O^-, H_2N, N^+, NH_2, N, N

(B)

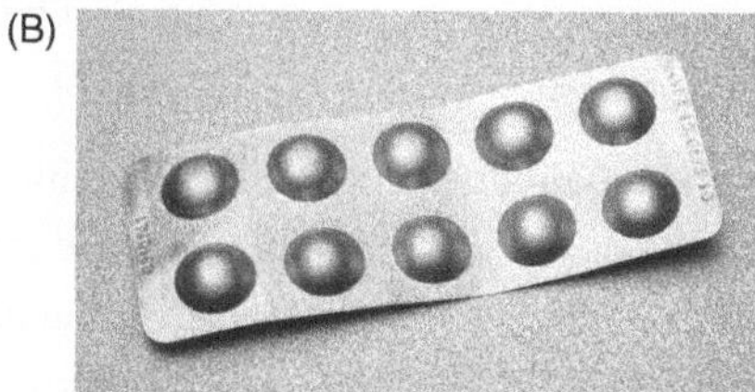

(C)

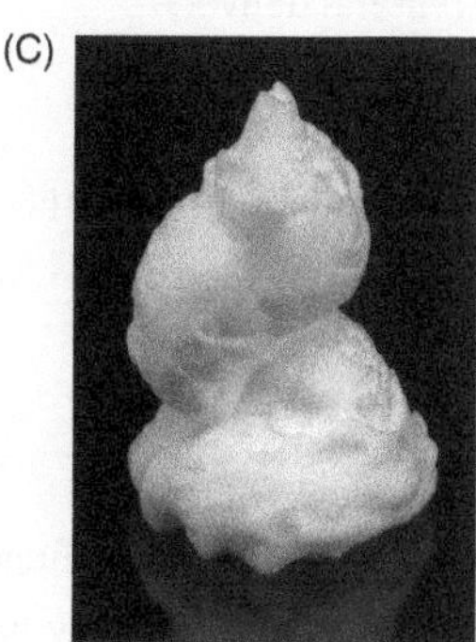

The application of minoxidal foam to the scalp as a treatment for hair loss is an example of **local delivery**, as the targeted receptors are at the site of administration. Where possible, local delivery is always preferred as it increases the likelihood of the API interacting with the intended target. Systemic delivery and local delivery are not exclusive terms, however, and a locally delivered medicine may well exhibit systemic effects. Thus, some minoxidil will end up in the bloodstream after application of Rogaine™ foam to the scalp, although not normally in pharmacologically significant quantities.

In addition to foams, you may have personally encountered medicines in a wide range of other physical states for application to the skin, including creams, gels, and aerosols. These all belong to an important class of materials called disperse systems. You will see that these systems can have a variety of structures and that their use as dosage forms is not just restricted to applications for the skin.

For more information on disperse systems and the dosage forms that belong to this classification, please refer to Chapter 10.

KEY POINT

Systemic delivery is where the body's circulatory system is used to transport an API from the site of administration to the biological target. Local delivery is where the site of action of a drug is located at the site of administration.

We have established that there are various ways in which an API can be delivered to the target and they may be classified as:

- Enteral delivery.
- Parenteral delivery.
- Topical delivery.

A basic understanding of these terms is required at this stage.

Enteral delivery

If you have ever been unfortunate enough to suffer from intense pain, then you may have purchased or been prescribed co-codamol tablets. This is an OTC **analgesic** containing the APIs codeine and paracetamol. The oral administration of tablets is an example of **enteral delivery**, as the API is ultimately absorbed through the gastrointestinal tract (GIT) into the bloodstream. Enteral delivery is not just restricted to oral administration, however, and this classification includes rectal **suppositories** that are designed to be absorbed in the terminal region of the GIT.

In order for absorption from the GIT to occur, the API must leave the **hydrophilic** environment of the gastrointestinal fluid and enter the **hydrophobic** environment of the cell membranes that line the GIT. This is an example of a phase transition called partitioning.

For more information on partitioning, please refer to Chapter 8.

Orally delivered APIs that are absorbed within the GIT are carried by the hepatic portal vein into the liver where their pharmacological activity may be lost due to chemical modification. This is called **first-pass metabolism** and it can reduce the API's concentration in blood before it enters the systemic circulation, reducing the **bioavailability** of the API.

Parenteral delivery

The IV infusion of propofol (Figure 1.3), is an example of **parenteral delivery**, as it involves piercing of the skin. Some parenteral dosage forms are not injections and these are summarized in Chapter 13, along with the most commonly encountered types of injection, including IV.

For more information on parenteral dosage forms, please refer to 'Parenteral administration' in Section 13.5.

Patient discomfort can arise if liquids for injection are not **isotonic** with physiological fluids. This is an issue that can be understood by taking into account the colligative properties of the API and excipients.

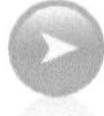

For more information on the colligative properties of fluids, please refer to Chapter 11.

Topical delivery

The application of minoxidal foam to the scalp is an example of **topical delivery**, as the medicine is applied to an external surface of the body. A **transdermal patch** is another example of topical delivery, the API being absorbed from the patch through the skin. A popular use of this dosage form is to deliver a controlled dose of nicotine to patients who are attempting to give up smoking. Topical delivery also includes medicines that are applied to the eye and **mucous membranes** of, for example, the mouth and nasal passages.

KEY POINT

Enteral delivery occurs when the drug is absorbed through the gastrointestinal tract. Parenteral delivery is a route of administration that normally involves the piercing of the skin. Topical delivery is where a medicine is applied to the external surfaces of the body, including the skin, mucous membranes and respiratory tract.

SELF CHECK 1.3

Consider these four example dosage forms and routes of administration:

1. An anaesthetic suppository to relieve haemorrhoids.
2. An analgesic tablet to treat a headache.
3. An anaesthetic injected into the gum before dental work.
4. An analgesic injected intravenously after major surgery.

Assign the most appropriate description to these four examples from this list:

A. Parenteral and local delivery.
B. Enteral and local delivery.
C. Parenteral and systemic delivery.
D. Enteral and systemic delivery.

1.3 The choice of dosage form

Like minoxidil (Figure 1.5), the API fentanyl is available in more than one dosage form. Fentanyl lollipops and patches (Figure 1.6) may be prescribed and the drug can also be formulated as a liquid for IV infusion. These three dosage forms can all offer pain relief, fentanyl being a potent analgesic. For any API, only one dosage form will exert the greatest therapeutic effect per unit dose in treating a particular medical condition. This may not, however, be the preferred choice for a particular patient.

A patient's characteristics, culture, and medical condition are always considered when a dosage form is chosen. Young children and elderly patients, for example, can have difficulty ingesting tablets so liquid dosage forms may be preferred. Furthermore, patients with impaired memory or motor skills may have trouble adhering to dosing schedules or using medicinal devices such as droppers, syringes, and inhalers. The culture in which the patient spent their formative years can also play a role in the choice of dosage form. In some countries, rectal suppositories are routinely prescribed to systemically treat fevers, whereas this suggestion might be politely declined in other nations.

The severity of the medical condition will also influence the selection of dosage form. Thus, a patient resistant to the idea of a suppository for a light fever might consider rectal drug delivery to treat severe migraines. Similarly, increasingly invasive routes of administration, such as IV infusions, will become more palatable as the pain caused by the medical condition increases. In the treatment of severe conditions,

FIGURE 1.6 Different dosage forms of the API fentanyl: (A) a lollipop, and (B) a patch

Source: (A) This file is licensed under the Creative Commons Attribution-Share Alike 3.0 Unported license. Credit: Crohnie. (B) Copyright Charlie Long

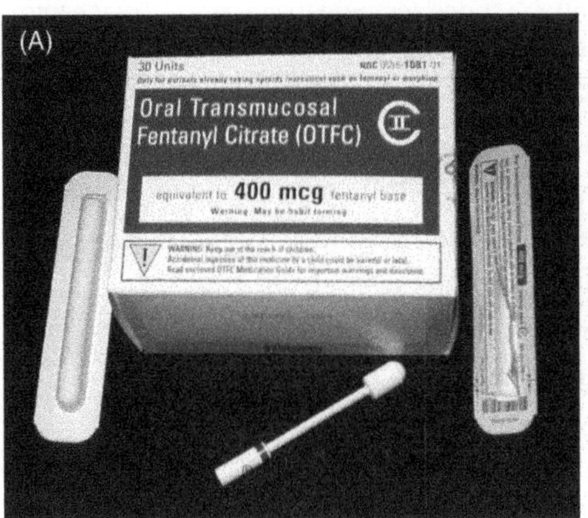

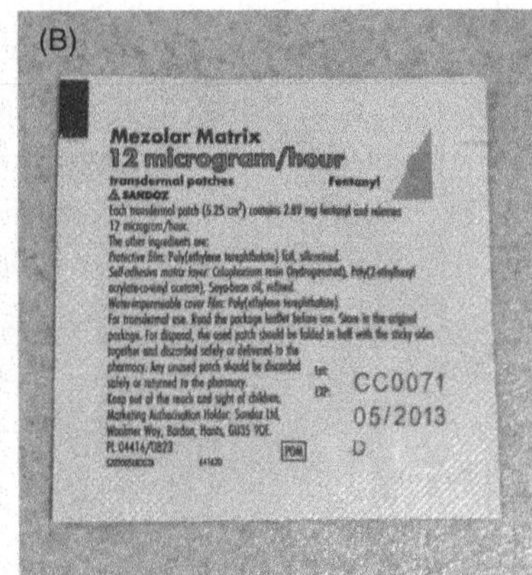

a patient will also be more likely to accept any adverse side-effects, such as hair loss during chemotherapy.

For more information on dosage form selection, please refer to Section 8.1 'Which medication is most appropriate?' of the *Pharmacy Practice* book within this series.

KEY POINT

A patient's characteristics, culture, and medical condition are always considered when a dosage form is chosen.

The physicochemical properties of the API and excipients

Of particular interest within pharmaceutics are the physicochemical properties of the API and excipients, as these will determine whether a particular dosage form and associated route of administration are viable. In some cases, it may be possible to chemically modify the API without significantly impairing its pharmacological effect in order to improve delivery. Thus, the analgesic fentanyl is weakly basic and it is used in this form within transdermal patches (Figure 1.6B). The base will react with citric acid to form a salt, fentanyl citrate. The use of this chemical form of API is preferred in lollipops for reasons discussed in Chapter 8.

For more information on the delivery of fentanyl please refer to 'Drug absorption across skin' in Section 8.7.

The physical modification of an API is sometimes necessary and this can be very subtle. Thus, some APIs are found to have poor bioavailability when incorporated within a tablet as the **crystalline** form. This can be addressed by using the alternative **amorphous** form of the API and this is discussed in Chapter 2.

For more information on the use of crystalline and amorphous forms of APIs within dosage forms, please refer to Section 2.2.

It is common to carefully select excipients with desirable physiochemical properties to improve the pharmacological activity of dosage forms and you will find numerous examples throughout this book. An API might not be sufficiently soluble to be presented as an aqueous solution for oral delivery, for example, so it may be formulated as a **suspension**. This requires the use of excipients to stabilize the suspension.

For more information on the use of excipients to stabilize suspensions, please refer to 'Suspensions and nanosuspensions' in Section 10.2.

Aside from oral administration, other routes of delivery place different demands on an administered medicine. Regardless of the route, pharmaceutics requires an understanding of the physicochemical properties of APIs and excipients so that the way in which they dictate how a medicine can be formulated may be fully appreciated.

KEY POINT

The physicochemical properties of the API will determine whether a particular dosage form and route of administration are viable.

KEY POINT

Pharmaceutics includes the chemical and physical modification of dosage forms in order to optimize their pharmacological effect.

SELF CHECK 1.4

Why might an elderly patient be prescribed an API in the form of an oral liquid, rather than as tablets or an inhaler?

1.4 Why do I need to study pharmaceutics?

The term 'pharmacist' typically conjures up an image of a dispensing chemist within a community pharmacy. As a pharmacy student, therefore, you might question the need for an understanding of the science that underpins dosage form design. Of course, not all pharmacists work in a dispensing setting. Industrial pharmacists, for example, work within pharmaceutical companies to research new APIs and develop improved manufacturing techniques. Furthermore, a number of specialist pharmacy roles exist in which pharmaceutics is also an important aspect. These include, for example, those requiring the preparation of non-standard medicines.

There are a number of reasons why the practice of pharmacy relies on a sound understanding of pharmaceutics:

- It provides a rationale for the inclusion of the various excipients listed on the packaging of a medicine, so that patient queries can be professionally handled. The pharmacist needs an appreciation of the properties of those excipients, and any impact that they may have on a person.
- Pharmacists should also be able to answer questions about why one dosage form has been preferred over another, e.g. a syrup instead of a tablet. Moreover, for a particular type of medicine, e.g. oral tablets, they should be able to justify why one formulation has been preferred. This might be, for example, to decrease the frequency with which the medicine needs to be administered in the case of a patient with impaired memory.
- As part of their **pharmaceutical care**, a pharmacist should be able to give informed advice regarding the storage and administration of medicines, in relation to the specific type of dosage form and formulation that has been prescribed.
- Patients who have deviated from the prescribed dosing procedure will require specific assistance. For example, if a patient cuts a coated tablet in half, will it remain stable prior to administration and exert a desirable pharmacological effect? Patients who have difficulty swallowing may ask whether they can crush or suck tablets and a pharmacist should be able to provide an informed response.
- A pharmacist may sometimes be required to request **extemporaneously prepared medicines** for individual patients that would be otherwise unavailable. These so-called 'specials' may be compounded by a dedicated unit within a large hospital. An understanding of formulation can assist the preparation unit and help to field patient queries.

Ultimately, a distinguishing feature of all pharmacists is their intimate knowledge of medicines, including both their formulation and dosage form. This knowledge promotes the correct storage and use of medicines, ensuring safe and effective delivery. A dispensing pharmacist, therefore, completes the professional aspect of an API's journey to the biological target, a journey initiated by the formulation of a dosage form from its constituent API and excipients by a pharmaceutical scientist.

For more information on pharmaceutical care, please refer to Chapter 8, 'Pharmaceutical care' of the *Pharmacy Practice* book of this series.

For more information on extemporaneously prepared medicines please refer to 'Preparation of extemporaneously dispensed items' in Section 5.8 of the *Pharmacy Practice* book of this series.

KEY POINT

All roles within pharmacy rely on an understanding of pharmaceutics, including those within both dispensing and industrial settings. An understanding of pharmaceutics enables patient queries about the storage and use of medicines to be handled in a professional manner. As part of pharmaceutical care, a dispensing pharmacist promotes the safe and effective delivery of an API to the intended biological target.

1.5 Pharmaceutical measurements

The study of pharmaceutics involves the consideration of the physicochemical properties of dosage forms. One of the achievements of pharmaceutics, and science in general, has been the development of mathematical models that afford a quantitative understanding of the natural world through these properties; for example, see the BBC TV series, *The Code* (2011). As with any discipline, there are established conventions that must be followed if one is to communicate ideas effectively. This is, if one likes, the 'language' of a subject. In pharmaceutical chemistry, for example, there are established rules for the naming of organic molecules.

For naming conventions of organic molecules, please refer to Chapters 1 and 4 of the *Pharmaceutical Chemistry* book of this series.

Within pharmaceutics, an important principle is that a physicochemical property expressed as a numerical value has no meaning if units are not stated. Thus, stating that a paediatric paracetamol formulation for oral delivery has a concentration of '24' provides no useful information whatsoever. Clearly, if a pharmacist were to misjudge a drug concentration from a failure to unambiguously record units, then this could have critical consequences. Regrettably, history records that fatalities have resulted from the dispensing of medicines that had unintended concentrations (see Integration Box 1.2).

The concentration of paracetamol in a paediatric suspension might typically be 24 mg mL^{-1}. It is worth taking a moment to consider this statement of concentration as it raises some general points. In this context, 'm' is used to indicate 'milli', a prefix within the metric system that is used to denote a factor of 10^{-3}, or one-thousandth. Common metric prefixes are usually lowercase, although all factors of 10^6 and above are capitalized (Table 1.1).

TABLE 1.1 **Metric prefixes**

Prefix	Symbol	Magnitude	Meaning
Giga-	G	10^9	1 000 000 000
Mega-	M	10^6	1 000 000
kilo-	k	10^3	1000
hecto-	h	10^2	100
deka-	da	10	10
deci-	d	10^{-1}	0.1
centi-	c	10^{-2}	0.01
milli-	m	10^{-3}	0.001
micro-	μ	10^{-6}	0.000 001
nano-	n	10^{-9}	0.000 000 001

INTEGRATION BOX 1.2

The importance of stating units: deodorized tincture of opium (DTO)

Although used extensively in the past, opium solutions are no longer prescribed regularly for pain relief. In addition to both morphine and codeine, opium includes emetic compounds that induce vomiting. These chemicals are removed in the preparation of *deodorized tincture of opium* (DTO). In the past, the letter 'D' in this acronym has been mistakenly taken to stand for 'diluted'. In practice, DTO is 25 times stronger than the diluted standard, known as *paregoric tincture of opium* (Figure 1.7). The former has been used in error over the latter, resulting in at least one fatality. Historical guidance for pharmacists has recommended that the use of the term DTO is avoided and that liquid medications containing opium clearly state the concentration on the label.

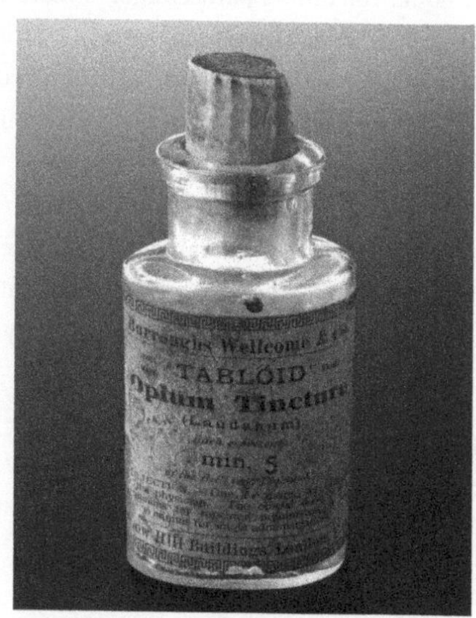

FIGURE 1.7 **A bottle containing paregoric tincture of opium**
Source: Reproduced with permission from the Wellcome Trust

In the unit 'mg mL^{-1}', the symbol 'g' represents grams and 'L' represents litres. As measures of mass and volume, they are derived from the set of **SI units**. This is also true of the units used to measure the pharmaceutically important quantities that we will see throughout this book (Table 1.2).

TABLE 1.2 **Pharmaceutically important quantities and their units**

Quantity	Symbol	Unit	Expressed in SI base unit(s)
Length	l	metre, m[a]	m
Mass	m	kilogram, kg[a]	kg
Time	t	second, s[a]	s
Temperature	T	kelvin, K[a]	k
Amount of substance	n	mole, mol[a]	mol
Length	l	angstrom, Å	10^{-10} m
Volume	V	litre, L	10^{-3} m^3
Volume	V	decimetre cubed, dm^3	10^{-3} m^3
Force	F	newton, N	kg m s^{-2}
Surface tension	γ	newtons per metre, N m^{-1}	kg s^{-2}
Energy	E	joules, J	kg m^2 s^{-2}
Pressure	p	pascal, Pa	kg m^{-1} s^{-2}
Dynamic viscosity	η	pascal second, Pa s	kg m^{-1} s^{-1}

[a]An SI base unit.

The preferred unit for a pharmaceutical quantity may be different from that expressed using SI units. This may be because typical amounts expressed in SI may be inconveniently high (or small). Thus, 5×10^{-6} m^3 of a liquid containing paracetamol is more readily expressed as 5 mL. In some instances, logarithms might also be used to produce numbers within a convenient range. Thus, the concentration of hydrogen ions in the small intestine is typically around 1×10^{-8} mol dm^{-3}. This is more conveniently expressed as **pH** 8, the corresponding logarithmic quantity. Pharmaceutics demands that we clearly state our chosen units of measurement, and that we are able to correctly convert between units.

For more information on pH, please refer to Section 6.3.

KEY POINT

A physicochemical property expressed as a numerical value has no meaning if units are not stated. The failure to unambiguously record units can have critical consequences within pharmacy practice. It is essential to be able to correctly convert between common units.

SELF CHECK 1.5

How many cm^3 are there in 1 m^3?

SELF CHECK 1.6

A bottle contains 250 aspirin tablets weighing 81.25 g. Express this mass in kg and mg.

CHAPTER SUMMARY

- Medicines can be formulated in a range of dosage forms, but all are composed of an active pharmaceutical ingredient (API), mixed with one or more excipients.
- Excipients are pharmacologically inactive but have a significant impact on the performance of a medication.
- The route of administration of a medicine is the path by which it is taken into the body.
- An API must first dissolve in a physiological fluid before ultimately interacting with the biological target that plays a role in the medical condition being treated.
- Systemic delivery is where the body's circulatory system is used to transport a drug, whereas in local delivery the site of action of a drug is located at the site of administration.
- Enteral delivery occurs when the drug is absorbed through the gastrointestinal tract.
- Parenteral delivery is a route of administration that normally involves the piercing of the skin.
- Topical delivery is where a medicine is applied to the external surfaces of the body, including the skin, mucous membranes and respiratory tract.
- The physicochemical properties of the API will determine whether a particular dosage form and route of administration are viable.
- Pharmaceutics includes the chemical and physical modification of APIs and the careful selection of excipients in order to optimize the pharmacological effect of dosage forms.
- All roles within pharmacy rely on an understanding of pharmaceutics, including those within both dispensing and industrial settings.
- A physicochemical property expressed as a numerical value has no meaning at all if units are not stated.

FURTHER READING

Atkins, P.W. and de Paula, J. (2009). *Physical Chemistry* (9th edn). Oxford: Oxford University Press.

This book presents a clear and succinct guide to the technical aspects of physical chemistry, including those that are relevant to the study of dosage form.

Aulton, M.E. (ed.) (2007). *Aulton's Pharmaceutics: The Design and Manufacture of Medicines* (3rd edn). Edinburgh: Churchill Livingstone.

A text that provides a good coverage of pharmaceutics, including advanced topics that are considered at higher levels.

Florence, A.T. and Attwood, D. (2011). *Physicochemical Principles of Pharmacy* (5th edn). London: Pharmaceutical Press.

This book presents some good explanations of the underlying scientific processes that are pertinent to pharmaceutics.

Monynihan, H. and Crean, A. (2009). *The Physicochemical Basis of Pharmaceuticals*. Oxford: Oxford University Press.

This text is written in an accessible style and provides the reader with a solid understanding of the physicochemical aspects of drug design.

2 Solids

BARBARA CONWAY

Drugs are most frequently given orally in solid dosage formulations. The **physicochemical** characteristics of the **active pharmaceutical ingredient (API)**, as well the other ingredients added to a formulation and the manufacturing method used to make them, all play a role in governing how the drug will behave in the body. The most common solid **dosage forms** are tablets and capsules, which have been used since the nineteenth century and are unit dosage forms usually containing an accurate dose of a drug. There are many different types of solid dosage forms designed to fulfil specific requirements but they are generally intended for oral administration and for **systemic delivery**.

Physicochemical characteristics are simply those properties of a substance relating to physical chemistry or physics. They include:

- Molecular formula.
- Molecular weight.
- Physical state.
- Appearance, colour, and odour.
- Evaporation rate.
- **Density**.
- Particle size.
- **Solubility**.
- **Acid dissociation constant**.
- **Boiling point** and **melting point**.
- **Vapour pressure**.
- **Partition coefficient**.

You will learn how these characteristics relate to the properties of the API. They provide vital information that allows pharmacists and pharmaceutical scientists to make informed design choices and deductions about drug action in formulations and in the body. This forms a vital part of the drug development process called **preformulation**, which is covered in more detail later in the book.

For more information on the acid dissociation constant, please refer to Section 6.5.

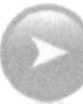
For more information on boiling point, melting point, and vapour pressure, please refer to Section 7.1.

For more information on the partition coefficient, please refer to Section 8.2.

For more information on preformulation please refer to Section 13.4.

Learning objectives

Having read this chapter you are expected to be able to:

- Describe the basic properties of solids.
- Describe the solid state, crystallinity, polymorphs, and solvates and their relevance to pharmaceutical formulation.
- Define simple solubility terminology and influencing factors.
- Outline the basic concepts governing the formulation of solid dosage forms.
- Identify the role of common excipients in solid dosage formulations.
- Describe what different solid dosage forms are available and how they are used.

2.1 Properties of solids

All pharmaceutically relevant materials have constituent particles (molecules and ions). There are three main states of matter: solid, liquid, and gas. Each of the three states has different physical characteristics, mainly concerning volume and shape. These are determined by the kinetic energy of the molecules and attractive forces that determine the physical characteristics of each state. Materials can transform between the various states of matter. In the solid state, matter maintains a fixed volume and shape; in liquids, matter maintains a fixed volume but adapts to the shape of its container; and in gases, matter expands to occupy whatever volume is available. At normal temperatures, most drugs are solids and maintain their original shape unless they are compressed, as happens during tablet formation.

For more information on liquids and gases, please refer to Chapter 3 and Chapter 4, respectively.

KEY POINT

All pharmaceutically relevant solids have constituent particles that are molecules and any associated ions.

The particles in solids are in fixed positions and are held together in close proximity by intermolecular forces. The particles may vibrate around their ordered positions, but no net movement or molecular rotation is possible. If more energy is supplied, such as an increase in temperature, the particles will gain energy, disrupt the order, and a **phase transition** can occur. The solid normally becomes a liquid that, with additional energy, will change to a gas. Some solids, with high vapour pressures, can transform directly from the solid to the gaseous state in a process called **sublimation**.

For more information on phase transitions, please refer to Section 7.1.

KEY POINT

Solids have a definite shape and volume as the particles are held in fixed positions and in close proximity by intermolecular forces.

Intermolecular forces

A knowledge of intermolecular forces is required for understanding the fundamental principles in pharmaceutics. Intermolecular forces (those which occur between molecules) are relatively weak compared to intramolecular forces (those which occur within molecules) and exist between molecules when they are sufficiently close to each other.

FIGURE 2.1 **Model of hydrogen bonds (labelled 1) between molecules of water in ice**

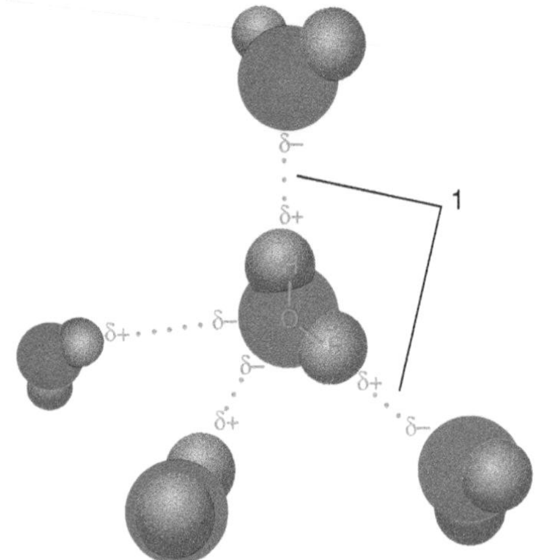

A hydrogen bond is the attractive, electrostatic interaction between a hydrogen atom and an electronegative atom such as nitrogen, oxygen, or fluorine (Figure 2.1). The hydrogen bond is a strong electrostatic dipole–dipole interaction. However, it also has some features of covalent bonding: it is directional and usually involves a limited number of interaction partners.

Van der Waals forces are non-ionic interactions between dipoles that arise because of an imbalance of charge across a molecule. They include:

- Dipole–dipole interactions (Keesom forces).
- Dipole-induced dipole interactions (Debye forces).
- Induced dipole-induced dipole interactions (London forces).

In solids, dipoles align so that the negative pole of one molecule points towards the positive pole of a neighbouring molecule, resulting in a lattice formation. Hydrogen bonds tend to be stronger interactions than van der Waals interactions and the distances between hydrogen bonded atoms are shorter than the sum of van der Waals radii. London forces are present in all materials and they explain why atomic materials, such as argon, can exist as liquids at very low temperatures.

For more information on intermolecular forces, please refer to Section 2.5 'Intermolecular forces' of the *Pharmaceutical Chemistry* book within this series.

KEY POINT

Intermolecular forces include hydrogen bonding and van der Waals forces. Hydrogen bonds tend to be stronger than van der Waals forces, and have similar characteristics to covalent bonds.

SELF CHECK 2.1

Which one of the following is not a property of all solids? (a) Definite shape. (b) Definite mass. (c) Definite colour. (d) Definite volume.

SELF CHECK 2.2

Which one of the following happens as a liquid freezes to become a solid at the melting point? (a) Enthalpy change is endothermic. (b) The temperature falls. (c) There is a decrease in particle order. (d) The molecules lose freedom.

2.2 Crystalline and amorphous solids

Within the solid state, the majority of materials have some level of short- and long-range order and these are described as **crystalline**. Those that do not have any overall order are referred to as **amorphous**. Both types of material are encountered within dosage forms.

KEY POINT

Solids may be classified as crystalline or amorphous.

Crystalline solids

A crystalline material is formed when the component molecules, atoms or ions, are arranged in a defined order and this order is then repeated throughout the entirety. They have sharp, well-defined melting points that can be determined when enough energy has been put into the system to break down the lattice structure. You may be familiar with the fixed geometric arrangement of the Na^+ and Cl^- ions in sodium chloride shown in Figure 2.2 in a repeating **unit cell**.

Within the lattice, each sodium ion is surrounded by six chloride ions and each chloride ion is surrounded by six sodium ions. The ions are bound by the electrostatic interaction of oppositely charged ions to form a lattice. We can classify crystals according to their shape, there being seven lattice systems (Figure 2.3). Sodium chloride is an example of a cubic crystal lattice. The majority of drugs form triclinic, monoclinic or orthorhombic unit cells.

KEY POINT

Crystals are composed of a regularly repeating unit cell that results in both short- and long-range order. We can group crystals according to their seven basic lattice systems: cubic, tetragonal, orthorhombic, hexagonal, trigonal (rhombohedral), triclinic, and monoclinic.

FIGURE 2.2 Sodium chloride crystal lattice

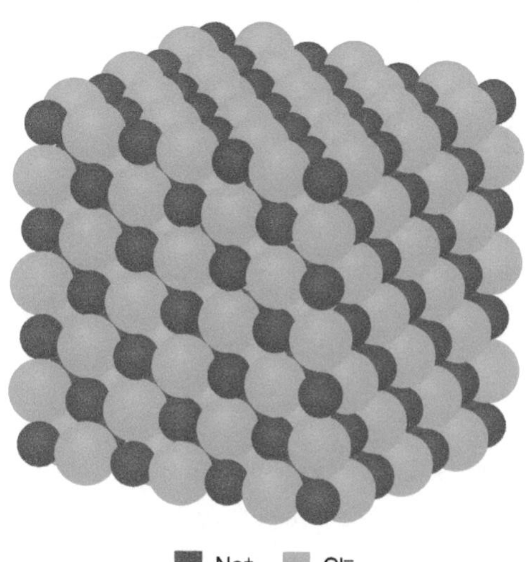

Crystal formation

Crystals are formed in several stages. First, nucleation needs to occur. This is the formation of a small mass, either of the drug molecules or deliberately added seed crystals. After nucleation, the crystals can grow into visible particles. Crystals are formed by inducing a change from the liquid to the solid state; for example, by cooling to below the melting point. They can also be formed by precipitation from a **supersaturated solution** (Box 2.1) by evaporation, cooling, or addition of an **antisolvent**.

The crystals can grow (or precipitate) out of a solvent with different sizes and numbers of faces, despite having the same unit cell. Crystals can be different shapes and this is important to know for the processing of drugs. For example, a needle-like crystal would have a larger surface area than a cuboid crystal and may dissolve more quickly, but flow properties could be compromised. A powdered solid that flows well is easier to manipulate during manufacture.

BOX 2.1

Supersaturated solutions

A supersaturated solution is one that contains more of the dissolved material than could be dissolved by the solvent under normal circumstances. Although not of practical use in dosage forms, due to their limited stability, the phenomenon of supersaturation can be important during manufacturing.

Saturation can be achieved by changing temperature or pressure and the concentration of solute is at its highest possible value at equilibrium. A saturated solution containing undissolved solid exists in dynamic equilibrium, as molecules are dissolving from the solid and crystallizing from the solution all the time. These two processes have the same rate, so the overall concentration (solubility) remains constant. A supersaturated solution is inherently unstable as it is not at equilibrium, but the rate of crystallization is very small so that the system is **metastable**.

FIGURE 2.3 The seven basic crystal unit cell systems

Seven crystal unit cell systems			
		Axes length	Angles between axes
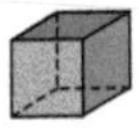	Cuboid	All equal	All 90°
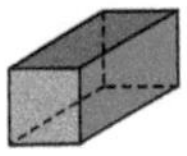	Tetragonal	Two equal One unequal	All 90°
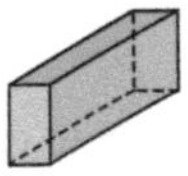	Orthorhombic	All unequal	All 90°
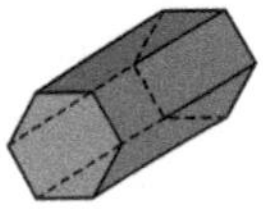	Hexagonal	Three equal One unequal	One 90° Three 60°
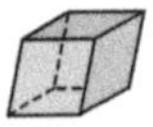	Trigonal	All equal	None 90°
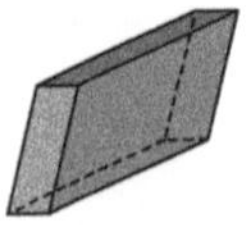	Triclinic	All unequal	None 90°
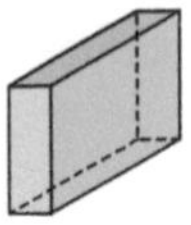	Monoclinic	All unequal	Two 90°

Amorphous solids

An amorphous, or non-crystalline, solid does not have the long-range order of a crystal and the molecules are in a random arrangement. You can see the difference in Figure 2.4, which shows the difference between the amorphous and crystalline forms of silicon dioxide (SiO_2). Although atoms in the amorphous solid are rigidly fixed, they are not in the orderly pattern of the crystalline form.

The amorphous form of a solid is usually more soluble than the crystalline form because minimal energy is required to break up the lattice and we can take advantage of this to improve drug **dissolution** and absorption. It is a challenge to keep the drug in the amorphous form during processing and specialized formulations may need to be used.

KEY POINT

An amorphous solid does not have the long-range order of a crystal. If the API is an amorphous form, it is usually more soluble than the corresponding crystalline form and this can be advantageous in drug delivery.

SELF CHECK 2.3

Name four of the seven basic crystal unit cell systems.

FIGURE 2.4 Amorphous (A) and crystalline (B) silicon dioxide

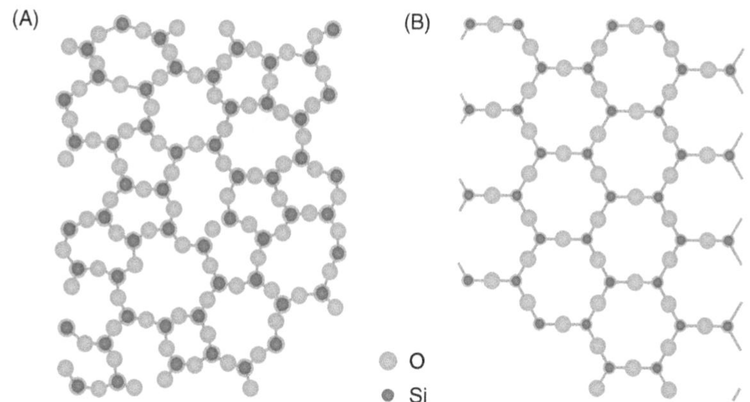

2.3 Polymorphism

Polymorphs are crystalline forms of the same substance but they have different structures at a molecular level. They are chemically the same but the crystals have different packing patterns. Polymorphs are found in around one in three organic compounds, and some drugs have many different crystalline forms. For example, 11 polymorphs of the antiepileptic drug phenobarbitone have been identified. They usually form when the conditions during crystallization are changed. **Enantiotropic** polymorphs can convert from one form to another under changing conditions, such as temperature or pressure. For compounds having **monotropic** polymorphism, only one form is stable at all conditions and other **metastable** forms will convert to the preferred form eventually. We need to identify, understand, and be able to quantify this inherent instability in drugs.

The most common example quoted for polymorphism is carbon, with diamond and graphite being polymorphic forms. Diamond is formed under high temperature and pressure. This form is hard and does not deform easily under compression, whereas in graphite, the carbon sheets can easily slip over each other when a force is applied. It is this property of graphite that enables it be used as the 'lead' in a pencil. At surface air pressure (one atmosphere), diamond is not as stable as graphite. The decay of diamond is thermodynamically favourable but the activation energy is large. Diamond does not decay into graphite under normal conditions, therefore, and is described as metastable.

For more information on activation energy, please refer to Section 12.3.

Different polymorphs have distinctive appearances, and the changes in mechanical properties between different polymorphs can cause them to behave differently when being processed. Differences in physical properties can also include:

- **Melting point.**
- **Solubility.**
- **Density.**
- **Crystal habit.**
- **Dielectric constant.**
- **Vapour pressure.**

Because the physical properties of polymorphs differ, this will influence the optimum formulation and have a large effect upon **bioavailability**.

Providing the polymorphs are stable enough to exist in isolation, different crystal lattices can be identified using X-ray diffraction crystallography, as they will each have distinct electron scattering patterns. For all new chemical entities (NCEs), or potential new drug candidates, it is important that there is a thorough polymorph screening process. Manufacturers need to be sure that they are using the same polymorphic form throughout, this usually being the most stable form.

KEY POINT

Polymorphs are different crystalline forms of the same substance. They are chemically the same but have different packing patterns. Different polymorphs have distinctive physical properties that will affect the preferred formulation and the bioavailability of the drug.

It is sometimes preferable to use a less stable polymorph of a drug if the most stable form is very poorly soluble in water. If the metastable form is used, it dissolves faster and this can lead to improved bioavailability. If you look at Figure 2.5, you can see that the equilibrium solubility achieved will be the maximum solubility of the stable polymorph, as the drug is ultimately converted to this form, but that the initial dissolution rate is higher. This means there will be more of the drug available for absorption (see Integration Box 2.1 for an example).

When a dosage form uses a metastable polymorph, this is a risk that must be fully controlled and quantified. All appropriate steps must be taken to minimize conversion to the stable polymorph during manufacture and storage. Unforeseen changes can be induced during processing; for example, when crystals are ground or milled to reduce the particle size. **Milling** of digoxin, a drug used in low doses for heart conditions such as atrial defibrillation, for example, can cause conversion to the amorphous form.

FIGURE 2.5 Typical solubility profiles for metastable and stable polymorphs

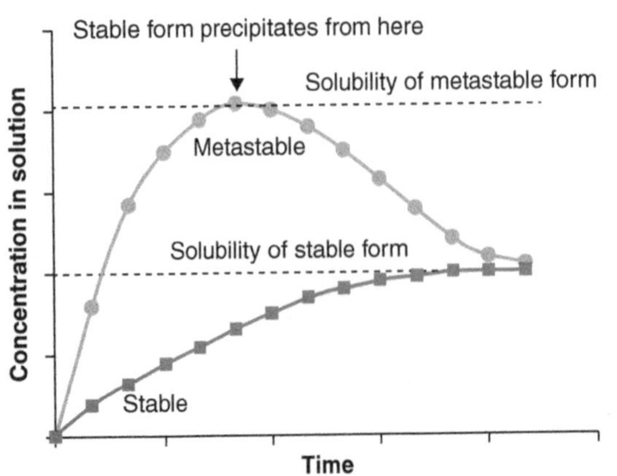

KEY POINT

At fixed conditions, one polymorph will be the most thermodynamically stable. The other forms are then referred to as metastable polymorphs. Metastable polymorphs of an API can lead to improved bioavailability, but steps must be taken to ensure that they do not convert to the more stable form before administration.

INTEGRATION BOX 2.1

Chloramphenicol and metastable polymorphs

The antibiotic, chloramphenicol palmitate, has three crystalline forms:

- A, the stable polymorph,
- B, a metastable polymorph, and,
- C, a very unstable polymorph that cannot be included in the dosage form.

The drug is given as an oral suspension and is hydrolysed to the active form in the body. The blood levels are represented schematically in Figure 2.6 following administration of a suspension of form A, form B, and a 50:50 mixture of both. The extent of absorption increases with increased B in suspension, as this has

FIGURE 2.6 Representative blood levels of chloramphenicol following administration of chloramphenicol palmitate suspensions

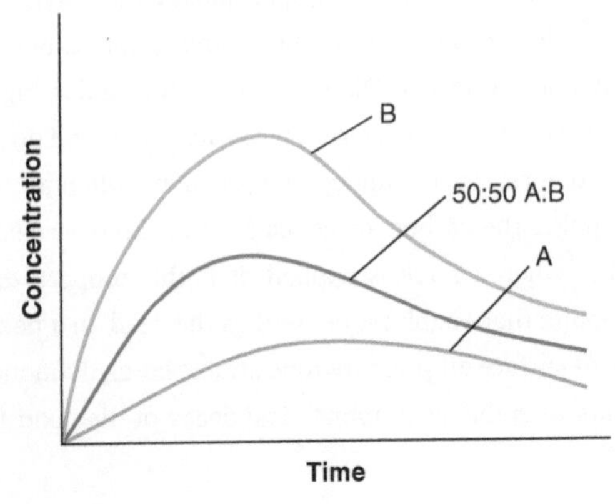

rapid dissolution *in vivo*. The stable A form dissolves slowly and is hydrolysed slowly, so absorption is limited.

As it has increased bioavailability, the metastable form B is used in chloramphenicol palmitate suspensions. Strict quality control measures ensure that the metastable form is not converted to the stable form on storage and there are specified limits for the amount of form A that can be present.

TABLE 2.1 **Aqueous solubility of anhydrous theophylline and theophylline hydrate**

Temp/°C	Solubility/mg mL^{-1}	
	Hydrate	Anhydrous
25	6.25	12.5
35	10.4	18.5
45	17.6	27.0
55	30.0	38.0

Taken from Eriksen (1964).

Crystal hydrates

Sometimes molecules of the solvent used for crystallization can be incorporated into the crystal lattice of a solid and these are called **solvates**. Usually, it is not acceptable to have solvent molecules associated with the drug because of toxicity concerns. Of more relevance in pharmacy is when the solvent is water; these are called **hydrates** and the form without water is the anhydrous form. Water is usually incorporated into the crystal in exact molar ratios, so 1 mole of drug will contain 1 mole of water (monohydrate) or 2 moles of water (dihydrate), etc.

Hydrates, like polymorphs, have different properties from the anhydrous form and they are sometimes referred to as **pseudopolymorphs**. The water can have a major role in intermolecular bonding, being an integral part of the crystal lattice, or it can be lost from the structure without a major impact on the lattice structure because it sits in voids or spaces in the lattice. Hydrates can have different melting points, solubilities and bioavailabilities. As the hydrated form already contains water and this can form hydrogen bonds between the components, the lattice is held more tightly and requires more energy to dissolve. Most hydrates, like the anti-asthmatic drug theophylline in Table 2.1, have higher melting points, lower solubilities, and lower dissolution rates than the equivalent anhydrous form.

KEY POINT

Hydrates are crystals containing water. They are described as pseudopolymorphs because they have different physical properties to the anhydrous form.

SELF CHECK 2.4

Chloramphenicol palmitate has three crystalline forms, A, B, and C. Which one of the following statements is false?

(a) B is the most stable polymorph.

(b) There is a limit test for levels of form A present in the oral suspension.

(c) A has a slow hydrolysis rate and little is absorbed.

(d) B has a rapid dissolution time *in vivo*.

(e) C is so unstable it cannot be included in a dosage form.

2.4 Solubility

A solution is formed when a solid solute dissolves in a solvent, typically water. When a solution contains solute at the limit of its solubility at any given temperature and pressure, the solution is said to be **saturated**. The solubility may be expressed quantitatively:

- Weight concentration, e.g. g L^{-1} or % w/v.
- Molarity, mol dm^{-3}.
- Milliequivalents.
- Mole fraction.

All these concentration units are interconvertible.

For more information on concentration units, please refer to 'Units of concentration' in Section 3.4.

In the **pharmacopoeiae**, the solubility of an API is often classified by using terms such as soluble, poorly soluble, etc., and a guide to these values can be seen in Table 2.2. Often APIs are not very soluble in water and there are a number of strategies we can use to help improve their solubility and bioavailability, such as salt formation if the API is a weak acid or base.

For more information on salt formation, please refer to Chapter 6.

KEY POINT

Soluble APIs are generally desirable as they have correspondingly high bioavailabilities. Acidic and basic APIs that are not very soluble in water may be converted to the corresponding salt to improve solubility.

Factors influencing solubility

In order to start the dissolution process, a liquid solvent needs to make good contact with the surface of the solid, a process called wetting. Hydrophobic drugs are not wetted easily and even when they are wet, the solubility is low. The **contact angle** is used to measure **wettability** of solid surfaces.

TABLE 2.2 **Solubility terminology**

Solubility at 20 °C	Approximate volume of solvent per gram of solute / mL
Very soluble	<1
Freely soluble	1–10
Soluble	10–30
Sparingly soluble	30–100
Slightly soluble	100–1000
Very slightly soluble	1000–10 000
Practically insoluble	>10 000

For more information on contact angle and wettability, please refer to Section 9.2.

When an amorphous solid is exposed to a gas (for example, water vapour), it can absorb the vapour into the bulk. If the solid is crystalline, it is usually limited to adsorption to the surface, but some substances can absorb enough water vapour to dissolve themselves. This is called **deliquescence**. The humidity of the environment can therefore have an impact on the solid-state stability of solids. Materials that take on water are called **hygroscopic** and must be protected from changes in the environment by the packaging either of the bulk material or the formulated product.

For more information about hygroscopic compounds, please refer to Chapter 5 'Alcohols, phenols, ethers, organic halogen compounds, and amines' of the *Pharmaceutical Chemistry* book within this series.

An ideal formulation should be hydrophilic enough to allow wetting but not so hygroscopic that it results in stability problems. Different additives can be incorporated into the formulation to control this.

Once a solid is added to a solvent, the rate of dissolution can be described by the Noyes–Whitney equation. Dissolution of solid particles is proportional to the surface area and therefore to the particle size. If the particle size is reduced, there is a larger surface area available for dissolution. This method is used to improve the absorption of poorly soluble drugs.

For more information on the Noyes–Whitney equation, please refer to 'Dissolution and the Noyes–Whitney Equation' in Section 7.1.

Griseofulvin is a very poorly soluble drug taken orally and used to treat fungal infections. It requires a high dose to be effective and particle size reduction (or micronization) has been shown to increase solubility (Figure 2.7). Formation of a **eutectic mixture** of 55% w/w griseofulvin with 45% w/w succinic acid increases the solubility even further. These mixtures can also be formulated as a crystalline solid solution, where a solid solute is molecularly dispersed in a solid solvent. The water-soluble solid solvent dissolves *in vivo*, leaving a fine solution of the drug, which can improve bioavailability.

FIGURE 2.7 Dissolution of griseofulvin
Source: Chiou and Niazi (1976)

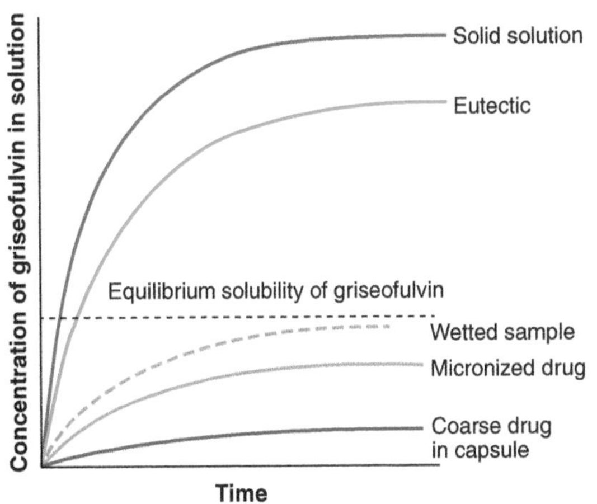

For more information on solid solutions, please refer to Section 10.2.

KEY POINT

Hydrophobic drugs have generally poor solubility as they are not readily wetted. Solubility can be improved by reducing particle size, and this includes the formation of solid solutions of an API within a solid solvent.

The van't Hoff equation

It is not uncommon to use eutectic mixtures in dosage forms because they have low melting points and are predicted to have high solubilities by the van't Hoff equation:

$$\ln(x_S) = \frac{-\Delta H^{\theta}_{fus}}{R} \cdot \left[\frac{T_m - T}{T_m \cdot T}\right]$$

where

x_S = Solubility of solute as **mole fraction.**
T_m = **Melting point** of solute in K.
T = Temperature of solution in K.
ΔH^{θ}_{fus} = **Standard enthalpy of fusion** in J mol^{-1}.
R = **Gas constant**, 8.314 J K^{-1} mol^{-1}.

Box 2.2 shows an application of this equation.

BOX 2.2

Application of the Van't Hoff equation to determine solubility

We can estimate the mole fraction solubility of naphthalene in benzene at 20°C (293 K) given that the enthalpy of fusion is 19 kJ mol^{-1} and its melting point is 80°C (353 K):

$$\Delta H^{\theta}_{fus} = 19\,\text{kJ mol}^{-1} = 19\,000\ \text{J mol}^{-1}$$

$$\ln(x_S) = \frac{-\Delta H^{\theta}_{fus}}{R} \cdot \left[\frac{T_m - T}{T_m \cdot T}\right]$$

$$\ln(x_S) = \frac{-19\,000}{8.314} \times \left(\frac{353-293}{353 \times 293}\right)$$

$$\ln(x_S) = -1.33$$

$$x_S = 0.27$$

This value is the amount of naphthalene that will dissolve in benzene, expressed as a mole fraction of naphthalene. This value assumes that this mixture behaves in an ideal manner.

For more information on enthalpy changes, please refer to Section 5.3.

The van't Hoff equation is derived by assuming the system being studied behaves as an **ideal solution**; that is, the presence of the solute has no effect on the forces existing between solvent molecules and vice versa. Consequently, the enthalpy change associated with the formation of an ideal solution from a pure solvent is zero. This behaviour is seldom encountered in practice but the concept allows development of equations and models, such as the van't Hoff equation.

Look at Figure 2.8. When temperature is increased, you can see how the solubility, shown as $\ln x_S$, is predicted to increase with temperature for a particular solid of fixed melting point. This is consistent with our experience. Thus, sugar dissolves more readily in hot tea than in cold water.

The van't Hoff equation can also be applied to study the solubilities of an ideal series of different compounds at fixed temperature. In this case, as the melting point of each compound increases, then the

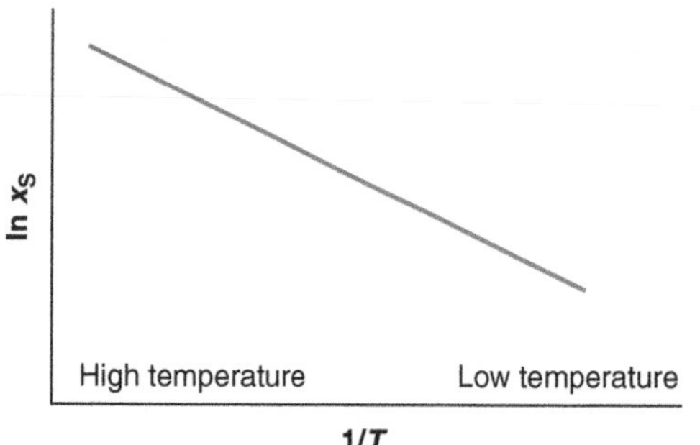

FIGURE 2.8 Predicted relationship between solubility and temperature for the ideal solutions

solubility is predicted to decrease. This behaviour is shown by a series of sulphonamide drugs (Table 2.3) and is evident in other series of compounds that are structurally similar.

As the van't Hoff equation is developed from considerations of ideal solutions, it has limitations when applied to real solutions. Factors other than melting point can have a stronger influence on solubility as seen in Table 2.4. Despite a decrease in melting point for the structurally related preservatives, parabens, there is a decrease in solubility. This is due to the impact of chain length of the substituents on the hydrophobic character, as measured by the **partition coefficient**, log *P*.

TABLE 2.3 Relationship between melting point and aqueous solubility at 20 °C for a series of sulfonamides

Compound	T_m/°C	Solubility/mg mL^{-1}
Sulfathiazole	173–175	0.588
Sulfapyridine	191–193	0.286
Sulfamerazine	234–238	0.200
Sulfadiazine	252–256	0.077

TABLE 2.4 Relationship between aqueous solubility at 20 °C and melting point for a series of parabens esters

-parabens ester	T_m/°C	Solubility/ mg mL^{-1}	Log *P*
Methyl	125–128	2.50	1.85
Ethyl	115–118	0.75	2.33
n-propyl	95–98	0.50	2.87
n-butyl	68–69	0.15	3.44

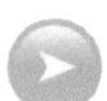

For more information on partition coefficient, please refer to Section 8.2.

KEY POINT

The van't Hoff equation predicts that solubility increases with temperature, and decreases as the melting point of the solute increases. The equation assumes ideal behaviour and does not take into account other factors that may affect solubility, e.g. hydrophobicity.

SELF CHECK 2.5

By application of the van't Hoff equation, determine the solubility of thymol in salol (phenyl salicylate) as a mole fraction at 40 °C. The standard enthalpy of fusion is 17.3 kJ mol^{-1}. Thymol has a melting point of 51.5 °C. (R=8.314 J mol^{-1} K^{-1}).

2.5 Solid dosage forms administered via the digestive tract

Tablets are the most common solid oral dosage form and they can range from relatively simple, single, **immediate-release** dosage forms to complex **modified-release** systems. In addition to the API, tablets usually contain a number of other ingredients called **excipients** (Table 2.5). In general, tablets offer the following advantages to both patients and manufacturers compared to other dosage forms:

- Easy to handle.
- Variety of manufacturing methods.
- Can be mass-produced at low cost.

- Consistent quality and dosing precision.
- Can be self-administered.
- Enhanced mechanical, chemical, and microbiological stability (particularly when compared to liquid dosage forms).
- Tamper-proof.
- Lend themselves to adaptation for other profiles, e.g. coating for modified-release.

Tablets are a popular dosage form because of their simplicity. For the patient, their uniformity of dose, blandness of taste, and ease of administration help to ensure **patient compliance**.

The purpose of the formulation and the identification of suitable excipients are of the utmost importance in the development of a successful solid formulation; that is, one of acceptable size, taste, and appearance. A well-designed formulation should contain, within defined limits, the stated quantity of active ingredient and it should be capable of releasing that amount of drug at the intended rate and site.

Compressed and layered tablets

The most common type of tablet is designed to be swallowed whole and they are prepared by compressing blends of **powders** or **granules**. If powder particles are cohesive, they have a tendency to clump together. This can be a problem when powders are moving through processing equipment, such as a tablet press, and can be addressed by granulation. A typical complete manufacturing process for a tablet product includes:

- Weighing.
- Milling.
- Granulation and drying.
- Blending and lubrication.
- Compression.
- Coating.

Tablets need to be strong enough to withstand damage during manufacture, transport, and handling.

Each processing step involves several process parameters. For a given formulation, all processing steps must be thoroughly evaluated so that a robust manufacturing process can be defined.

Stresses, such as heat and moisture, can lead to stability problems in susceptible formulations. **Direct compression (DC)** is a simple process and is more economical and less stressful to ingredients than, for example, the granulation process. However, not all formulations can be prepared by direct compression. This is determined by the physical properties of the ingredients and the quality of raw materials, and these must be carefully controlled. It can be difficult to form directly compressed tablets containing high-dose and poorly compactible drugs.

Granulation is the process of forming particles into larger grains with a diameter of 0.2–4.0 mm. Although

TABLE 2.5 Some common excipients used in tablets and their functions

Excipient	Role	Examples
Diluents or fillers	To make tablets of a size suitable for handling	Lactose, mannitol, calcium carbonate, sorbitol, microcrystalline cellulose
Binders (adhesive)	To ensure powders stick together during granulation or compression	Polyvinyl pyrrolidone (povidone, PVP) Hydroxypropylmethylcellulose (HPMC)
Glidants	To improve how the powder or granules flow	Colloidal silica, talc
Lubricants	To reduce friction between the solid and the die wall and between particles	Magnesium stearate, sodium lauryl sulphate
Disintegrants	To facilitate breaking apart of the tablet when it is in contact with fluid	Starch, sodium starch glycollate, cross-linked polyvinyl pyrrolidone
Adsorbents	To hold fluids in an apparently dry state	Fumed silica, microcrystalline cellulose
Colourants	To make the tablet more appealing and aid identification	Iron oxide, natural pigments
Flavour modifiers	To mask unpleasant tastes	Mannitol, aspartame

these aggregates can then be used as a dosage form, more commonly they are used to facilitate the pharmaceutical manufacturing process. When mixed with other excipients, granules can improve compaction properties enabling the successful production of tablets and capsules. Granulation can also improve flow properties and reduces the tendency for segregation or separation of the powders in the mix due to a more even particle size and bulk density. Granules can be produced by either dry or **wet granulation** methods, based on the stability of the API and excipients. Wet-granulation is not suited to moisture-sensitive APIs, for example.

A layered tablet, comprising two or even three layers, can be made when physical separation of ingredients is desired due to their incompatibility or to produce a repeat-action product. This formulation can also be designed to provide an immediate and a slow-release component. The technique involves using a preliminary compression step to produce a relatively soft tablet core, which is then placed in a larger die containing coating material. Further coating material is added and the content compressed. A similar light compression is used for the production of layers and a final main compression step used to bind the layers together.

KEY POINT

Direct compression (DC) involves the formation of tablets by applying a force or compressing a powdered API and excipients without the prior physical modification of this material. Wet or dry granulation may be required for poorly compactible powders that are not suited to direct compression.

Coated tablets

Tablets are often coated to protect the drug from the external environment, to mask bitter tastes, to increase physical strength or to make swallowing easier. There are several different types of coated tablets:

- Sugar coated.
- Film coated.
- Gelatin coated.
- Enteric coated.

Coatings can also be used for aesthetic or commercial purposes, improving product appearance and identity.

A sugar coating is useful in protecting the drug from the environment (for example, against oxidation) and it is also useful for taste-masking and identification. The sugar coating is water soluble and dissolves after swallowing but its use has declined in recent years due to its relative expense. It is a bulky coating, often requiring a waterproofing layer containing shellac and a subcoating process with polymers such as polyvinylpyrrolidone (PVP) to help prevent micro-cracks forming. The tablets can then be smoothed, coloured, and polished. It can add up to 50% to the weight and size of a tablet but the tablets have a smooth and elegant appearance.

Film coatings, although most often applied to tablets, can also be used to coat other formulations, including capsules. It results in the same general characteristics as sugar coating but the associated weight gain is significantly less, typically up to only 5%. Film coating is easier to automate than sugar-coating and it has capability to use organic solvents, if required. Celluloses are often used as film-forming polymers but usually require addition of a compatible plasticizer to reduce the brittleness of these thin coatings. The coating dissolves when the tablet is swallowed and the tablet core is then exposed.

Recent developments include the use of gelatin and non-animal derived coatings for tablets. It is easy to see if there is any damage to the coating and the coats can be designed with different colours for branding and identification purposes. They are reported to be preferred by patients due to their ease of swallowing and superior taste- and odour-masking properties.

Enteric coated tablets show delayed release of the drug, so the tablet passes unchanged through the stomach and into the intestines. Enteric means pertaining to the intestines and comes from the same Greek origin as enteral and parenteral (administration by a route other than the digestive tract). The coating becomes soluble at the higher pHs found in the lower part of the intestines (some can even target the colon) and the tablet core is then exposed.

For more information on routes of administration, please refer to Section 13.5.

KEY POINT

Tablets are often coated to protect the drug from the external environment, to mask bitter tastes, to increase mechanical strength or to make swallowing easier.

Modified-release tablets

To achieve and maintain effective drug levels in the body, it is often necessary to administer immediate-release formulations several times daily. This can be inconvenient for the patient and can lead to missed doses (poor compliance). There can be sequential peaks and troughs in drug levels as shown in Figure 2.9. Drug blood levels above the minimum toxic concentration can cause unwanted side-effects, while levels that fall below the minimum effective concentration will not have the desired effect. The goal is to maintain drug concentrations within this window in order to have the optimum therapeutic effect.

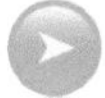

For more information on the effect our bodies have on administered drugs, please refer to Section 1.5 of *Therapeutics and Human Physiology* within this series.

Modified-release tablets are designed to deliver the drug, either locally or systemically, at a pre-determined rate for a specified duration. This approach can lead to a reduction in the number of times a dosage form needs to be given per day, especially useful for those drugs with a short **half-life**. This can reduce toxic side-effects arising from high drug levels in the body and improve **patient compliance** by keeping the plasma concentration within the desired therapeutic range.

The rate of drug release can be determined for different formulations and in extended release formulations, typically, the drug levels are maintained over a longer period of time (Figure 2.10). This is in contrast to delayed-release or enteric coated formulations, which only have a delay in the onset of release.

The API can be released from modified release formulations by diffusion or by dissolution. **Diffusion-controlled release** systems can have a reservoir or a matrix design. In reservoir systems, the API is contained completely within a rate controlling membrane as shown in Figure 2.11.

To get from inside the device to the outside environment, the drug must move across the membrane by diffusion. When used for oral delivery, these systems tend to be pellets or multiple-unit systems, rather than single-dose units. These can pass more evenly through the GI tract. When swallowed, physiological fluids from the external environment can diffuse across the membrane and dissolve the drug, thus establishing a concentration gradient. The API can then diffuse down such a gradient, through pores in the membrane

FIGURE 2.9 Variation of plasma concentrations following oral delivery of a single immediate-release tablet

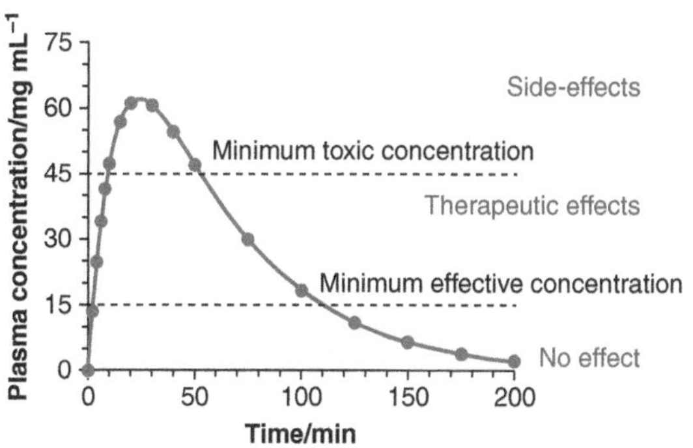

FIGURE 2.10 Schematic of the cumulative drug release from immediate-release, delayed-release, and extended-release formulations

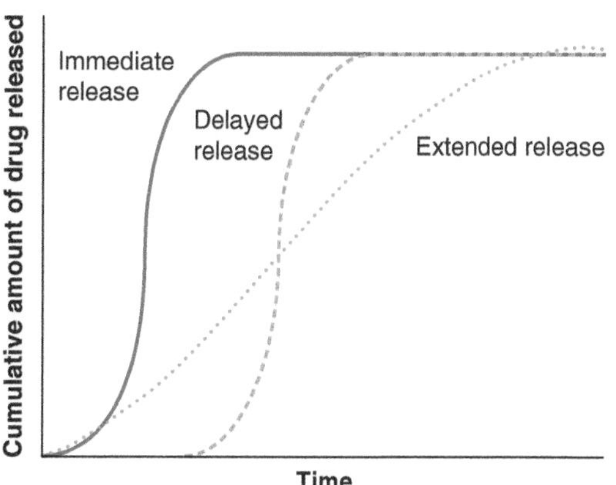

FIGURE 2.11 Reservoir-controlled drug delivery device

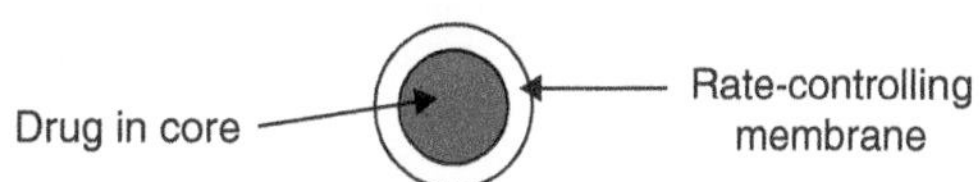

or through the membrane itself, and partition into the GI tract. Providing an excess of solid drug is maintained within the reservoir, zero-order kinetics can be maintained. This means that the release rate remains constant and is not influenced by the amount of drug released from the formulation.

For more information on zero-order kinetics, please refer to 'Zero-order reactions' in Section 12.2.

In matrix systems, which you can see in Figure 2.12, the drug is evenly or homogeneously dispersed throughout a water-insoluble polymer, an example of a **dispersion**. After swallowing, drug located at the surface of the device is dissolved and reaches the external environment by diffusion, creating a layer of API-saturated solution around the tablet. The rate of API release then decreases over time as the drug has further to diffuse to reach the external environment. If the tablet matrix itself can also dissolve or erode over time, the drug can be released by a mixture of diffusion and erosion processes and the kinetics can become quite complex.

In **dissolution-controlled release** systems, the drug can be incorporated into a slowly dissolving matrix or a slowly dissolving coating. Indeed, enteric coated formulations can be categorized in this way.

In osmotic pump delivery systems, the drug reservoir, either a solid or solution, is surrounded by a semipermeable membrane that allows water in but the drug can only be released through a pre-drilled hole.

For more information on osmotic pump delivery, please refer to Section 11.5.

For drugs with a narrow **therapeutic index**, such as nifedipine, diltiazem, and theophylline, it is recommended that the dosage form is specified when prescribing a drug, as even small changes in release profiles can lead to differences in bioavailability with a risk of underdosing or side-effects. This topic is explored further in Case Study 2.1.

KEY POINT

Tablets include immediate-release dosage forms and modified-release systems. Modified-release systems include diffusion-controlled, dissolution-controlled, and osmotic pump systems. Diffusion-controlled release systems can have a reservoir or a matrix design.

FIGURE 2.12 Matrix drug release showing (A) non-eroding and (B) eroding systems

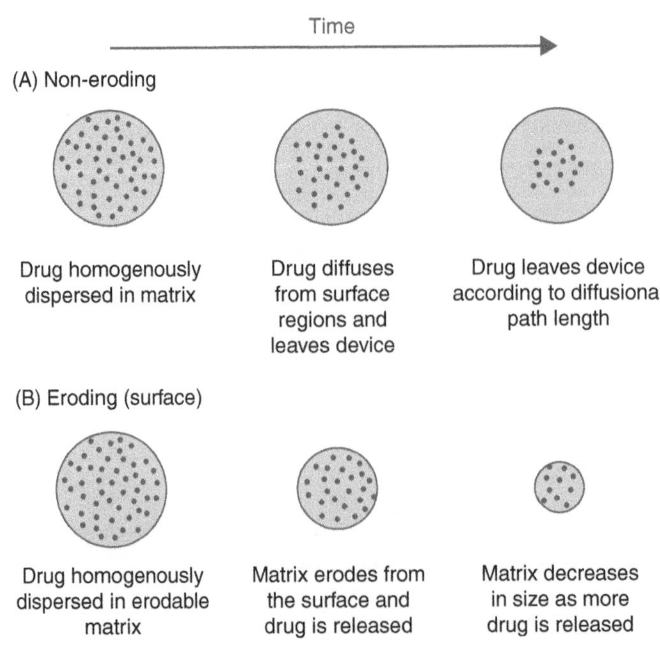

CASE STUDY 2.1

Naina was diagnosed with hypertension two years ago. She has been receiving repeat prescriptions for the last 6 months for diltiazem 120 mg twice daily. She has always received the same make of tablet, Adizem SR 120 mg, but this time she has received a capsule, Dilzem SR 120 mg.

REFLECTION QUESTIONS

1. What is meant by SR in the names of the formulations?

2. Both products contain the same amount of the same API but the brand name is different. Does it matter if she takes the Dilzem SR or should she go back and ask for Adizem SR? If so, should she approach the pharmacist or the prescribing doctor?

Answers

1 Sustained (or slow) release. This indicates that Adizem is a modified-release formulation.

2 For drugs with a narrow therapeutic index, it is recommended that the modified-release formulation is prescribed by brand name, so the release kinetics and the bioavailability are the same. She should approach the doctor as the brand name should be specified on the prescription.

Oral-disintegrating tablets

The market for **orally disintegrating** or orodispersible tablets (ODTs) has been growing rapidly, particularly for those having difficulty swallowing tablets, such as the elderly and children. They are referred to using a range of different titles: fast-dissolving, orodispersible, and fast-melting. They are useful in cases of persistent nausea or for those who have little or no access to water. Other advantages include product differentiation and market expansion; applications exist in the veterinary market for oral administration to animals, for example.

ODTs disintegrate and/or dissolve rapidly in the saliva without the need for water, within seconds to minutes. Some tablets are designed to dissolve in saliva remarkably quickly, within a few seconds, and are true fast-dissolving tablets. Others contain agents to enhance the rate of tablet disintegration in the mouth, and are more appropriately termed fast-disintegrating tablets, as they may take up to a minute to completely disintegrate. Increased bioavailability using such formulations is sometimes possible if there is sufficient absorption via the membranes in the mouth (**buccal** mucosa) prior to swallowing. However, if the amount of swallowed drug varies, there is the potential for inconsistent bioavailability. The fairly complex nature of manufacture and scale-up contribute to a relatively high manufacturing cost.

Chewable tablets

Chewable tablets are designed to be mechanically disintegrated in the mouth. Advantages mainly concern patient convenience and acceptance because they can be taken without water, although enhanced bioavailability is also claimed. This can be due to a rapid onset of action as disintegration is more rapid and complete compared to standard formulations that must disintegrate in the GI tract. This dosage form is an appealing alternative for children and elderly consumers.

A limitation with this system is that many APIs have an unpleasant bitter taste that can reduce compliance among patients. Iron salts in vitamin formulations, for example, can impart a rusty flavour and some antihistamines, such as promethazine HCl, can have a bitter aftertaste. As such, we may need to use taste-masking strategies to provide acceptable patient tolerance and to ensure patient adherence to their pharmaceutical regimen; these are often flavouring agents as mentioned in Table 2.5.

KEY POINT

Orally disintegrating tablets spontaneously break down rapidly in the mouth, while chewable tablets are designed to disintegrate through mechanical action.

Effervescent tablets

Effervescence is the reaction of acids and bases in water to produce carbon dioxide and **effervescent tablets** are dissolved or dispersed in water before administration. Advantages of effervescent formulations over conventional formulations are that the drug is usually already in solution before administration and can therefore have a faster onset of action. Although the solution may become diluted in the gastrointestinal (GI) tract, any precipitation should be as fine particles that can be redissolved more easily. Variability in absorption can also be reduced.

Formulations can be made more palatable (better tasting) and there can be improved tolerance after ingestion. Thus the types of drugs suited to this formulation method are those that are difficult to digest or are irritant to mucosal tissue of the GI tract. Vitamins and analgesics, such as paracetamol and aspirin, are common effervescent formulations. The inclusion of buffering agents can help with improving the stability of pH-sensitive drugs.

KEY POINT

Effervescent tablets are those that release carbon dioxide when in contact with water.

Lozenges

Lozenges are tablets that dissolve or disintegrate slowly in the oral cavity to release drug into the saliva. Occasionally they may be presented on a stick similar to a lollipop. They are easy to administer to paediatric and geriatric patients and are useful for maintaining extended activity within the mouth. They can contain a variety of ingredients depending on their application. Anaesthetics, antiseptics, and antimicrobials intended for local administration can be added to a sweetened, flavoured base. Alternatively, they can be used for **systemic delivery** if the drug is well-absorbed through the buccal lining or is swallowed. More traditional drugs used in this form include phenol, sodium phenolate, benzocaine, and cetylpyridinium chloride. Decongestants and antitussives are in many over-the-counter (OTC) lozenge formulations and there are also lozenges that contain nicotine (as bitartrate salt or as nicotine polacrilex resin), flurbiprofen (for inflammation), or mucin (for treatment of a dry mouth).

Compressed lozenges (or troches) differ from conventional tablets in that they are non-porous and do not contain disintegrant. As the formulation is designed to release drug slowly in the mouth, it must have a pleasant taste, smoothness, and **mouth-feel**. Chewable lozenges are popular with the children since they are 'gummy-type' lozenges. Most formulations are based on the glycerinated gelatin suppository formula, which consists of glycerin, gelatin, and water. These lozenges are often highly fruit-flavoured and may have a slightly acidic taste to cover the acrid taste associated with glycerin.

KEY POINT

Lozenges are designed to dissolve or disintegrate slowly in the mouth.

Tablets for buccal and sublingual delivery

Buccal and **sublingual** tablets dissolve in the mouth and Figure 2.13 shows where they are placed:

- Buccal tablets are placed either in the cheek area, or above the teeth.
- Sublingual tablets are placed under the tongue.

These routes of administration avoid the harsh conditions of the GI tract and are useful for drugs that are subject to high **first-pass metabolism**. Tablets placed under the tongue usually dissolve quickly and have a fast onset of action (e.g. nitroglycerin tablets), allowing a rapid intervention. Normal gels and creams are not particularly useful for retention in the mouth, as the continual production of saliva washes them away. We can add bioadhesives to buccal tablets to try and extend retention of the formulation at the site. Common uses

FIGURE 2.13 Placement of buccal and sublingual tablets

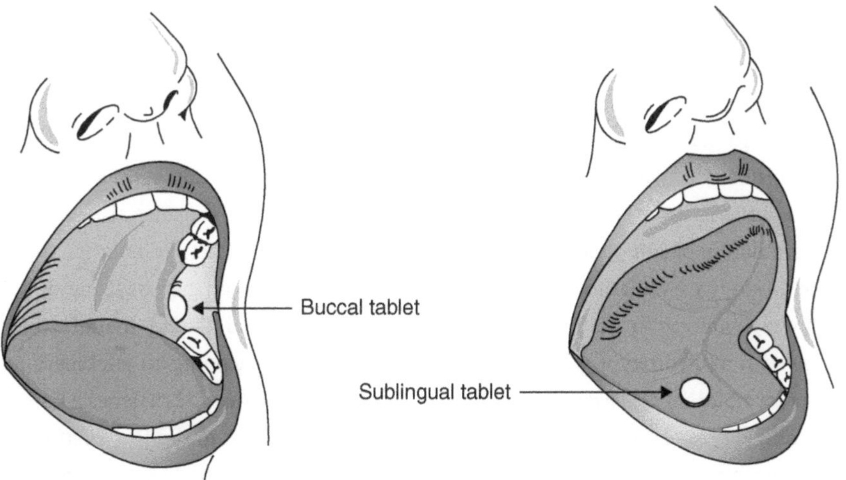

are for nausea (e.g. prochlorperazine) and nicotine replacement.

KEY POINT

Buccal and sublingual tablets avoid the harsh conditions of the GI tract and provide useful routes of administration for drugs that are subject to high first-pass metabolism.

Powders

The term powder is used to describe the physical form of a dry solid comprising finely divided particles. Many drugs or excipients are in powder form prior to processing into a dosage form. We also use the term to describe a particular dosage form and a pharmaceutical powder is made up of solid, dry, free, and quite fine particles. They can contain just the active ingredient or, more usually, excipients are added. Effective mixing of any different ingredients in a powder and prevention of segregation is very important.

As solid preparations tend to be more stable than liquids, this dosage form is useful for products that have a short half-life once in solution or suspension. Antibiotics, especially those for children, are often supplied as a dry powder to the pharmacy and the pharmacist reconstitutes them into a liquid just prior to dispensing. The patient can complete the course within the stability window (often 1–2 weeks) for the liquid product.

Drugs given as a powder can have a faster dissolution than normal immediate release tablets as there is no need for them to go through disintegration. The powders can be supplied in glazed paper wrappers, which are then packed into a box, but they are not suitable for very potent drugs, which would have little bulk; it is more common to administer these in a capsule if a tablet is not suitable. Powders must be stored in a dry place.

KEY POINT

Powdered dosage forms are useful for products that have a short half-life once in solution or suspension.

SELF CHECK 2.6

Beechams Powders contain two active ingredients, aspirin and caffeine, and other excipients.

How are they intended to be taken (what are the 'directions for use')?

Look up the Summary of Product Characteristics (SPC) for Beechams Powders and find the list of other excipients. Identify the likely main role for each of these in the formulation.

Capsules

Capsules are solid oral dosage forms in which the drug is enclosed within a hard or soft shell. The shell is normally made from gelatin and results in a simple, easy-to-swallow formulation with no requirement for a further coating step. They can be either hard or soft depending on the nature of the capsule shell, with soft capsules being manufactured using a flexible, plasticized, gelatin film. Hard gelatin capsules are usually rigid, two-piece capsules that are manufactured in one procedure and packed in another totally separate operation. The formulation of soft gelatin capsules is more complex but all steps are integrated.

There is a growing interest in using non-animal derived products, such as hydroxypropylmethyl cellulose (HPMC), for formulation of the capsule shells to address cultural, religious, and dietary requirements. Although the challenges of powder blending, homogeneity, and lubrication exist for capsules as for tablets, they are generally perceived to be a more flexible formulation as there is no requirement for the powders to form a robust compact. This means that they may also be more suitable for delivery of granular and bead-like formulations, these being fragile formulations that could be crushed by the normal compaction step. They are useful for taste-masking and are commonly employed in clinical trials as it is relatively straightforward to formulate both the placebo and active drug so that they have an identical appearance.

For more information on clinical trials and placebos, please refer to Section 13.7.

Capsules are generally a more expensive dosage form than an equivalent tablet formulation, due to the increased cost of the shells and the slower production rates. Even with modern filling equipment, the filling speeds of capsule machines are much slower than tablet presses. However, costs may be reduced by avoiding a granulation step. Although smoother and easier to swallow, capsules also tend to be larger than corresponding tablet formulations, potentially leading to retention in the oesophagus. Humidity needs to be considered during manufacture and storage, with moisture leading to stickiness and drying out (desiccation) causing brittleness. Cross-linking of the polymeric gelatin in the formulation can also lead to **dissolution** and **bioavailability** concerns.

KEY POINT

Capsules are dosage forms in which the drug is contained within a shell, normally gelatin.

SELF CHECK 2.7

Name four types of coated tablet.

SELF CHECK 2.8

Name three types of modified-release system.

2.6 Solid dosage forms administered by other routes

Solid dosage forms are often tablets for oral administration, but not exclusively so. **Dry powder inhalers (DPIs)** consist of an aerosol of fine, solid powder dispersed in a propellant gas. They are used to deliver APIs to the respiratory tract for the prevention and treatment of pulmonary conditions, and can also be used to deliver drugs systemically to other sites.

Powders for reconstitution are solid, sterile powders that can be manufactured in their final packaging; for example, an ampoule. It is intended that you reconstitute the powder before administration. If for parenteral use, then a prescribed volume of sterile diluent, often **water for injection**, is added and a solution or a suspension is formed in the container. The final product must still comply with the regulations and requirements for other injectables and is used immediately to avoid degradation.

Dusting powders are for topical use and are usually for lubrication; for example, talc. They must be sterilized if applied to open wounds to make sure they do not introduce infections. They can contain antibiotics or antifungal drugs for treatment of skin conditions.

For more information on liquid solutions for parenteral administration, please refer to 'Liquid dosage forms for parenteral delivery' in Section 3.5, and for dry powder inhalers, see 'Aerosol powder devices' in Section 4.5.

Suppositories are solid or semi-solid, dosage forms designed for rectal, vaginal, and urethral delivery. They can be used in treatments through either systemic or local action. Rectal suppositories usually contain the API within a cocoa butter or polyethylene glycol base. Many types of product have been designed for vaginal administration with creams, gels, and **pessaries** being most popular, although powders and tablets have also been used. Despite the effectiveness of systemic vaginal absorption, most products administered by this route are for the treatment of localized infections, especially *Candida albicans* (e.g. Canestan® vaginal tablets) and can contain a bioadhesive to help them remain longer at the site.

Depots and implants

A depot dosage form is designed to remain in place within the body for several days or weeks. While some depot injections are formulated using oily liquids or suspensions, **implants** are solid, sterile drug-delivery products, which are usually formed by compression or moulding. This type of dosage form is used routinely in the delivery of contraceptive drugs.

Implants can be cylindrical or pellets and they are normally placed into the layer of fatty tissue beneath the skin. This is called subcutaneous (SC) delivery and the implant is usually injected by a trained person. They are then left in place to release the API over extended periods. When the release period reaches an end, they can be removed and this gives an advantage over other depot dosage forms. Others implants are made from biodegradable polymers that break down in the body and do not require a removal step.

KEY POINT

In addition to the common oral route, solids may also be delivered through the respiratory tract, topically, parenterally, and via the rectum, vagina, and urethra.

CHAPTER SUMMARY

- At normal temperatures, most drugs are solids and maintain their original shape unless they are compressed, as happens during tablet formation.
- A crystalline material is formed when the constituent particles are arranged in a defined order and this order is then repeated, in units, throughout the entirety.
- The amorphous form of a solid is usually more soluble than the crystalline form because minimal energy is required to break up the lattice and we can take advantage of this to improve drug dissolution and absorption
- Molecules are arranged differently in different polymorphic forms; this can have a large effect upon formulation and bioavailability.
- Hydrates, like polymorphs, have different properties from the anhydrous form.
- For an ideal series of compounds, if the melting point is increased, then the solubility decreases.
- The rate of dissolution of solid particles is proportional to the surface area and, therefore, to the particle size.
- The major solid, oral dosage form is the tablet, which, in addition to the API, usually contains a number of excipients.
- To achieve and maintain effective drug levels in the body, it is often necessary to administer immediate-release formulations several times daily.

- Modified-release tablets are designed to deliver the drug, either locally or systemically, at a pre-determined rate for a specified duration.
- Tablets are often coated to protect the drug from the external environment, to mask bitter tastes, to increase strength, or to make swallowing easier.
- Buccal and sublingual pathways avoid the harsh conditions of the GI tract and are useful routes for delivery of drugs that are subject to high first-pass metabolism.
- Solid dosage forms are predominantly used for oral delivery, but are not restricted to this route.

FURTHER READING

Florence, A.T. and Attwood, D. *Physicochemical Principles of Pharmacy*, (5th edn). London: Pharmaceutical Press, (2011).

The first chapter in this book has more detail on crystal structures, crystal habit and implications for pharmaceutical development

Pudipeddi, M. and Serajuddin, A.M. Trends in solubility of pharmaceutical polymorphs and hydrates. *Journal of Pharmaceutical Sciences.* (2005); 94: 929–39.

This review article is a useful overview of the extent of polymorphism in drug substances and the impact on solubility London

Sinko, P.P. *Martin's Physical Pharmacy and Pharmaceutical Sciences*, (6th edn). Baltimore: Lippincott, Williams and Wilkins, (2010).

Chapter 22 in this book is particularly good for oral solid dosage forms and contains a useful section on mechanical properties

The British Pharmacopoeia. London: British Pharmacopoeia Commission, The Stationary Office, (2013).

The Pharmacopoeia is an official compendium containing monographs, useful definitions and standards for all types of preparations, including solid dose formulations

Pharmaceutical Excipients, available from Medicines Complete at www.medicinescomplete.com.

This reference source contains information about hundreds of different excipients and their roles in the formulation of dosage forms

REFERENCES

Eriksen, S.P. *American Journal of Pharmaceutical Education*, (1964); 28: 47.

Chiou, W.L. and Niazi, S. *Journal of Pharmaceutical Sciences*, (1976); 65: 1212.

3

Liquids

MATTHEW ROBERTS

Pharmaceutically, liquids are used extensively as a range of different **dosage forms** for the delivery of therapeutic agents via a number of routes. Liquid medicines offer advantages including ease of administration, dose uniformity, and dose flexibility.

An understanding of the chemical and physical properties of liquids is essential when developing liquid dosage forms. We will see that most liquid medicines are combinations of several ingredients mixed together to optimize the properties of the finished product.

Learning objectives

Having read this chapter you are expected to be able to:

- Define liquids in terms of their chemical and physical properties.
- Describe the key properties of liquids.
- Explain the difference between Newtonian and non-Newtonian liquids.
- Recall the meaning of the terms *dynamic viscosity* and *kinematic viscosity*.
- Describe different types of liquids, namely: solution, suspension, and emulsion.
- Recall the categories of excipients commonly used in liquid medicines.
- Recall the routes of administration used for liquid medicines and the types of liquid formulations delivered via these routes.

3.1 Structure of liquids

Liquids are one of the three states of matter. They have particles that are able to move relatively freely, whilst being attracted by intermolecular forces, including van der Waals interactions and hydrogen bonding. All pharmaceutically relevant liquids have constituent particles that are molecules and ions. Liquids are able to take on the shape of any container and have a volume that remains relatively constant, even under pressure. Figure 3.1 shows how molecules within a liquid are closely associated with each other and assume the shape of the beaker.

As the molecules within a liquid are relatively tightly packed, liquids are usually similar in density to solids and are far denser than gases. Liquids and solids can both be referred to as condensed matter, whilst liquids and gases are known as fluids, as they are both able to flow. The ability of liquids to flow is an advantage when it comes to measurement, as we can use volumetric techniques to accurately measure amounts of liquids. This ability also aids manufacturing, as liquids can be easily stirred, poured, and transferred between vessels.

FIGURE 3.1 Representation of the arrangement of molecules within a liquid

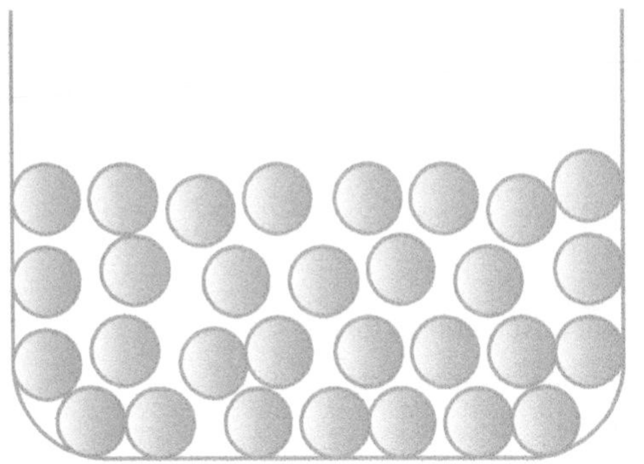

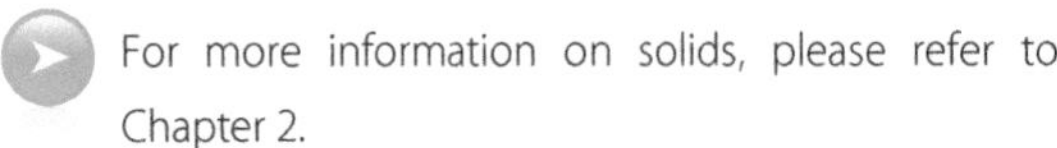

For more information on solids, please refer to Chapter 2.

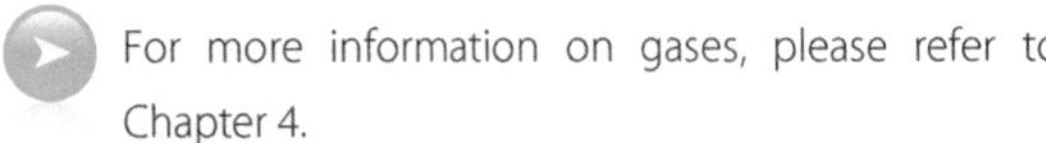

For more information on gases, please refer to Chapter 4.

KEY POINT

All pharmaceutically relevant liquids have constituent particles that are molecules and ions. The particles within a liquid are bound together firmly but not rigidly. Liquids are similar in density to solids, but far denser than gases, and have a fixed volume. They adopt the shape of their container.

The particles within a liquid are bound together firmly but not rigidly and have limited freedom to move around and slide over each other. **Kinetic theory** predicts that, as temperature increases, both molecular vibrations and the average distances between the molecules increase. A liquid reaches its normal **boiling point** at the temperature at which the **vapour pressure** of the liquid is equal to the external atmospheric pressure (1 atm). At this point, the cohesive forces that bind the molecules closely together begin to break and the liquid undergoes a **phase transition** to a gas. This process is called **vaporization**. When temperature is decreased, the distances between the molecules become smaller. When the liquid reaches its **melting point**, the molecules will begin to lock into a very specific order. This process is called freezing and the bonds between particles become more rigid, changing the liquid into its solid state.

For more information on phase transitions, please refer to 'Phases, phase transitions, and phase equilibria' in Section 7.1.

KEY POINT

Phase transitions between solid and liquid occur at the melting point, and between liquid and gas at the boiling point.

Examples of the general use of liquids in everyday life include oils in the food industry, solvents in cosmetics, inks and dyes, or coolants and lubricants in machinery. Water is ubiquitous in biological systems and many common pharmaceutical liquids are water-based (aqueous).

SELF CHECK 3.1

(a) Name two types of intermolecular forces associated with molecules within a liquid. (b) What happens to the molecules within a liquid when (i) the temperature drops to the melting point, and (ii) the temperature rises to the boiling point?

3.2 Properties of static liquids

Liquids have a variety of different physical properties, which can be measured and manipulated when developing medicines. We will see that liquid **dosage forms** can range from mouthwashes, oral syrups, and suspensions, to injectable solutions, topical lotions, and shampoos. The physical appearance and properties of these products varies greatly.

Volume

Quantities of liquids are commonly measured in units of volume. These include the **SI unit** metre cubed (m^3) and its divisions, in particular the **decimetre cubed (dm^3)**, more commonly called the litre ($1\,dm^3 = 1\,L = 0.001\,m^3$), and the centimetre cubed, also called millilitre ($1\,cm^3 =$

FIGURE 3.2 Representation of 1 litre (1 dm^3) and 1 millilitre (1 cm^3) volumes

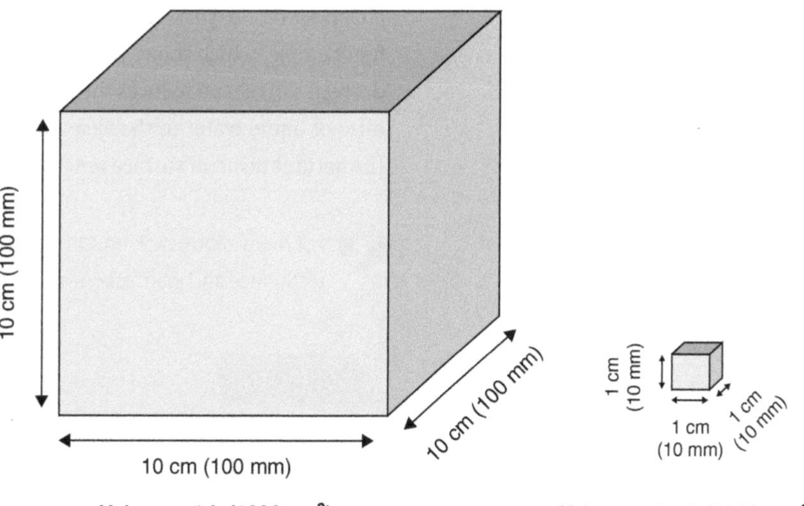

1 mL=0.001 L=1×10^{-6} m^3). Figure 3.2 illustrates the difference between the two common volumetric measurements of a litre and a millilitre. The volume of a liquid is fixed by its temperature and pressure. Liquids generally expand when heated, and contract when cooled.

A range of equipment may be used for the accurate measurement of the volume of pharmaceutically relevant liquids:

- Measuring cylinders for quantifying a range of liquid volumes.
- Volumetric flasks for the precise measurement of single volumes.
- Pipettes for the precise measurement and transfer of liquids.
- Burettes for measurement and control when transferring liquids during titrations.

Standard volumetric laboratory apparatus are shown in Figure 3.3.

KEY POINT

Liquids generally expand when heated and contract when cooled.

KEY POINT

A volume of 1 dm^3 is equivalent to 1 litre and it occupies 1000 cm^3, 1000 mL or one-thousandth (1×10^{-3}) of a metre-cubed (m^3).

FIGURE 3.3 Standard laboratory apparatus for the measurement of liquid volumes: (A) measuring cylinder, (B) volumetric flask, (C) pipette, and (D) burette

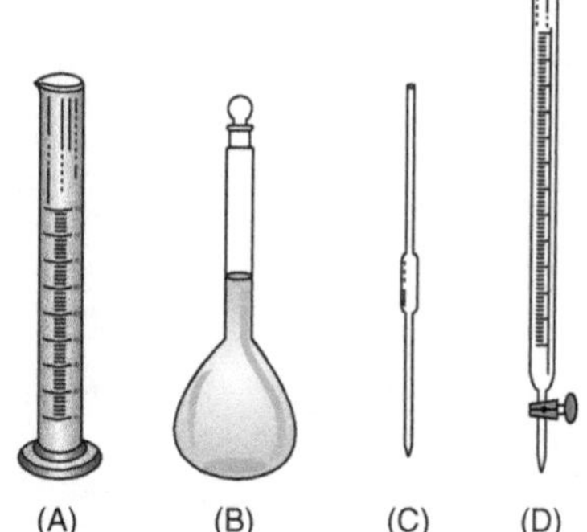

Density

The **density** (Greek letter rho, ρ) of a liquid is obtained by dividing its mass by its volume:

$$\rho = m/V$$

Knowledge of the density of liquids is important as it has a direct influence on other fundamental properties such as **viscosity**. Density is expressed in SI units as kilogram per metre cubed (kg m^{-3}). Water has a density of 998 kg m^{-3} at 20 °C, which is equivalent to 0.998 g cm^{-3}. The densities of some other pharmaceutically relevant liquids are shown in Table 3.1.

KEY POINT

Density is the mass of a substance per unit volume.

TABLE 3.1 The densities of some pharmaceutical liquids at 20 °C

Liquid	Density / g cm^{-3}
Ethanol	0.789
Water	0.998
Chloroform	1.483
Glycerol	1.261

Surface tension

The phenomenon of **surface tension** is caused by the **cohesive forces** between liquid molecules. Everyday examples of surface tension can be seen when objects that are denser than water, such as a needle or a paperclip, float on the surface of water. Look at Figure 3.4, for example, which shows the formation of a spherical droplet. This shape reduces the surface area to volume ratio of liquid water to the absolute minimum, and is the natural result of surface tension.

For more information on surface tension please refer to 'Surface and interfacial tension' in Section 9.1.

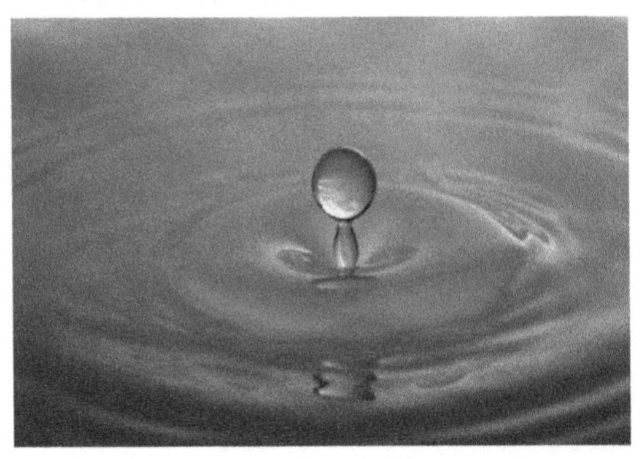

FIGURE 3.4 A spherical droplet of water
Source: iStockphoto/BanksPhoto

KEY POINT

The phenomenon of surface tension explains why liquid droplets prefer to adopt a spherical shape.

SELF CHECK 3.2

What are the following volumes when expressed in litres?

(a) 25 cm^3

(b) 250 mL

(c) 2.5 dm^3

SELF CHECK 3.3

If a liquid has a density of 1.35 g cm^{-3}, what volume, in cm^3, will 27 g of the liquid occupy?

3.3 Properties of flowing liquids

Liquids, like gases, are fluids and are able to flow. This may be described as **lamellar flow**, when the liquid moves in parallel layers that do not interact with each other. For example, blood flow in most of the circulatory system is laminar. In **turbulent flow**, the movement of the fluid at a particular point is constantly changing in both speed and direction. In the circulatory system, turbulent blood can sometimes occur due to the presence of an obstruction caused by disease.

For more information on lamellar and turbulent flow, please refer to 'Flow' in Section 4.2.

Viscosity measures the resistance of a liquid to flow. Relatively viscous liquids, such as honey or oil, will have less fluidity than less viscous liquids, such as milk or water. The viscosity of liquids normally decreases as temperature increases, as the molecules within the liquid are able to move more freely and therefore flow more readily.

An understanding of viscosity is essential when formulating liquid medicines. Manufacturers must be able to reproduce the same consistency and smoothness of the product in every batch that is made. Pharmaceutical liquids have a range of viscosities and,

FIGURE 3.5 **Examples of liquid formulations with different viscosities: (A) a mouthwash and (B) a linctus**
Source: (A) iStockphoto/Juanmonino and (B) iStockphoto/DNY59

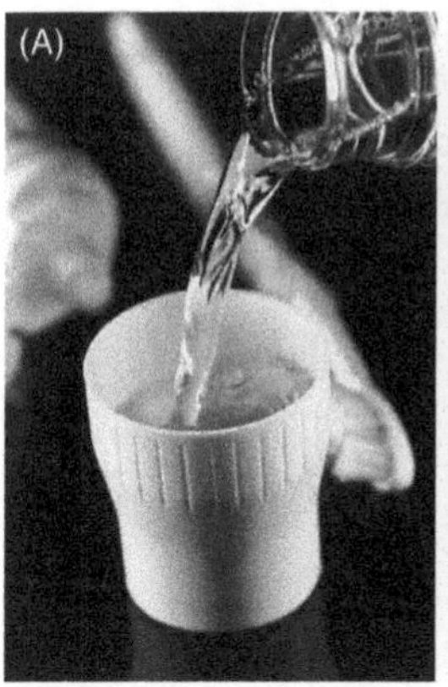

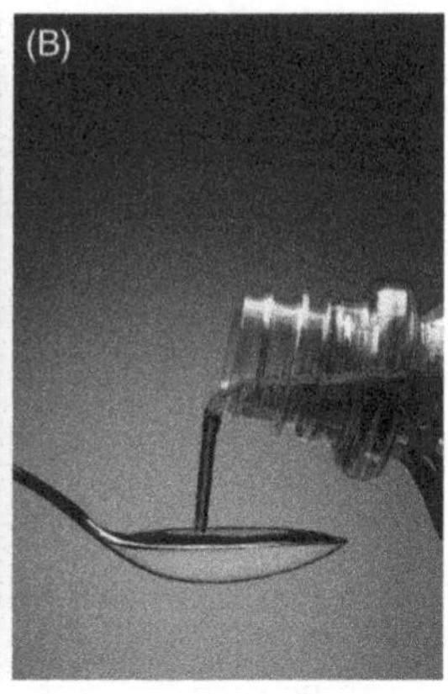

in many cases, it is a key property of the formulation. For example, the antibacterial mouthwash and cough linctus shown in Figure 3.5 have very different flow characteristics. The lower viscosity of the mouthwash enables it to be rinsed around in the oral cavity. The higher viscosity of the linctus enables more effective relief when swallowed by prolonging the time in contact with affected area and it allows for easier delivery using a measuring spoon.

The viscosity of **otic** preparations is important to ensure ease of administration and also the retention of the preparation at the site of administration. **Ophthalmic** preparations, such as eye drops or contact lens wetting solutions, must provide lubrication to the eye on blinking, but must not flow away from the surface of the eye too rapidly. This is a fine balance that requires optimization of the viscosity of the solution. Pharmaceutical liquid formulations for parenteral use generally have a relatively low viscosity to avoid difficulties during administration and pain at the site of injection.

Clearly, the viscosity of liquid dosage forms is of direct interest within pharmaceutics. Some APIs affect the viscosity of physiological fluids and this is, therefore, of indirect interest. An example API is discussed in Case Study 3.1.

For more information about otic, ophthalmic, and parenteral delivery please refer to Section 13.5.

Dynamic viscosity (η)

A liquid flows when subjected to **shear stress** (δ), which is the force applied per unit area. Different layers within the liquid flow at different rates and this deformation is measured as **strain** (γ) or shear rate. Viscosity measures the resistance of a liquid that is being deformed by shear stress. Water and most gases are described as **Newtonian** fluids because they exhibit constant viscosities, regardless of how fast they are stirred or mixed. When shear stress is plotted against strain, a linear relationship will be observed for Newtonian liquids (Figure 3.6). Other liquids may

CASE STUDY 3.1

Dilip Patel is suffering from painful leg cramps. His doctor tells Dilip that he has a condition called intermittent claudication caused by poor circulation. The doctor prescribes tablets containing pentoxifylline, which is a type of drug that acts by reducing blood viscosity.

REFLECTIVE QUESTIONS

1. Does the medicine that Dilip has been prescribed produce a local effect or a systemic effect?

2. Explain how the drug that Dilip has been prescribed can improve his blood circulation?

Answers

1 Systemic effect – the medication is delivered in the form of tablets, which are to be taken orally. The drug is absorbed into the bloodstream from the gastrointestinal tract.

2 Blood consists of plasma and particles such as red blood cells and its viscosity is about five times greater than that of water. Viscosity measures the resistance of a liquid to flow and the medicine prescribed to Dilip acts by reducing blood viscosity, thus improving blood flow and improving the circulation of blood in his legs and thereby providing relief from his painful cramps.

FIGURE 3.6 Types of liquid behaviour

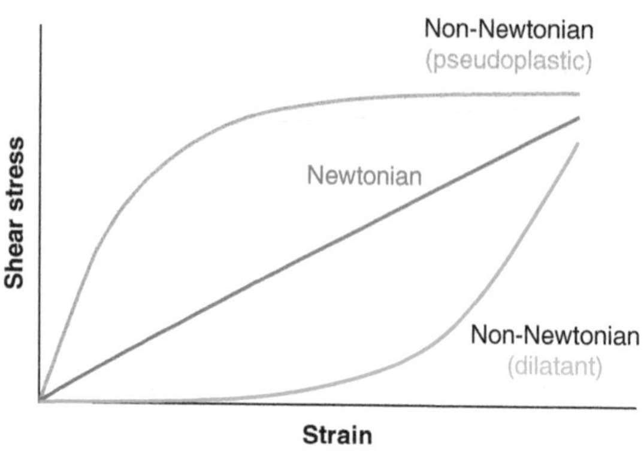

show **non-Newtonian** behaviour and exhibit non-linear stress-strain profiles.

The ratio of shear stress to strain is known as the **dynamic viscosity** (Greek letter eta, η):

$$\eta = \delta / \gamma$$

The **SI unit** of **dynamic viscosity** is the pascal-second (Pa s), where 1 Pa s is equivalent to 1 kg $m^{-1}s^{-1}$. If a fluid with a viscosity of 1 Pa s is placed between two plates, and one plate is pushed sideways with a shear stress of 1 Pa, it moves a distance equal to the thickness of the layer between the plates in a time of 1 s. The dynamic viscosities of some pharmaceutical liquids, expressed in millipascal-second units (mPa s), are shown in Table 3.2 (also see Box 3.1).

KEY POINT

Viscosity is a measurement of a liquid's resistance to flow and must be considered in the design of liquid dosage forms. Dynamic viscosity is the measure of the resistance to flow of liquid under an applied force and it is constant for Newtonian liquids. It has SI units of pascal-seconds (Pa s). Some pharmaceutically relevant dispersions exhibit non-Newtonian behaviour, where the viscosity of the liquid depends on the applied force.

TABLE 3.2 The viscosity of some pharmaceutical liquids at 20 °C

Liquid	Dynamic viscosity/mPa s
Chloroform	0.58
Water	1.00
Ethanol	1.20
Glycerol	1490

BOX 3.1

Centipoise

Dynamic viscosity is often expressed in the physical unit of the *poise* (P), named after Jean Louis Marie Poiseuille, or more commonly as *centipoise* (cP). One poise is equivalent to 0.1 pascal-second (Pa s). It follows that:

$$1\ \text{cP} = 1\ \text{mPa s} = 0.001\ \text{Pa s}$$

Water at 20 °C has a viscosity of 0.001 Pa s or 1.00 cP.

Non-Newtonian fluids

As can be seen in Figure 3.6, non-Newtonian fluids exhibit a non-linear relationship between shear stress and shear rate and may be described as follows:

- Pseudoplastic: viscosity *decreases* with increasing strain, so-called shear-thinning.
- Dilatant: viscosity *increases* with increasing strain, so-called shear thickening.

Pseudoplastic liquids become less viscous as they are stirred or mixed and a minimum viscosity is approached at high shear stresses. Common examples of pseudoplastic liquids include paints and ketchup, which can be made to flow by the application of force but regain their higher viscosity once the force is removed. Pharmaceutical materials that exhibit pseudoplastic behaviour include aqueous **dispersions** of polymers such as methyl cellulose and polyvinyl pyrrolidone, which may be used to modify the viscosity of liquid formulations.

For more information about dispersions, please refer to Section 10.1.

Materials that exhibit dilatant behaviour are less common, but can be seen in highly concentrated dispersions. At high shear rates, particles aggregate and cause an increase in resistance to flow; for example, a concentrated mixture of corn flour and water.

Other types of non-Newtonian fluids undergo time-dependent changes in viscosity. These include **thixotropic** materials, which become less viscous over time when a constant shear stress is applied and **rheopectic** materials, which become more viscous over time when a constant shear stress is applied.

Kinematic viscosity (ν)

The ratio of dynamic viscosity to the density (Greek letter rho, ρ) of the liquid is characterized by the **kinematic viscosity** (Greek letter nu, ν), and may be calculated as follows:

$$\nu = \eta / \rho$$

As the SI unit of dynamic viscosity (Pa s) is equivalent to kg $m^{-1}s^{-1}$ and the SI unit of density is kg m^{-3}, we can express the kinematic viscosity in units of m^2s^{-1} (also see Box 3.2).

Viscosity measurement

We can measure viscosity with instruments known as viscometers and rheometers. For Newtonian liquids, viscosity is a constant over a wide range of shear rates and we may use a viscometer. Non-Newtonian liquids without a constant viscosity cannot be described by a single number and exhibit a variety of different correlations between shear stress and shear rate. A rheometer is used for these liquids as they require more parameters to be set and measured (Box 3.3).

One of the most common instruments for measuring kinematic viscosity is the glass capillary viscometer (sometimes referred to as the U-tube viscometer), which measures the flow of a liquid through a capillary under the influence of gravity. A diagram of a glass capillary viscometer is shown in Figure 3.7. The liquid being examined is transferred to the viscometer through tube L, until it fills the bulb A and reaches the mark G. The liquid is then forced through capillary R under pressure to a point above the mark E. When the pressure is released the time taken for the liquid to fall from E to F is measured.

The kinematic viscosity (ν) of the liquid can then be found from the expression:

$$\nu = Ct$$

Where t is the time taken in seconds for the liquid to fall and C is the instrument constant, determined by measuring the time taken for a liquid of known viscosity to fall.

C can then be determined using:

$$C = \nu / t$$

It follows that if kinematic viscosity is expressed in units of m^2s^{-1} and time in seconds, then the instrument

BOX 3.2

Centistoke units

In addition to SI units, kinematic viscosities are commonly expressed in units of stokes (St), named after George Gabriel Stokes:

$$1\ \text{St} = 10^{-4}\ m^2s^{-1} = 1\ cm^2s^{-1}$$
$$1\ \text{cSt} = 10^{-6}\ m^2s^{-1} = 1\ mm^2s^{-1}$$

Water at 20 °C has a kinematic viscosity of about 1 centistoke (cSt).

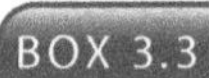

BOX 3.3

Rheology

Rheology is the study of the flow of liquids and semi-solids in response to an applied force. A rheometer is an instrument that measures changes in the rate of strain relative to the rate of stress applied. Rheometers that control the applied shear stress or shear strain are called rotational rheometers. They are used pharmaceutically to characterize non-Newtonian fluids such as emulsions, suspensions, and other **disperse systems**.

For more information on disperse systems, please refer to Section 10.4.

FIGURE 3.7 A diagram of a glass capillary viscometer

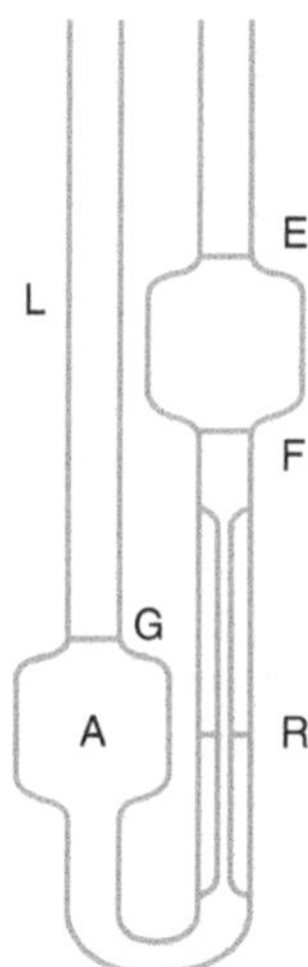

constant will have units of m^2s^{-2}. The value of C is dependent on the radius of the glass capillary.

KEY POINT

Kinematic viscosity is the ratio of a liquid's dynamic viscosity to its density. It has SI units of $m^2\ s^{-1}$.

An alternative method for determining the viscosity of many pharmaceutically relevant liquids is to use a falling sphere viscometer. Stokes' law states that the force retarding a sphere moving through a viscous fluid is directly proportional to the velocity of the sphere, the radius of the sphere, and the viscosity of the fluid. This law is the basis of the falling sphere viscometer (Figure 3.8), in which the fluid is stationary in a vertical glass tube. A steel sphere of known size and density is allowed to descend through the liquid in the viscometer.

The time taken for the sphere to travel through the central portion of the viscometer is recorded; for example, from the 175 mm mark to the 25 mm mark in Figure 3.8. Within this section, the sphere travels at a constant velocity known as the terminal velocity. This arises when the force of gravity on the sphere is equal to the resistive force due to the liquid viscosity. If the sphere travels a distance s over time t then we can calculate the terminal velocity (u):

$$u = s/t$$

In the case of the viscometer shown in Figure 3.8, $s = 150$ mm. Knowing the terminal velocity (u), the acceleration due to gravity (g), the diameter (d) and density of the sphere (ρ_s), and the density of the liquid (ρ_l), the kinematic viscosity (ν, mm^2s^{-1}) of the liquid may be calculated using the following equation:

$$\nu = [d^2 g(\rho_s - \rho_l)F]/[0.18\,u\rho_l]$$

The acceleration due to gravity, g, normally has a value of 9.81 m s^{-2}. F is a correction factor, also known as the Faxen term, and is calculated based on the diameters of the viscometer (D) and the sphere (d). Providing D is at least 10 times larger than d, and only the middle half of the viscometer tube is used to determine the velocity of the sphere, F may be calculated using the following equation:

$$F = 1 - (2.1(d/D))$$

FIGURE 3.8 A diagram of a falling-sphere viscometer

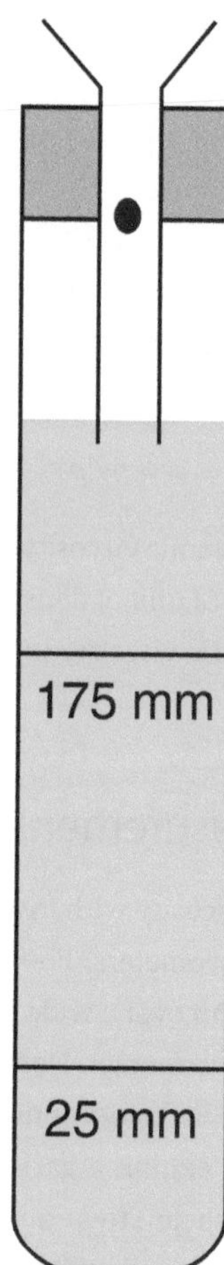

The Faxen term is a unitless quantity that is required to account for the additional resistance that the walls of the viscometer exert on the motion of the sphere.

KEY POINT

Viscosity can be measured using a viscometer or a rheometer.

SELF CHECK 3.4

What is the difference between a Newtonian and a non-Newtonian liquid?

SELF CHECK 3.5

What is the kinematic viscosity of liquid, in m^2s^{-1}, which has a density of 1.5 g cm^{-3} and a dynamic viscosity of 2.3 cP?

SELF CHECK 3.6

The instrument constant of a glass capillary viscometer was determined by the investigation of a liquid with a kinematic viscosity of 2 mm^2s^{-1}. This liquid takes 300 s to flow through the viscometer. (a) What is the instrument constant of this viscometer? (b) What is the kinematic viscosity of a liquid which takes 450 s to flow through the same viscometer?

SELF CHECK 3.7

A steel sphere of 0.2 cm diameter and density 8 g cm^{-3} takes 30 s to fall a distance of 15 cm through a liquid of density 1.4 g cm^{-3} in a viscometer with a diameter of 4 cm. (a) Given that the diameter of the viscometer is more than 10 times larger than the diameter of the sphere, determine the Faxen term for this viscometer. (b) Assuming g=981 cm s^{-2}, what is the kinematic viscosity of the liquid?

3.4 Types of liquids

A typical liquid dosage form is composed of the **active pharmaceutical ingredient (API)** contained within a liquid vehicle, the solvent, along with other excipients. We can broadly classify solvents into two categories: **polar** and **non-polar**.

Water is the most common solvent used in dosage forms and it has a polar nature. The water molecule forms an angle, with hydrogen atoms at the tips and oxygen at the vertex. Since oxygen has a higher electronegativity than hydrogen, the oxygen atom has a partial negative charge (δ^-), whereas hydrogen atoms have a partial positive charge (δ^+). An object with such a charge difference is called a dipole, meaning two poles. By convention, the direction of the dipole moment points towards the negative pole, the oxygen atom. The charge differences cause water molecules to be attracted to each other (the relatively positive areas being attracted to the relatively negative areas) and to other polar molecules. This attraction contributes to hydrogen bonding, and explains many of the properties of water, such as solvent action. Look at Figure 3.9 and see how the structure of a water molecule creates a dipole.

FIGURE 3.9 The chemical structure of water

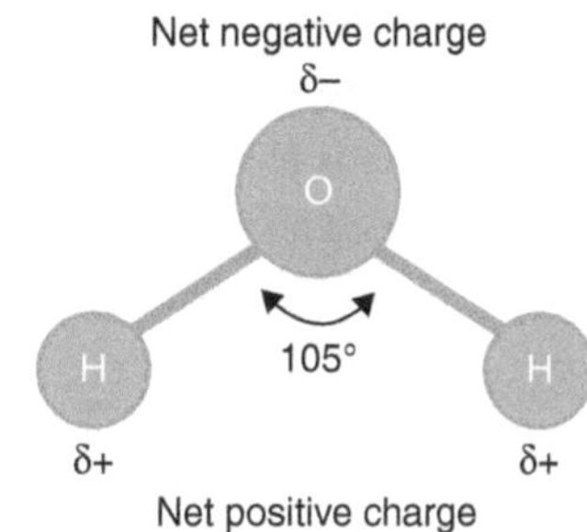

Substances that mix well and dissolve in water are called *hydrophilic* ('water-loving'), while those that do not mix well with water are known as **hydrophobic** ('water-fearing'). The ability of a substance to dissolve in water is determined by whether or not the substance can overcome the strong attractive forces between the molecules of water. When an ionic or polar compound enters water, it becomes surrounded by water molecules and we refer to this process as hydration. The relatively small size of water molecules typically allows many water molecules to surround one molecule of solute. The regions of each water molecule that bear a partial negative charge are attracted to positively charged regions of the solute, and vice versa.

For more information on hydrophobicity, please refer to Section 8.1.

KEY POINT

Water is the most common solvent used in dosage forms. It has a polar nature.

Solutions

A solution may be defined as a single **phase** (homogenous) system where one or more ingredients (solute) are dissolved in a vehicle (solvent). The solute is molecularly dispersed throughout the solvent and cannot be extracted by filtration. When a solid, liquid or gaseous solute dissolves in a solvent, both substances interact with each other in a process called **dissolution**. When a solid dissolves, solvent molecules disrupt the arrangement of solute molecules and **entropy** is increased, making the solution more thermodynamically stable than the solute alone. This arrangement is mediated by the respective chemical properties of the solvent and solute, such as their hydrogen bonding ability and dipole moment. The ability of a solute to dissolve into a solvent is known as **solubility**. It is important to emphasize that solubility refers to the amount of a solute that can dissolve in a solvent and the rate of dissolution refers to how long it takes for the solute to dissolve. Although highly soluble materials tend to dissolve quickly, some materials are soluble in water but take can take several hours to dissolve. An example of the latter is hypromellose, a cellulose polymer used in eye drops and other pharmaceutical formulations. Gas solutes have limited pharmaceutical application.

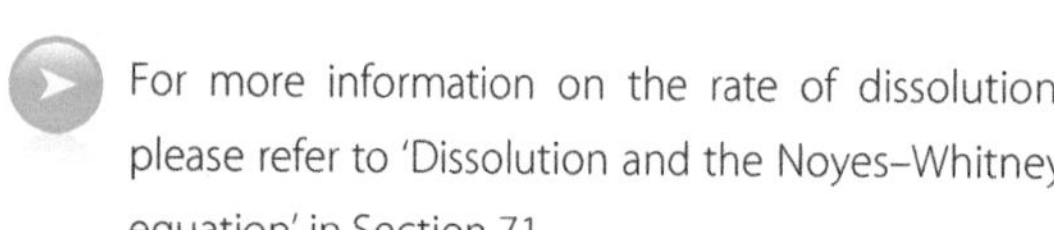

For more information on the rate of dissolution, please refer to 'Dissolution and the Noyes–Whitney equation' in Section 7.1.

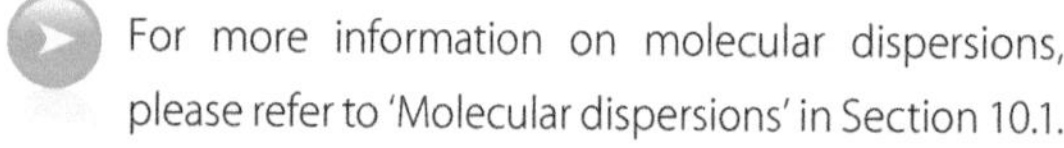

For more information on molecular dispersions, please refer to 'Molecular dispersions' in Section 10.1.

For more information on entropy, please refer to 'Entropy of a system' in Section 5.4.

For more information on the solubility of solids, please refer to Section 2.4.

When discussing combinations of two or more liquids in solution, we refer to **miscibility** rather than solubility. **Miscible** liquids readily mix together in any ratio without separating into two phases, whilst **immiscible** liquids do not mix readily and do not, therefore, form a solution but may be formulated as an **emulsion**. A familiar mixture of miscible liquids is alcohol and water, used as a base for liniments or as a solution for sterilizing work surfaces.

For more information on emulsions, please refer to 'Emulsions' in Section 10.2.

Solid solutes are by far the most common in solution dosage forms and their solubility is dependent on the solvent and influenced by other factors, such as temperature. The concentration of the solution can be expressed in a variety of units:

- Molarity, M or mol dm^{-3}.
- Molality, mol kg^{-1}.
- %(w/v), %(v/v), and %(w/w).
- ppm and ppb.
- Mole fraction.
- Milliequivalents (mEq).

These units are interconvertible, although other information may be required, e.g. the molecular mass of the solute or its valency (see Box 3.4).

In general, ionic and polar substances, such as acids, alcohols, and salts, are relatively soluble in water, and non-polar substances, such as fats and oils, are not. Non-polar molecules stay together in water because it is energetically more favourable for the water molecules to hydrogen bond to each other than to engage in van der Waals interactions with non-polar molecules.

An example of an ionic solute is table salt, NaCl. Upon addition to water, sodium chloride separates into Na^+ cations and Cl^- anions that are transported away from their crystalline lattice and into solution. An example of a non-ionic solute is sugar. The water dipoles make hydrogen bonds with the polar regions of the sugar molecule (OH groups) and allow it to be transported into solution.

KEY POINT

A solution may be defined as a single-phase (homogenous) system, where a solute is dissolved in a solvent. Solution concentrations can be expressed using molarities (mol dm^{-3}) or a variety of other units.

Suspensions and emulsions

Suspensions and **emulsions** are both examples of **disperse systems**. Suspensions are heterogeneous systems

BOX 3.4

Units of concentration

You may have already encountered solution concentrations expressed as molarities (M), where 1 M=1 mol dm^{-3}. The molar concentration of a solute, [S], is given by:

$$[S]=n/V$$

Where n is the number of moles of solute and V is the volume of the *solution* in dm^3.

Molality is distinct as it measures the number of moles of solute per kilogram of solvent. At low concentrations, molarities and molalities are similar for aqueous solutions, as water has a density close to 1 kg L^{-1}.

Solution concentrations may also be expressed as a percentage: %(w/v), means percentage weight–volume, is used to represent the mass of solute in grams per 100 mL of solution. Thus, 0.04%(w/v) chlorphenamine maleate, used in the treatment of hayfever and other allergies, will contain 2 mg per 5 mL spoonful. %(v/v), means percentage volume–volume and might be preferred when considering solutions formed by two miscible liquids. A 70%(v/v) alcohol solution contains 70 mL of ethanol per 100 mL of solution. Less commonly, solution concentrations can be expressed as %(w/w) or percentage weight–weight. A 1% (w/w) solution contains 1 g of the soluble component per 100 g of solution.

Parts per million (ppm) and parts per billion (ppb) are terms used to express the concentration of very dilute solutions as the mass of solute per 10^6 or 10^9 total mass of solution, respectively. Thus, a solution that is 1000 ppb is equivalent to 1 ppm. This is more convenient than writing the concentration as %(w/w), which is effectively equivalent to 'parts per hundred':

$$1000\text{ ppb}=1\text{ ppm}=1\times10^{-4}\%(\text{w/w})$$

For solutions, an equivalent (Eq) is defined as the number of moles of a dissolved substance that will either:

- Accept or donate one mole of hydrogen ions (H^+) in an acid–base reaction
- Accept or donate one mole of electrons in a redox reaction.

As values are often small, milliequivalents (mEq) are often be used. A solution that contains 1 mM of Mg^{2+} ions, for example, would have a magnesium concentration of 2 mEq/L, given that this metal has a valency of 2.

The mole fraction of a component in a mixture is a number within the range 0 and 1 that equals the fraction of the total number of moles (n) that the component contributes to the mixture. For an aqueous solution, the mole fractions of the solvent and solute (S) are given by:

$$x_{H_2O}=\frac{n_{H_2O}}{n_{H_2O}+n_S} \qquad x_S=\frac{n_S}{n_{H_2O}+n_S}$$

where solid particles are dispersed throughout a liquid continuous phase. Emulsions are mixtures where immiscible liquid droplets are dispersed within a second liquid phase. In each case, stabilizing agents may be added to improve the stability of these dispersions.

For more information on suspensions, please refer to 'Suspensions and nanosuspensions' in Section 10.2.

KEY POINT

Suspensions and emulsions are examples of dispersions; fine particles of solid, or droplets of liquid, are dispersed throughout a liquid continuous phase.

SELF CHECK 3.8

Given that the relative molecular mass of NaCl is 58.5, what is the molarity of a 0.9 % (w/v) saline solution?

SELF CHECK 3.9

Drug A has an aqueous solubility of 50 mg mL^{-1}, drug B has an aqueous solubility of 500 g L^{-1} and drug C has an aqueous solubility of 500 µg mL^{-1}. List the three drugs in order of decreasing solubility.

3.5 Liquid dosage forms

Liquid dosage forms can be classified according to the route of delivery, the most common ones being oral and parenteral. Liquid dosage forms may also be applied directly to the skin (topical) or eye (ocular), inserted into the nose (nasal) or ear canal (otic), or delivered as an **aerosol** form via the respiratory tract.

For more information on aerosols, please refer to 'Pharmaceutical aerosols for respiratory drug delivery' in Section 4.5.

KEY POINT

The most common routes of delivery for liquid dosage forms are oral and parenteral.

All pharmaceutical liquids contain excipients, and each serves a variety of functions in liquid formulations (Table 3.3). When formulating liquid medicines, it is essential to ensure that all excipients included are physically and chemically compatible with every other component of the formulation.

KEY POINT

All pharmaceutical liquids contain excipients and they serve a variety of functions.

Liquid dosage forms for oral delivery

The delivery of liquid medicines via the oral route has many advantages. These include:

- Ease of administration to patients who have difficulty in swallowing (e.g. infants and elderly).
- Fast absorption of the drug from the gastrointestinal tract leading to rapid therapeutic benefit.
- Possibility of masking the unpleasant taste of many drugs.

TABLE 3.3 Excipients used in liquid medicines

Excipient	Role	Example(s)
Vehicles	Liquid in which the API is dissolved or dispersed	Purified water
Co-solvents	Enhance API solubility in the vehicle	Ethanol, glycerol, propylene glycol
Surfactants	Enhance API solubility in the vehicle	Cetrimide, sodium lauryl sulphate, triethanolamine
Preservatives	Limit the presence of microorganisms in the formulation	Parabens, phenyl mercuric nitrate, sodium benzoate, benzalkonium chloride
Viscosity modifiers	Control the viscosity of the formulation	Cellulose polymers, polyvinyl pyrrolidone, alginic acid, xanthan gum
Buffers	Regulate the pH of the formulation	Citric acid, sodium citrate
Antioxidants	Enhance API stability	Sodium sulphite, ascorbic acid, butylated hydroxytoluene
Chelating agents	Enhance API stability	Disodium edetate, phosphoric acid
Sweeteners	Enhance the palatability of oral liquid formulations	sucrose, saccharin, aspartame, sorbitol
Flavourings	Enhance the palatability of oral liquid formulations	Lemon oil, orange oil, peppermint, menthol
Colourants	Enhance the aesthetic appearance oral liquid formulations	Chosen to complement the flavour

The disadvantages associated with oral liquid medicines are:

- Many APIs are chemically unstable in the presence of water.
- The mass of the product means they are expensive to transport and inconvenient for patients to carry.

For more information on drug stability please refer to Chapter 12.

Pharmaceutical solutions (and suspensions) for oral administration provide systemic absorption of the drug via the digestive tract. They are non-sterile dosage forms, however, there are limits on the number and type of microorganisms permitted to be present within the formulation. Pathogenic bacteria such as *Escherichia coli* must not be present and as oral liquids are multiple dose formulations, inhibition of the growth of less harmful microorganisms is also required. Preservatives are excipients that have antibacterial and antifungal properties and these are included in most oral liquid medicines to prevent the growth of microorganisms.

In oral solutions, the API and all of the excipients are dissolved in a suitable vehicle, which is usually purified water. Typically, the other excipients included in an oral solution are preservatives, antioxidants, viscosity modifiers, and flavourings/colourants. Oropharyngeal formulations (mouthwashes), are normally aqueous solutions designed to treat infections and inflammation of the oral cavity and may also be considered as oral solutions, although they are not swallowed.

Syrups and linctuses are examples of oral solutions that are intended to be swallowed, the drug being dissolved in a viscous, highly concentrated aqueous solution of sugar (e.g. sucrose) or artificial sweeteners (e.g. sorbitol). Linctuses are normally produced for the treatment of throat irritations and most cough medicines fall into this category. Elixirs are clear, aqueous, oral solutions containing high concentrations of alcohol and other co-solvents that improve the solubilization of the formulation ingredients.

Oral **suspensions** include many of the same excipients as oral solutions, but as the API is dispersed in a suitable vehicle (rather than being dissolved in solution), oral suspension formulations are inherently unstable.

KEY POINT

Liquid dosage forms for oral delivery are useful for treating patients who have difficulty in swallowing, although many APIs are chemically unstable in the presence of water.

Liquid dosage forms for parenteral delivery

Parenteral delivery involves the injection of a sterile solution, suspension, or emulsion system containing the therapeutic agent, directly into the body. The three common routes of parenteral delivery are:

- **Intravenous** (IV), where the formulation is administered directly into a vein.
- Intramuscular (IM), where the formulation is delivered directly into a muscle in the buttocks, the thigh, or the upper arm.
- Subcutaneous (SC), where the formulation is administered into the layer of fatty tissue beneath the skin.

IV products must be aqueous solutions that do not precipitate in the bloodstream, whilst parenteral suspensions and oil-based parenteral solutions can only be administered via the IM or SC routes. These types of formulations ensure that the active pharmaceutical ingredient (API) persists at the site of injection for extended periods and they are referred to as depot injections.

Formulations delivered via the IV route will have an immediate therapeutic action, whilst absorption of drugs from IM and SC routes is slower. Small-volume parenteral liquids (up to 10 mL) may be administered by any route but large-volume (up to 500 mL) parenteral liquids must be administered intravenously. This includes total parenteral nutrition (TPN) products which contain electrolytes and nutrients for patients who cannot take food orally.

The main drawback of IV administration is the need for training to ensure correct targeting of the injection and that the drug is administered to the vein at the correct rate. Formulations for SC delivery may be self-administered, the most common example being the self-delivery of insulin in the treatment of diabetes. SC administration is also preferred when there are problems accessing a vein for IV delivery.

Parenteral liquid formulations must be sterile and free from microorganisms that elicit a fever (known as pyrogens). Parenteral liquids for IV administration must also be *isotonic* to avoid damage to cells due to **osmotic pressure**. The vehicle for all aqueous parenteral liquids is known as **water for injection** (WFI), which is purified water prepared by distillation or **reverse osmosis** that meets specifications in terms of appearance, pH, and purity, and is free from pyrogens. Other excipients included in parenteral liquid formulations may include buffers, co-solvents, surfactants, antioxidants, chelating agents, and compounds to maintain the isotonicity, such as sodium chloride or dextrose. Preservatives are not necessary if the formulation is a single-dose product that has been sterilized.

For more information on osmotic pressure and reverse osmosis, please refer to 'Osmosis' in Section 11.1.

KEY POINT

Parenteral suspensions and oil-based parenteral solutions can only be administered via the IM or SC routes. IV dosage forms must be aqueous solutions that do not precipitate in the bloodstream.

Sterilization

Sterilization is the destruction or removal of all viable microorganisms. When pharmaceutical liquids are sterilized in their final container or packaging, then this is referred to as **terminal sterilization** and there are four traditional techniques:

- Moist heat.
- Dry heat.
- Ionizing radiation.
- Gaseous sterilization.

A fifth sterilization technique, filtration, is a **non-terminal sterilization** process.

In everyday life, boiling is a common way of purifying water but it is not a method of sterilization, as higher temperatures are required to destroy all microorganisms. Sterilization of pharmaceutical materials, equipment, and products by the use of heat is regular practice.

Moist-heat sterilization is usually performed in autoclaves and uses a combination of temperature, steam, and pressure to achieve sterility. The pressure inside the autoclave is increased to allow higher temperatures to be reached and the steam enables efficient transfer of heat. As a result, shorter exposure times can be employed during moist-heat sterilization processes and typical conditions are 121 °C for 15 minutes. Thermostable formulations, such as aqueous solutions, may be sterilized via this method, as well as dressings and glassware items such as bottles and ampoules.

Dry-heat sterilization is performed in ovens and, as it is a less efficient method of sterilization than moist heat, the temperatures used are usually higher and the exposure times are usually longer. Typical conditions are 170 °C for 1 h or 160 °C for 2 h. It is a useful technique for materials that are sensitive to moisture or impermeable to steam, and is used to sterilize some powders and oil-based liquid formulations.

Gaseous sterilization involves exposing materials or products to an appropriate gas, such as ethylene oxide, which has antimicrobial properties. Gaseous sterilization may be employed when the use of heat is not feasible and, due to the ability of the gas to penetrate porous materials, is often used to sterilize surgical accessories and medical devices.

For more information on gaseous sterilization, please refer to 'Sterilization' in Section 4.3.

Exposure of pharmaceutical products to ionizing radiation, such as electromagnetic radiation (γ-rays), is a less common form of terminal sterilization due to the requirement of specialist equipment and high cost. However, ionizing radiation may be used to sterilize materials or products that cannot be sterilized by heat, as it does not cause a significant increase in temperature.

Filtration may be used as an efficient and inexpensive way of removing microorganisms from solutions instead of destroying them using terminal sterilization techniques. Filters of pore diameter 0.22 μm are used to sterilize temperature-sensitive (thermolabile) solutions, such as parenterals and eye drops, by removing all bacteria and fungi (although viruses may not be removed due to their smaller size).

Regardless of the method of sterilization used, strict aseptic techniques must be employed during the manufacture of all sterile products. This includes such precautions as the use of specialized areas with a filtered air supply, routine cleaning and disinfecting procedures. In addition, all personnel must wear sterile clothing to avoid contamination of the product.

KEY POINT

Sterilization is the destruction or removal of all viable microorganisms and it may be terminal or non-terminal. Parenteral, nasal, ocular, and rectal delivery routes all require solutions to be sterile and isotonic.

Liquid dosage forms for other routes of delivery

There are many examples of liquid preparations for **topical** application to the skin. Lotions are usually aqueous solutions or suspensions from which water evaporates to leave a thin uniform coating of powder. This process that soothes and cools the skin and is useful in treating acutely inflamed areas. Liniments are alcoholic or oily solutions or emulsions designed for application to unbroken skin.

Liquids for application to the skin in small amounts are called paints and are formulated with a solvent such as alcohol or acetone, which evaporates quickly to leave a film on the skin containing the drug. Collodions are similar preparations to paints that leave a strong flexible film that can be used to seal small cuts or wounds. Shampoos are liquid formulations specifically intended to treat conditions affecting the scalp.

Eye drops are the most common solution formulations for the ocular delivery of an API. They must be sterile and are usually small-volume liquids that are formulated to be **isotonic** with body fluids. The main advantages of ocular drops are that they are applied directly to the problem site and, with practice, they can be administered effectively by the patient.

For more information on isotonicity, please refer to 'Isotonicity' in Section 11.3.

Nasal preparations are aqueous-based systems that are usually dropped or sprayed into the nasal cavity for the treatment of localized symptoms of congestion, allergic rhinitis (hayfever), or infection. Systemic delivery may also be achieved due to the large surface area and highly vascularized nature of the nasal cavity. Products for the systemic treatment of conditions such as migraine, diabetes, and smoking cessation are available as nasal solutions. Nasal solutions must be isotonic and buffered to pH 5.5–6.5 to maintain the natural function of the nasal passage.

Otic dosage forms can be aqueous or non-aqueous and are usually solutions for the local treatment of infection, pain, or inflammation within the ear. Otic solutions are usually applied to the ear canal in the form of drops and may include an anaesthetic and an agent to soften the ear wax.

Enemas are solutions administered rectally to irrigate or ensure clearance of the bowel (evacuation). They may also be used for both the **local** and **systemic** delivery of APIs. For example, the rectal delivery of the systemically-acting drug aminophylline minimizes the unwanted gastrointestinal reactions associated with oral therapy. Enemas can be aqueous or oil-based solutions and should be isotonic.

SELF CHECK 3.10

An oral liquid formulation contains the following excipients: water, ethanol, methyl paraben, methyl cellulose, sodium metabisulphite, and sodium saccharin. Which of the excipients perform the following roles within the formulation?

(a) Preservative.

(b) Sweetening agent.

(c) Viscosity modifier.

(d) Co-solvent.

(e) Antioxidant.

SELF CHECK 3.11

Name two routes of drug delivery for liquid medicines where the formulations must be sterile.

CHAPTER SUMMARY

- Liquids are one of the three principal classes of matter, similar in density to solids and having the ability to flow like gases.
- Molecules in a liquid move relatively freely whilst being attracted by intermolecular forces.
- Viscosity is a measure of the resistance of a liquid to flow.
- Newtonian liquids exhibit constant viscosities, regardless of the forces acting on them.
- Non-Newtonian liquids exhibit a non-linear relationship between stress and shear force.
- Dynamic viscosity (η) is expressed in pascal-second (Pa s) or centipoise (cP).
- Kinematic viscosity (ν) is the ratio of the dynamic viscosity of a liquid to the density of a liquid and is expressed in metre squared per second (m^2s^{-1}) or centistokes (cSt).
- Liquid dosage forms include solutions, suspensions, and emulsions.
- Solutions are homogenous systems where one or more solutes are dissolved in a solvent.
- Liquid medicines contain a variety of excipients.
- Liquid medicines are delivered via a number of different administration routes that will influence whether they need to be sterile and/or isotonic.

FURTHER READING

Jones, D. Chapter 5 Parenteral formulations in *FASTtrack: Pharmaceutics—Dosage Form Design*. Pharmaceutical Press, London, (2008), pp 103–33.

Provides a useful summary of parenteral formulations and sterilization processes.

Marriott, C. Chapter 4 Rheology in *Aulton's Pharmaceutics: The Design and Manufacture of Medicines*, (3rd edn). London: Churchill Livingstone, (2007), pp 42–58.

Gives a thorough overview of the rheological properties of fluids and their measurement.

Moynihan, H. A. and Crean, A. M. Chapter 2 Pharmaceutical solutions in *The Physicochemical Basis of Pharmaceuticals*. New York: Oxford University Press, (2009), pp 22–55.

A complete account of solutions and solubility relevant to pharmaceutics.

Gases

4

BEN FORBES

A number of therapeutic agents are gases that are inhaled into the **respiratory tract** for **local action** or **systemic action** through absorption into the circulatory system. There are also pharmaceutical **dosage forms** used in drug delivery that include an internal or external gas phase, e.g. aerosols and foams. These dosage forms offer advantages such as the ease of administration and control over the amount of therapeutic agent delivered.

An understanding of the chemical and physical properties of gases is essential when developing medicines that include volatile agents or utilize a gaseous phase. This chapter provides an introduction to the properties of gases, transitions between the solid or liquid and gaseous states, and examples of the practical applications of gases and gas-based pharmaceutical dosage forms in pharmacy.

Learning objectives

Having read this chapter you are expected to be able to:

- Define gases in terms of their chemical and physical properties.
- Describe the key properties of gases.
- Manipulate the ideal gas law and explain the difference between ideal and non-ideal gas behaviour.
- Explain the meaning of the terms vapour pressure and partial pressure.
- Understand the applications of gases and vaporization in the formulation and manufacture of pharmaceutical products.
- Recognize how product stability may be affected by gases.
- Describe the different types of drug delivery systems that utilize gases, namely: vapours, aerosols, and foams.
- Appreciate the routes of administration used in aerosol medicine and the types of formulations delivered via these routes

4.1 The gas laws

Matter is categorized into three states of increasing complexity: **gases**, **liquids**, and **solids**. The major distinguishing feature of material in the gaseous state is that it has no surface (and hence no boundary) and will fill completely any vessel or space. Gases are particularly sensitive to changes in temperature and pressure. The general gas laws, which are described below, apply to **ideal gases** from which it may be inferred there are limitations to the behaviour of gases in practice (non-ideal or '**real gases**'). According to the

kinetic theory of matter, gas molecules are presumed to undergo completely random movement. In the ideal gas model:

- Particles are taken to occupy negligible volume.
- Forces between molecules are considered to be insignificant.
- Collisions with other particles and the walls of the container are completely elastic (i.e. no kinetic energy is lost).

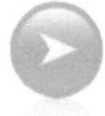

For more information on solids and liquids, please refer to Chapter 2 and to Chapter 3 respectively.

For more information on kinetic theory, please refer to 'Heat' in Section 5.1.

Non-ideal gas behaviour (i.e. deviation from the behaviour predicted by the ideal gas model) is manifest mostly under boundary conditions; for example, when a gas approaches liquefaction or is at high pressure. A full consideration of non-ideal gas behaviour is beyond the scope of this book.

Ideal gas behaviour

For ideal gases at constant temperature, a simple inverse relationship exists between volume and pressure, i.e. as the pressure of a gas increases, the volume will decrease proportionately. This is known as **Boyle's Law** and is often written as:

$$p_1V_1 = p_2V_2 \quad (4.1)$$

where V_1 is the volume of gas when the pressure is p_1 and V_2 is the volume that will result from increasing the pressure to p_2.

The relationship between pressure and volume may be represented graphically (Figure 4.1). Such correlations are referred to as **isotherms**, as they relate to quantities measured at fixed temperature.

For ideal gases at a constant pressure, the volume of a gas is directly proportional to temperature. This property of gases can be expressed simply as Charles' Law:

$$V_1 / V_2 = T_1 / T_2 \quad (4.2)$$

where V_1 is the volume of gas when the **absolute temperature** is T_1 and V_2 is the volume that will result from a temperature of T_2.

FIGURE 4.1 Representation of Boyle's law: the relationship between volume and pressure for ideal gases
Source: Adapted from Atkins and de Paula (2009)

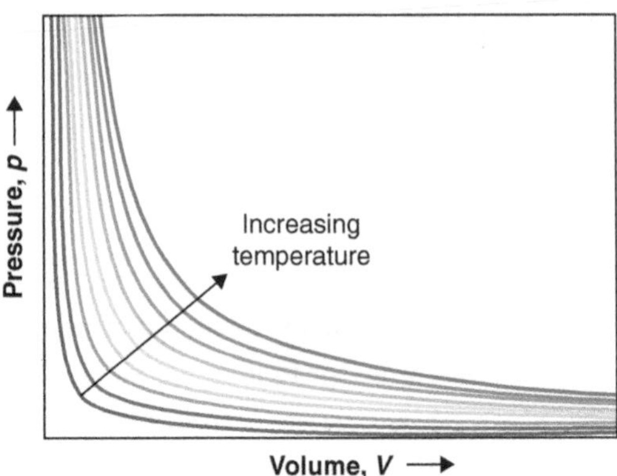

This dependence of volume on temperature explains why hot air rises, i.e. it expands upon heating and becomes less dense. The relationship between volume and temperature can be plotted as an **isobar** (Figure 4.2), the term 'isobar' being used as pressure is constant.

These laws can be combined to show the interdependency of pressure, volume, and temperature. This is demonstrated in the combined gas equation:

$$pV / T = \text{constant} \quad (4.3)$$

The value of this constant is dependent on the nature of the gas. However, if p (pressure in pascal; Pa) and T (temperature in kelvin; K) are the same, then V (volume in metre cubed, m^3) will be the same for different gases, as long as the same number of molecules (n) are present. Under Avogadro's law, this is determined by the molecular mass of the gas and hence there is a

FIGURE 4.2 Representation of Charles' law: the relationship between volume and temperature for ideal gases
Source: Adapted from Atkins and de Paula (2009)

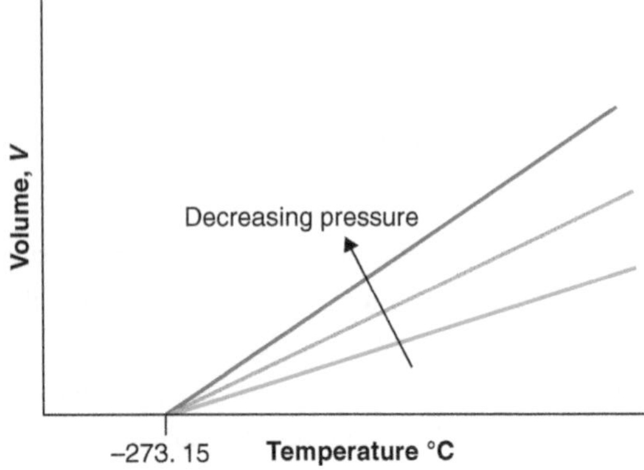

TABLE 4.1 Commonly used units for pressure. The presentation of standard atmospheric pressure in each unit is also shown

Unit	Symbol	p(atmospheric)
atmosphere	atm	1 atm
pascal	Pa	1.01325×10^5 Pa
bar	bar	1.01325 bar
millibar	mb	1013.25 mb
torr	Torr	760 Torr
millimetres of mercury	mmHg	760 mmHg

universal **gas constant,** R, which is the value of pV/T for one mole of an ideal gas.

The ideal gas equation is usually written as:

$$pV = nRT \quad (4.4)$$

The value of R is 8.314 m^3 Pa $K^{-1}mol^{-1}$. As the product of pressure and volume has equivalent units to energy, R may also be expressed as 8.314 J $K^{-1}mol^{-1}$.

The **SI unit** for pressure is the pascal (Pa) = 1 N m^{-2}. A comparison of commonly used units for pressure is provided in Table 4.1. **Standard temperature and pressure (STP)** is defined as 273.15 K (0°C) and 1×10^5 Pa (1 bar).

For more information on SI units, please refer to Section 1.5.

Real (non-ideal) gas behaviour

Ideal behaviour makes no allowance for the volume of the molecules in the gas or any attraction or repulsion. Thus any conditions that deviate from this, particularly the effect of van der Waals forces, will lead to non-ideal behaviour. In practice, this is most relevant at high pressure or low temperature, when the gas is closer to the point at which it will liquefy. In most conditions encountered in pharmaceutical applications, deviations from ideal behaviour will be small.

KEY POINTS

- An ideal gas is a theoretical model in which the constituent particles occupy negligible volume, do not exert forces, and have elastic collisions.
- Boyle's and Charles' Laws are embodied within the ideal gas equation,

$$pV = nRT$$

- If quantities are expressed in SI units, then the universal gas constant, R, has the value 8.314 J $mol^{-1}K^{-1}$.
- In general, real gases approximate to ideal behaviour under pharmaceutically relevant conditions.
- Real gases deviate significantly from the predictions of the ideal gas equation at high pressure and low temperature.

SELF CHECK 4.1

A sample of gas is held at constant temperature. If the gas is compressed so that the volume occupied is one-quarter of the original volume, how will the pressure change according to Boyle's Law?

SELF CHECK 4.2

What is the volume in centimetre cubed (cm^3) occupied by 2.60×10^{-2} mol of an ideal gas at STP?

4.2 The properties of gases

Partial pressure

The pressure, p, exerted by a gas is the result of collisions of the molecules of gas with the walls of the container. If two non-reactive gases, A and B, are combined, then the total pressure exerted by the mixture of gases is equal to the sum of the partial pressures of individual gases. Empirical observation of this phenomenon led to **Dalton's Law** of partial pressures and it applies to both ideal and real gases.

$$p = p_A + p_B \quad (4.5)$$

where p_A and p_B are respective partial pressures.

Individual partial pressures may be calculated if the **mole fraction** of gas, x_A, is known. Thus:

$$p_A = x_A p \quad (4.6)$$

For example, the mole fraction of nitrogen in air is typically 0.79. Given that normal atmospheric pressure is 1 atm, it follows that the partial pressure of nitrogen in air is 0.79 atm.

For more information on units of concentration, please refer to 'Units of concentration' in Section 3.4.

Vapour pressure

The term **vapour** is used to describe the gaseous form of a substance that exists below the **critical temperature** of that substance. The phenomenon of humidity illustrates this point. Humidity arises from water vapour in air that is at atmospheric pressure and ambient temperature. Vapours may provide a source of physical instability in products and environmental contamination during manufacture or storage (see Section 4.3). **Vapour pressure** arises when an equilibrium is established between a condensed state (liquid or solid) and a vapour phase within a **closed system**. This is highly dependent on temperature.

For more information on critical temperature, please refer to Section 7.2.

For more information on closed systems, please refer to 'Systems and surroundings' in Section 5.1.

For a mixture of miscible volatile solvents in a closed system, a vapour phase will be established at equilibrium. **Raoult's Law** describes the relationship between the partial vapour pressure of a component (A) in the vapour phase, and the mole fraction of the same component in the solution.

$$p_A = x_A p^*_A \quad (4.7)$$

where p^*_A is the vapour pressure recorded when $x_A = 1$, i.e. the vapour pressure above pure liquid A.

FIGURE 4.3 Vapour pressures of toluene–benzene mixtures at 79.6 °C illustrating Raoult's Law

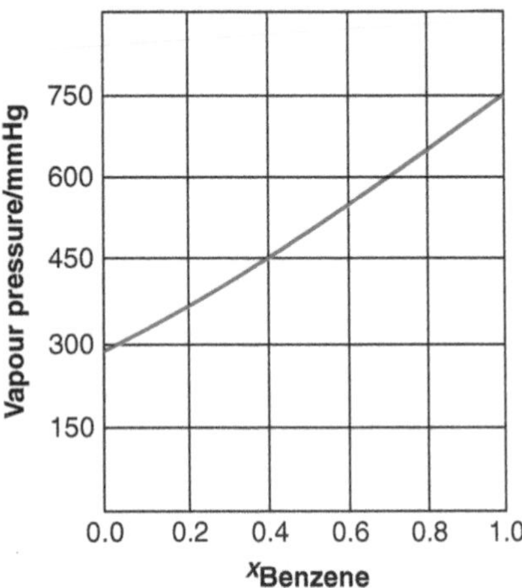

The term x_A in Raoult's law is the mole fraction of the component *in solution*, in contrast to Dalton's law (equation 4.6). In practice, closed systems that consist of two miscible volatile liquids often deviate from the predictions of Raoult's law due to the influence of intermolecular forces, giving rise to non-ideal behaviour. For pairs of components (A, B), where the energies of attraction between A and A, B and B, and A and B are equivalent, Raoult's law is upheld. The toluene–benzene system exhibits this behaviour (Figure 4.3).

For systems consisting of a solvent and a non-volatile solute, e.g. water and sodium chloride, the **vapour pressure** of the solvent is observed to fall as the mole fraction of solvent decreases, i.e. as more solute is added. This type of behaviour is an example of a **colligative property**.

For more information on lowering of vapour pressure, please refer to Section 11.1.

As pharmaceutical products are rarely single-component formulations, Raoult's Law is very useful. In the context of gases, it can be combined with Dalton's Law of partial pressures. The formulation of pressurized metered dose inhalers provides a good example of the application of these principles and is considered in Section 4.5.

Diffusion and permeability

All gases **diffuse** rapidly, i.e. they will quickly escape from an unsealed vessel and become distributed within the surrounding gas (typically air). **Graham's Law** states that the rate of diffusion of a gas is inversely proportional to the square root of its density. This means that a light gas will **diffuse** much more quickly than a heavier one. Density is directly proportional to molecular mass, therefore helium (He), with an atomic mass of 4, will diffuse more rapidly than oxygen (O_2), with a molecular mass of 32.

The diffusion or **permeability** of gas through packaging materials has practical implications for the stability of some pharmaceutical products. The permeability of pharmaceutical packaging is dependent upon the container material and thickness, the internal and external environments, and the closure. The ingress of water vapour may lead to hydrolytic degradation or physical instability; the ingress of oxygen may lead to oxidative degradation. The *United States Pharmacopoeia*, for example, has a schedule for permeation of water vapour into pharmaceutical packaging. This sets out standard tests for containers and stipulates what level of permeation is acceptable.

For more information on types of degradation, please refer to Section 12.1.

For more information on pharmaceutical packaging, please refer to Section 13.6.

Flow

Gases and liquids undergo fluid flow. The **viscosity** (η) and density (Greek letter rho, ρ) of a gas defines its propensity for lamellar (streamline), transitional or turbulent flow (Figure 4.4). This may be quantified by the **Reynolds number** (*Re*), for a gas flowing at constant velocity (v) through a tube of fixed diameter (d).

$$Re = \rho v d / \eta \quad (4.8)$$

A Reynolds number of less than 2000 indicates flow will be lamellar, whereas a value greater than 4000 indicates that flow will be turbulent. Between these values the flow is highly dependent upon the conditions, e.g. surface and angles of the tube through which the flow is occurring. A practical example of this is the use of Heliox as a medical gas (see Section 4.4).

For more information on viscosity, please refer to Section 3.3.

FIGURE 4.4 (A) Turbulent flow, (B) transitional flow, and (C) laminar flow

(A) Turbulent

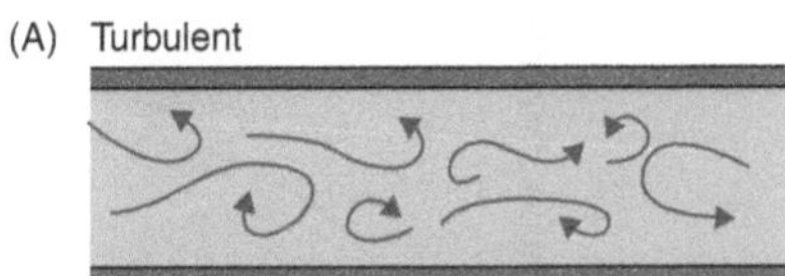

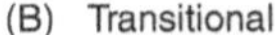

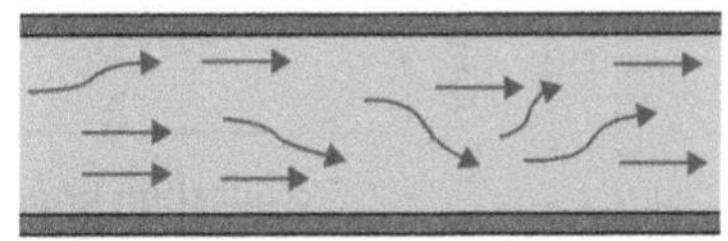

(C) Laminar

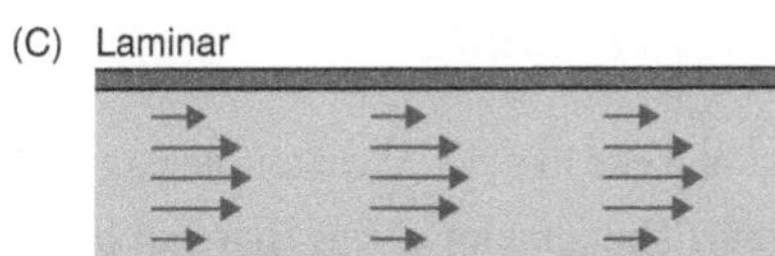

During fluid flow, pressure and velocity are interrelated by **Bernoulli's equation**. This predicts that an increase in flow results in a decrease in pressure. A **Venturi tube** features a constriction followed by an increase in bore that generates a pressure drop as flow increases through the constriction, which can be used to draw liquid droplets from a capillary tube. Within the field of fluid dynamics, this is known as entrainment and it is the principle upon which jet nebulizers work (see Section 4.5).

Adsorption

The **physisorption** of gases on to a solid surface is a rapid reversible process where molecules attach to the surface through weak, non-specific forces (van der Waals forces). The gas may be adsorbed to the surface as a **monolayer** or as a **multilayer**. Example adsorption isotherms are shown in Figure 4.5 and are produced by measuring the mass of gas or vapour adsorbed per mass of solid at a constant and different equilibrium pressures to produce an adsorption isotherm. Type I isotherms are indicative of single layer adsorption, while type II suggest multiple layer adsorption is occurring.

The measurement of surface area of a pharmaceutical powder is a good example of the application of these principles and is considered in Section 4.3.

For more information on surface adsorption, please refer to 'Liquid/solid systems' in Section 9.4.

FIGURE 4.5 Type I and type II isotherms for gas adsorption onto a solid powder

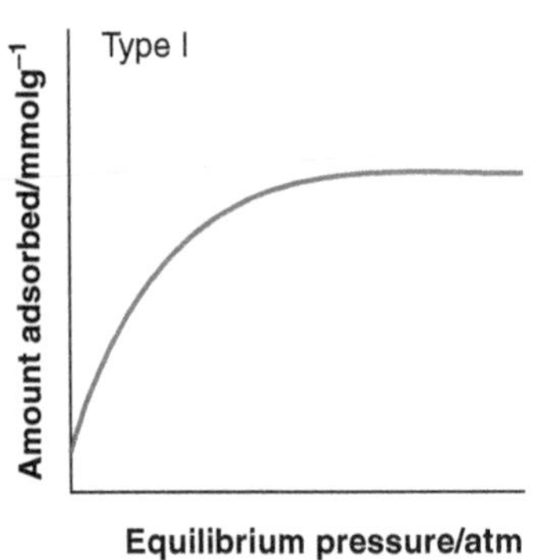

Solubility of gases

A solution of a gas in a liquid constitutes a two-component system. The amount of gas that can be dissolved in a solution depends upon both the gas and solvent involved, and is both temperature and pressure dependent. Unlike with many solid and liquid solutes, gas solubility is reduced by an increase in temperature; as shown by the appearance of bubbles upon warming a solution. Thus, heating may be used to remove gases that may lead to instability in liquid formulations. For example, air can be removed by boiling to prevent oxidative degradation or the precipitation of susceptible drugs under the influence of carbon dioxide. The effect of pressure on gas solubility is modelled by **Henry's Law**. This predicts a proportionate increase in the amount of gas dissolved as the external pressure is increased.

SELF CHECK 4.3

In a mixture of trichloromethane and acetone at 310 K, the mole fraction of acetone, x_A, was 0.680 and the recorded partial vapour pressure of acetone, p_A, was 27.1 kPa. If the vapour pressure above pure acetone, p^*_A, is 46.1 kPa, determine whether this system conforms to Raoult's law.

The solubility of anaesthetic gases in blood provides a clinical scenario where the factors affecting solubility are important (see Section 4.4). However, the complex interaction of these gases with blood and tissue is a complicating factor.

KEY POINTS

- Dalton's law states that the pressure of a mixture of gases is equal to the sum of the partial pressures of each component gas.
- Raoult's law predicts that the partial vapour pressure of a component will be proportional to the mole fraction of the same component in a mixture of miscible volatile solvents.
- Graham's Law states that the rate of diffusion of a gas is inversely proportional to the square root of its density.
- The diffusion of oxygen and water vapour is a consideration in the design of pharmaceutical packaging.
- The Reynolds number may be used to predict whether gas flow will be lamellar (streamline) or turbulent.

4.3 Pharmaceutical operations and product stability

The ability of gases and vapours to flow readily can be exploited in a number of pharmaceutical operations.

Measurement of surface area

Adsorption of gases is utilized in formulation science to measure the surface area and porosity of powders or other solid materials. The surface area of a powder may be measured by gas adsorption during **preformulation** optimization. The solid first requires degassing by heating or application of a vacuum. The application of an inert gas, typically nitrogen, at constant temperature and various pressures will generate adsorption isotherm profiles that are characteristic of the surface area and porosity of the material. The simplest profile is the type I adsorption isotherm (Figure 4.5). This corresponds to a rapid increase in adsorption with increasing pressure up to a limiting value corresponding to the formation of a complete monolayer. This type of profile is typical of **chemisorption**, where a specific reaction between the adsorbate and the solid surface occurs.

More commonly, multilayer adsorption resulting from physical adsorption of gas onto the surface of a non-porous material generates a type II isotherm (Figure 4.5). The Langmuir equation for type I isotherms or the Brunauer, Emmett, and Teller (BET) equation for type II isotherms can be used to derive the amount of molecules that form a complete single layer. This allows the specific surface area to be calculated from the effective surface area of one adsorbate molecule (e.g. 0.162 nm^2 for nitrogen). Methods for BET surface area determination are specified in the *United States Pharmacopoeia*.

For more information on the Langmuir and BET equations and isotherms, please refer to 'Liquid/solid systems' in Section 9.4.

Drying and lyophilization

Drying is a pharmaceutical operation that depends upon the evaporation of liquid. For molecules to evaporate, they must be located at the surface of the liquid, be moving in the right direction, and have sufficient kinetic energy to overcome liquid-phase intermolecular forces. Since the kinetic energy of a molecule is proportional to its temperature, evaporation proceeds more quickly at higher temperatures. As the faster-moving molecules escape, the remaining molecules have lower average kinetic energy and the temperature of the remaining liquid decreases. The application of energy, e.g. heat, and removal of the vapour promote drying. Large numbers of apparatus are available for the drying of pharmaceutical products, but the hazards of product instability or deformation must be considered when designing drying operations.

Lyophilization is a specialized form of drying in which the solvent is frozen then sublimed directly into the gas phase at a temperature below the melting point of the solvent. The process is enabled by low pressure generated via a vacuum pump. This benign method of drying is useful for retaining the structure and biological activity of biopharmaceuticals, e.g. therapeutic proteins, and vaccines.

Distillation

Distillation has many applications in pharmacy. It is defined as the boiling of a liquid mixture to establish a vapour phase in which a component of the original mixture is concentrated. According to Raoult's and Dalton's Laws (Section 4.2), it is always the more volatile component that will be present with the largest mole fraction in the gas phase. In a mixture of ethanol (**boiling point**, T_b = 78 °C) and water (T_b = 100 °C), for example, this will be the ethanol.

The boiling point is reached when the *vapour pressure* is the same as the atmospheric pressure acting on the bulk liquid. Consequently, boiling points are lower at higher altitudes, where atmospheric pressure is lower. At the boiling point, vapour is released in the bulk solution (seen as bubbles); this is in contrast to evaporation, which occurs at the surface of a liquid.

The composition of a vapour produced by heating a mixture of two liquids during distillation can be determined using a liquid–vapour phase diagram for a binary system. Condensation of the vapour produces the distillate and the mole fraction of each component in this liquid is determined by the composition of the original liquid mixture. Non-volatile solutes, such as sodium chloride, have zero vapour pressure and are not carried over into the distillate. Deviations from ideal behaviour often occur, including the formation of azeotropes. These are mixtures of a particular composition that cannot be purified further by distillation. Applications of distillation include the purification of alcohol–water mixtures and/or the concentration of the volatile components of herbal medicines.

For more information on liquid–vapour phase diagram for two-component systems, please refer to Section 7.5.

Sterilization

Sterilization can be achieved by antimicrobial gases such as ethylene oxide and formaldehyde. The gases are highly reactive and present hazards associated with their toxicity. Ethylene oxide also has a risk of explosion and sterilizing gases must be fully removed from products; formaldehyde requires a long airing time due to the persistence of adsorbed molecules at solid surfaces.

Vapour formation and instability

There are instances where the formation of vapours may be undesirable. **Vaporization** may be a source of product instability or a mechanism of environmental contamination. Volatile drugs, e.g. glycerol trinitrate tablets, or preservatives, e.g. chloroform, may be lost through gas-permeable packaging, inadequately sealed containers, or during use. **Sublimation** may result in the loss of the **active pharmaceutical ingredients (APIs)** that are not obviously volatile: loss of ibuprofen from solid dosage forms is a classic example of this. The sublimation of cytotoxic APIs has been identified as a potential source of the contamination in manufacturing environments and must be considered in risk assessments.

SELF CHECK 4.4

Why is a vacuum pump an essential component of lyophilization apparatus?

KEY POINTS

- Gases have a variety of roles in pharmaceutical operations, including the measurement of surface area.
- Lyophilization is a method of drying at low pressure that can retain the structure and activity of biopharmaceuticals.
- Distillation is a common technique in pharmaceutical processing and it is used for purifying and concentrating liquids.
- Gases have applications in sterilization of pharmaceutical materials.
- Some dosage forms contain components that may sublime and this has implications for manufacturing and packaging.

4.4 Gaseous therapy

Medical gases

Oxygen is used medically to treat **hypoxia**; for example, in respiratory failure or chronic obstructive respiratory disease. Oxygen may be stored on a large scale as liquefied gas (e.g. for use in hospitals), but is typically provided to patients as a compressed gas in cylinders with administration controlled through a high-pressure regulator. Oxygen concentrators are also available for home use. For many patients, supplemental oxygen is sufficient and may be provided through a nasal **cannula** or face mask. When using oxygen, the risk of fire should be considered; although not in itself flammable, oxygen will greatly enhance the burning of other fuels and ignition sources, e.g. cigarettes, should be kept away.

Mixtures of gases are always molecular **dispersions** and they can have pharmaceutical applications. Heliox is a mixture of 21% oxygen and 79% helium and has a significantly lower density compared to air (0.5 gL^{-1} versus 1.25 gL^{-1} at standard temperature and pressure). This mixture is used to reduce the work of breathing in patients with airway obstruction. Under the laws of fluid flow, the lower density results in less resistance to turbulent flow in larger airways, as well as increasing the tendency towards laminar flow. The effect of Heliox is less significant in smaller airways where laminar flow dominates.

For more information on molecular dispersions, please refer to 'Molecular dispersions' in Section 10.1.

Nitrous oxide (N_2O) is an **analgesic** and sedative with a rapid onset and offset of action. One application is for maintenance of light anaesthesia using suitable apparatus. Entonox is commonly used in analgesia and is a mixture of 50% N_2O and 50% oxygen, known colloquially as 'gas and air'. It is widely used in obstetrics by self-administration using an on-demand valve, and for relieving acute pain and discomfort in other settings, such as accident and emergency services.

The **critical temperature** of N_2O is 37 °C (310 K). Above this temperature, the gas cannot be liquefied, even by increasing pressure. This is evident from a phase diagram for nitrous oxide (Figure 4.6). Below the critical temperature, gaseous N_2O can be compressed to obtain the liquid. Above the critical temperature, increasing the pressure of gaseous N_2O will initially lead to the formation of a **supercritical fluid**, rather than a condensed phase.

For more information on critical temperature and supercritical fluids, please refer to 'Vapour pressure' in Section 7.2.

To create Entonox, nitrous oxide is combined with oxygen (added to prevent hypoxia during administration). The critical temperature of the gas mixture is lowered by the addition of oxygen. Entonox has a pseudocritical temperature of −6 °C (267 K), the prefix 'pseudo' being used to indicate a gas mixture. Thus, pressurized cylinders of Entonox must be stored above this temperature, otherwise the N_2O will liquefy. If this occurs, then a high concentration of O_2 will be delivered at first with little analgesic effect, but as the cylinder empties, the mixture will become progressively more potent and hypoxic as it approaches 100% N_2O. A cylinder that has been exposed to temperatures below −6 °C may be warmed for 5 minutes in a water bath set at normal body temperature or for 2 hours in a room at 15 °C. After heating, the cylinder should be inverted three times before use.

FIGURE 4.6 A phase diagram for nitrous oxide. Two isotherms illustrating the phase transitions resulting from increasing the pressure (A) below and (B) above the critical temperature are shown

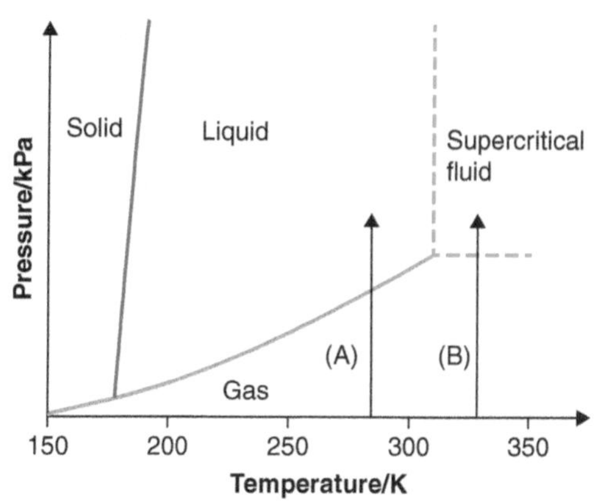

When compressed gases are provided in cylinders for medical use, pharmacists may need to advise patients regarding safe handling of cylinders and precautions for storage, preparation for use, leak testing, and operation.

Volatile liquids

A number of anaesthetic agents are volatile liquids, e.g. isoflurane, which is delivered via specifically calibrated vaporizers with doses delivered in oxygen or N_2O–oxygen gas mixtures, and adjusted according to patient response.

Non-prescription Inhalations

Steam and salt-water inhalation are the simplest non-prescription inhalations with a long history of medical use via a plethora of inhaler devices. Steam may be supplemented with essential oils, e.g. eucalyptus or menthol, which are popular remedies as mild expectorants and decongestants. The use of hot water enhances vapour release from the volatile oils, but care is recommended with the use of steam inhalation, especially in paediatrics, as cases of burns have been reported. An alternative presentation of volatile oils is in topical creams (i.e. chest rubs). Upon administration, these formulations benefit from an increase in temperature due to body heat, which increases the vaporization rate of volatile agents.

For more information on creams, please refer to 'Emulsions as dosage forms' in Section 10.7.

SELF CHECK 4.5

Explain why a cylinder of Entonox that has been stored at temperatures below −6 °C would need to be warmed before use.

KEY POINTS

- Some pure gases and gas mixtures have applications in therapy.
- Oxygen or Heliox may be used with patients who have breathing difficulties.
- Gases are used in clinical settings to induce anaesthesia, Entonox being a common example.
- Non-prescription formulations may be used as a vehicle for a volatile API for inhalation.

4.5 Gas-based dosage forms

Pharmaceutical aerosols for respiratory drug delivery

Aerosols for respiratory delivery are colloidal dispersions with a gaseous continuous phase, i.e. solid in gas or liquid in gas. In the liquid form, an API may be in suspension or dissolved in solution. Particles in therapeutic aerosols are **polydisperse**, i.e. the particle size is not constant. They should present a mass median aerodynamic diameter of less than 5 μm to be in the respirable range. Upon inhalation, aerosols will be drawn into the lung with rapid and turbulent flow in the upper airways. This gives way to slower laminar flow as the aerosol reaches the small airways. The size and density of the particles will determine where and how they deposit in the respiratory tract. Smaller particles will penetrate further into the lung, with the predominant mechanism by which they deposit being dependent on size:

- Inertial impaction for particles larger than 5 μm, generally within the upper airways. Smaller particles have less inertia and are more likely to be carried along in the flow of gas, rather than collide with the walls of the airway when its direction changes.
- Gravitational sedimentation for particles of 0.5–3 μm. This is where particles fall under the influence of gravity and are captured by an internal surface.
- Brownian motion for particles smaller than 0.5 μm in the alveoli. Small particles not subject to gravitational sedimentation may instead diffuse into the internal walls of the lungs.

For more information on colloidal dispersion, please refer to 'Colloidal dispersions' in Section 10.1.

Pressurized aerosols

Pressurized metered dose inhalers (pMDIs) are the most popular devices for inhaled drug delivery. The earliest metered dose inhalers were formulations of an API in solution or suspension in liquefied gas under pressure. The liquefied gas acts as a propellant through a rapid expansion (reversion to the gaseous state) when a dose is released from pressurization by a metering valve. Chlorofluorocarbons (CFCs) were the original gases used in pMDIs, although these are now largely replaced by hydrofluoroalkanes (HFAs).

For more information on chlorofluorocarbons, please refer to Chapter 5 'Alcohols, phenols, ethers, organic halogen compounds, and amines' of the *Pharmaceutical Chemistry* book within this series.

HFA 134a (trifluoromonofluoroethane) and HFA 227 (heptafluoropropane) are the most popular HFAs. Binary mixtures of these two gases display near-ideal behaviour regarding their vapour pressure, i.e. they generally obey Raoult's Law. This is important for their use in pMDIs, as vapour pressure determines particle size and hence the penetration into the lung and subsequent clinical effects of API delivered by these products.

For more information on ideal behaviour, please refer to 'Chemical potential and solute concentration' in Section 11.6.

When formulating liquids for use in pDMIs, the solubility of the API or properties of the propellant mixture can be adapted, if necessary, using co-solvents, e.g. ethanol or glycerol. As solubility in propellants is often poor, suspension formulations are frequently used and these require stabilizing agents, such as lecithin or oleic acid at low concentrations, to maintain dose uniformity. pMDIs are simple, effective economic presentations of an API that enable direct targeting to the respiratory tract. This allows for reduced dosing and, in turn, reduced systemic side-effects of agents, such as bronchodilators (e.g. beta receptor agonists, anticholinergic agents), and anti-inflammatory agents, such as corticosteroids. Despite their effectiveness, these formulations have some drawbacks that are related to their propellant-driven nature:

- A proportion of the dose is lost by impaction in throat due to the high velocity of emitted aerosol.
- Deposition of drug in the throat can lead to side-effects.
- Some patients are unable to coordinate the actuation of the device with inhalation.
- There is no visual indication that a dose has been delivered. For this reason, dose counters are fitted in some products.

Problems with coordination and high aerosol velocity can be overcome using spacer devices (holding chambers) into which the pMDI is actuated. Spacers reduce particle velocity and act as a reservoir from which the aerosol can be inhaled.

For more information on patient use of inhalers, please refer to Chapter 8 'Pharmaceutical care' of the *Pharmacy Practice* book within this series.

Aerosol powder devices

Dry powder inhaler (DPI) devices are breath actuated and avoid the coordination problems associated with pMDIs. Such devices employ API particles with sizes suitable for inhalation, but usually require **excipients** such as larger carrier particles (almost exclusively lactose). A wide variety of inhaler devices are available in both unit dose and reservoir formats. Both formats require an airflow and velocity to be generated through the **powder** bed upon actuation, which will liberate and disperse the fine powder API into an aerosol of respirable size. An ideal powder presentation will have these characteristics:

- It must be sufficiently free-flowing to achieve accurate manufacture. This requires homogeneity achieved through adhesion of fine API particles to larger carrier particles.
- It must have the ability to liberate the fine powder upon actuation. This requires the release (desorption) of the fine particles from the carrier particles.

Nebulizers

Nebulizers are less convenient for patients than the portable pMDI and DPI devices. Modern technology is increasingly addressing this challenge and recent developments include thermally generated inhalation aerosols (Integration Box 4.1). Nebulizers produce mists (liquid droplets in gas) and are generally available in two formats: jet and ultrasonic nebulizers. Jet nebulizers use high-velocity gas flow through a **Venturi tube** (Section 4.2; Figure 4.7) to draw liquid into the airflow. Here, it is sheared into particles with characteristics dependent on the properties of the gas and the solution, e.g. the velocity of the gas and the surface tension of the solution. The output from jet nebulizers includes solvent vapour and, because evaporation is an **endothermic** process, the temperature of the nebulizer solution decreases by 10–15 °C during operation. This change in temperature may alter formulation properties, such as **viscosity**, **surface tension**, and API **solubility**.

For more information on endothermic processes, please refer to Section 5.3.

FIGURE 4.7 **Entrainment of fluid in a gas flow by the Venturi effect**

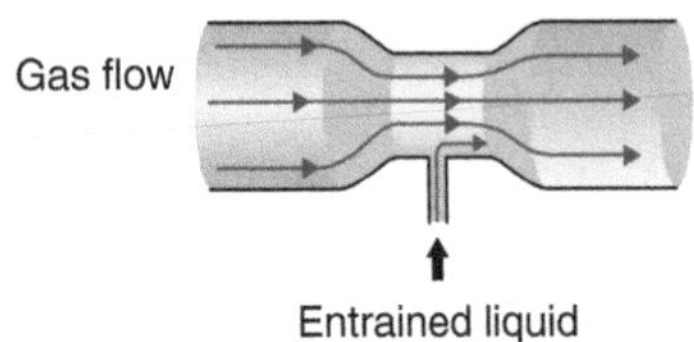

For more information on surface tension, please refer to Chapter 9.

Ultrasonic nebulizers use a piezoelectric crystal vibrating at high frequency to create surface conditions in the liquid that lead to the liberation of droplets to create the aerosol mist. The energy imparted to the solution increases the temperature of the nebulizer solution and has been found to denature some biopharmaceuticals such as deoxyribonuclease, which is used in the treatment of cystic fibrosis.

Nebulizer solutions are specialized liquids that must be stable and compatible with the airways when administered. Unlike liquids for **intravenous** delivery, for example, nebulizer solutions may not be **isotonic**, and deviate from physiological **pH**. The latter will be restored when the small droplets deposit in the fluid of the respiratory tract lining *via* buffer action.

For more information on pH, please refer to Section 6.3.

For more information on intravenous delivery, please refer to Section 13.5.

For more information on isotonicity, please refer to 'Isotonicity' in Section 11.3.

In addition to the API and solvent, nebulizer solutions contain excipients. Preservatives may be added to enhance shelf life, although caution is required as these may irritate the lungs. The need for preservatives can be avoided by presenting the solution as a sterile, single-unit dose. Formulation viscosity and surface tension may, in combination with nebulizer device characteristics, affect the formation of respirable droplets. Other excipents may therefore be used to modify these properties, although foaming must be avoided.

Non-inhalation aerosols

In addition to inhalation use, aerosols may be used to apply medicines to other sites of the body, e.g. for **topical**, nasal, or oral use. In these circumstances it is not

BOX 4.1

Thermally generated inhalation aerosols

Thermally generated aerosols provide an example of drug delivery in which the dosage unit (the inhaled aerosol particle) is generated through a dramatic material state transition of pure API at the point of use. These work by heating thin films of a solid thermostable API to elevated temperatures to generate vapours that condense rapidly into respirable particles of 1–3 μm mass median aerodynamic diameters. This is the pharmaceutical equivalent of the delivery of drugs by smoking, without the attendant dangers of inhaling harmful materials.

For example, a respirable form of the antipsychotic loxapine can be delivered using an excipient-free thermally generated aerosol. The delivery device is produced by coating loxapine in solution thinly onto a metal substrate upon which it dries in a crystalline powder layer. Upon heating of the metal to 450 °C, flash vaporization occurs. The pure loxapine vapour is collected using an airflow generated by inhalation, is rapidly cooled, and condenses to form the aerosol particle *in situ* during the inhalation procedure. The particles formed are **amorphous**, as opposed to the **crystalline** starting material, as a consequence of the speed of particle formation in the aerosol (particles typically form in less than 1 s). Although amorphous forms are generally less stable, these particles are formed only at the point of administration and generally have higher **dissolution** rates than crystalline solids. Upon inhalation of such aerosols by human volunteers, absorption is rapid with peak plasma loxapine concentration after 2 minutes.

For more information on crystalline and amorphous solids, please refer to Section 2.2.

necessary to use such fine droplet sizes and coarse dispersions may be acceptable. Examples include spray dressings that are able to coat wounds evenly with a sterile protective layer. An interesting application of aerosols is to generate topical analgesia through the refrigerant effect of propellant evaporation, e.g. the chloroethane 'cold sprays' often applied to injuries sustained during sports.

For more information on topical applications, please refer to Section 13.5.

For more information on coarse dispersions, please refer to 'Coarse dispersions' in Section 10.1.

Foams

Foams are gas-in-liquid presentations in which the gas is the disperse phase surrounded by liquid films. These dosage forms have many applications in nature and the cosmetic and food industries, e.g. shaving foams, ice cream, and other confectionary. In processing and manufacturing operations involving agitation of a liquid, foams can be problematic and anti-foaming agents may be required.

Foam-based pharmaceutical products are dynamic in that the foam is formed at the point of administration upon actuation of a device containing the formulation with a pressurized gas. Once formed, foams often have limited physical stability, but achieve their purpose of being easily and gently applied and providing good coverage at the site of administration for topical treatment. An example of their use is in anti-inflammatory and analgesic foams for rectal administration.

For more information on foams, please refer to 'Foams' in Section 10.2.

KEY POINTS

- Respiratory drug delivery includes the delivery of colloidal solid and liquid aerosols.
- Pressurized metered dose inhalers (pMDI) are the most popular devices for inhaled drug delivery and are actuated mechanically by the user.
- Problems associated with the use of pMDI inhalers can be overcome by the use of spacer devices.
- Dry powder inhaler (DPI) devices employ solid excipients as carrier particles to deliver an API through breath actuation.
- Nebulizers are traditionally less portable than DPIs or pMDIs and are available in two formats, jet and ultrasonic nebulizers.
- Thermally generated inhalation aerosols are not widely available but offer a novel route to nebulise thermostable APIs.
- Coarse aerosol sprays are acceptable for topical, oral and nasal use.

SELF CHECK 4.6

What are the distinctions between a pMDI and a DPI?

CHAPTER SUMMARY

- The properties of gases at pharmaceutically relevant conditions can be predicted using the ideal gas equation,

$$pV = nRT$$

- The pressure of any mixture of gases can be calculated as the sum of the component partial pressures, according to Dalton's Law.
- For ideal systems, the partial vapour pressure of a component above a mixture of volatile miscible liquids can be calculated using Raoult's Law.
- The rate of diffusion of oxygen and water vapour can be determined using Graham's Law and is a consideration when designing pharmaceutical packaging.

- Gases have a variety of roles in pharmaceutical operations, including surface area measurement, distillation, lyophilization, and sterilization.
- Pure gases and gas mixtures have pharmaceutical applications; for example, in assisting respiration, inducing analgesia, and as decongestants.
- Colloidal aerosols for respiratory delivery contain the API within the dispersed phase and may be delivered through a pressurized metered dose inhaler (pMDI) or dry powder inhaler (DPI).
- Aerosols not designed for inhalation, e.g. nasal sprays, are normally coarse dispersions.

FURTHER READING

Florence, A. T. and Attwood, D. *Physicochemical Principles of Pharmacy*, (5th edn). London: Pharmaceutical Press, (2011), pp 35–54.

Gives a fuller account of the gas laws and examples of their applications in pharmacy.

Taylor, K. Pulmonary drug delivery, Chapter 31 in *Pharmaceutics: the Science of Dosage Form Design*, (2nd edn). London: Churchill Livingstone, (2002), pp 473–88.

Gives a fuller account of the devices and formulations used for inhaled drug delivery.

Winfield, A. J. Medical gases, Chapter 20 in *Pharmaceutical Practice*, (2nd edn). London: Churchill Livingstone, (1998), pp 188–92.

Gives a fuller account of medical gases.

REFERENCE

Atkins, P. and de Paula, J. *Elements of Physical Chemistry*, (5th edn) (2009). Oxford: OUP.

5

Thermodynamics

LINDA SETON

Chemical and biological processes involve change. For example, milk turns sour when it is left out of the refrigerator. We can detect the chemical change by the smell given off by the sour milk and we can observe the physical change by its appearance: the white opaque liquid is replaced by clear liquid and white solid. We also understand that the fats in milk contain energy. If we drink fresh milk, our body's digestive system releases that energy for other biological and chemical processes. So, energy is converted from one form to another as chemical and biological processes take place.

Thermodynamics is the study of the transfer of energy during chemical and physical processes. It describes energy changes at a macroscopic level, i.e. those involving bulk substances, rather than energy changes at the molecular level. We need to know about chemical and biological processes because this knowledge helps us to fight disease, maintain health, manufacture goods (including medicines), and produce food. In order to understand and study the chemistry involved, we need to be able to understand the energy changes that occur, and also how processes are affected by their environment. The principles contained within this chapter are used to understand and control the processes used in the manufacture and formulation of drugs. They also aid our understanding of the stability of **active pharmaceutical ingredients (APIs)** and other products.

Learning objectives

Having read this chapter you are expected to be able to:

- Describe different types of system.
- State the laws of thermodynamics.
- Describe reactions as being either exothermic or endothermic.
- Calculate enthalpies of reaction using heats of formation or similar values.
- Describe the entropy changes that occur when a reaction takes place.
- Relate Gibbs free energy, entropy, and enthalpy.
- Understand the effect of temperature on the spontaneity of reaction and predict the temperature at which a reaction becomes spontaneous.
- Understand chemical equilibria and define the equilibrium constant for a reversible reaction.
- Predict the equilibrium constant of a reaction at one temperature if it is known at another.

5.1 Energetics of chemical and physical processes

All chemical reactions, and many physical processes, bring about a conversion of energy. We know that when wood burns on a fire, for example, energy is released to the surroundings and this keeps us warm. We know that when food is digested, energy is released into the body, which fuels other biological processes, such as cell manufacture. When we sweat, the fluid on the skin evaporates into the air. This change of state absorbs energy, which comes from the skin, and results in a cooling of the skin.

We may have an understanding of the term energy, but there are many ways to define energy depending on what is being studied. Moving particles, such as a tennis ball or a molecule of oxygen, have **kinetic energy**. When an object is elevated, such as a sledge at the top of a hill, it is said to have **potential energy**. The sledge has stored energy due to its position. This means that it can slide down the hill spontaneously, reducing its energy in the process. Chemical substances have both kinetic energy and potential energy. Kinetic energy arises from the movement of atoms, i.e. vibration of atoms in a solid, diffusion of molecules in a liquid. Chemical bonds and intermolecular forces give a substance potential energy. Therefore all substances have an inherent energy, known as the **internal energy**. This has the symbol, U, and is measured in joules.

Internal energy is an example of a **state function**. This means that the value of internal energy of a substance does not depend on the path it took to arrive at its current state. The value of internal energy depends only on the current status of the system. For example, two people might each weigh 80 kilograms. Body weight is a state function as it measures the current state of each person. Over the preceding month, the amount of exercise each person undertook and the amount of food they consumed might well be very different. These are, therefore, not state functions. We will revisit this point later and will encounter other examples of state functions.

> **KEY POINT**
>
> All chemical reactions, and many physical processes, bring about a conversion of energy.

> **KEY POINT**
>
> A state function is a property of a system that depends only on the current state of the system, not on the path the system took to reach that state. All substances possess internal energy, U, a state function that is the sum of the molecular kinetic and potential energies.

System and surroundings

In order to describe and study chemical processes, we need to be able to talk about them in a consistent way. To do this we define two important terms: system and surroundings. The **system** is the part of the Universe in which we are interested. It could be a reaction flask, a cell, an engine, etc. The system is usually contained within a physical boundary such as the glass wall of a reaction flask or a cell membrane. The **surroundings** is the name given to the environment outside the system. There is no physical boundary to this environment and so it is often defined as 'the rest of the Universe'.

Energy changes that occur in the system can be measured. Energy changes in the surroundings might be observed, but generally cannot be measured directly. There are different types of systems, which you can find out about by looking in Figure 5.1.

An **open system** can exchange heat and matter with the surroundings. An example is a cup of tea from which both heat and water vapour can escape. A **closed system** has a boundary that does not allow material to pass into or out of the system; however, heat can be transferred and the boundary is described as diathermic. A sealed bottle of water is an example of a closed system. An **isolated system** does not allow either matter or heat to be transferred through

FIGURE 5.1 Systems can be (A) open, (B) closed, or (C) isolated
Source: (A) Stockbyte, (B) Corbis

(A)

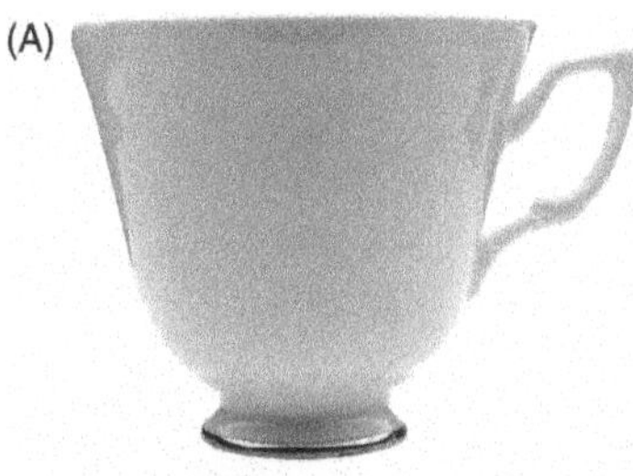

(B)

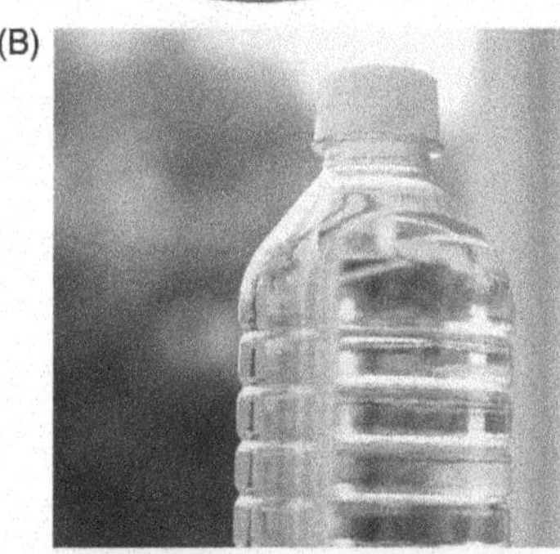

(C)

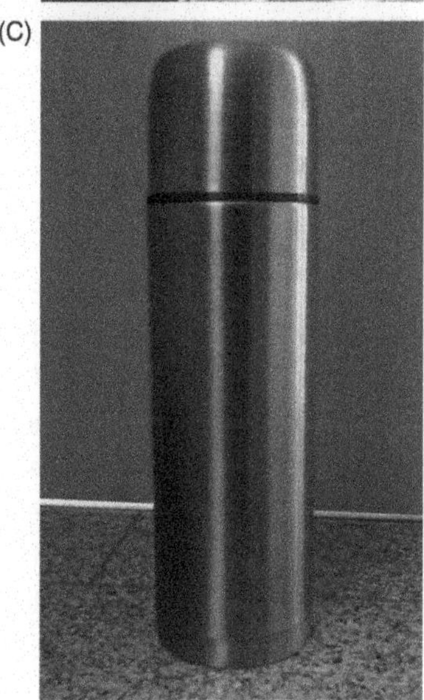

the boundary. A boundary that does not allow heat to be transferred is described as adiabatic. A sealed Thermos® flask is close to being an isolated system.

KEY POINT

The system is the part of the Universe that is being studied. The surroundings is the name given to the environment outside the system. Systems may be open, closed, or isolated, depending on whether matter and/or heat can be transferred between the system and surroundings.

Heat

In the example systems previously, we considered **heat (*q*)**. Heat is a measure of the transfer of energy from one object or substance to another, due to a temperature difference. Look again at Figure 5.1A. A hot cup of tea has a temperature of around 90°C. The molecules are moving randomly in the liquid. Heat is transferred through the boundaries (the ceramic wall of the cup and the liquid/air interface) to the air molecules surrounding the cup. The molecules in the air will become more energetic as a result and their movements will become faster. We perceive this as an increase in the temperature of the air. The molecules of the tea (which is mostly water) will become less energetic and move more slowly. The temperature of the tea will decrease. This process will continue until the tea and the surrounding air are at the same temperature, and there is no more net flow of heat. The tea and the air are then said to be at **thermal equilibrium**. At this point most people wouldn't want to drink the tea! Thermal equilibrium can be achieved between more than two objects. Look at Figure 5.2 and imagine you are holding the glass of iced water on a hot day. Although your hand and the iced water are not in direct contact, they are said to be in **thermal contact** because heat transferred from your hand

FIGURE 5.2 A glass of iced water will absorb heat from the surroundings
Source: Copyright Victor Blacus licensed under the Creative Commons Attribution-Share Alike 3.0 Unported, 2.5 Generic, 2.0 Generic and 1.0 Generic license

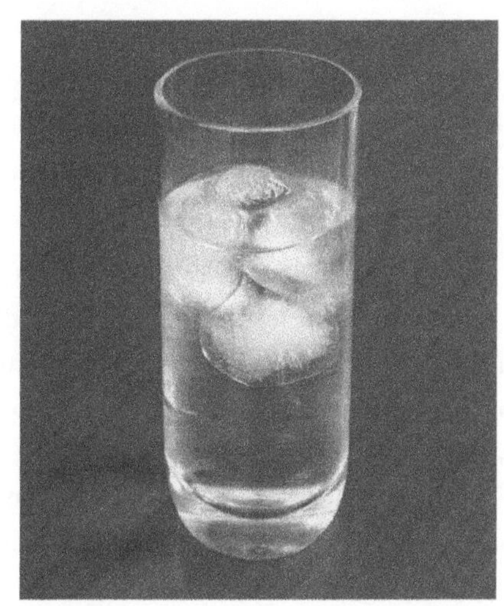

to the glass is then transferred from the glass to the water. You can feel this happening because your hand gets cold. Eventually, your hand, the glass, and the water will all be at the same temperature, the ice having melted, as it too was in thermal contact with your hand. Most people will drink the water before thermal equilibrium is reached. This illustrates the **Zeroth Law of Thermodynamics**, which states that when objects are in thermal contact with each other, heat will be transferred between them until they reach the same temperature.

Temperature is not the same as heat. Temperature is a manifestation of the motion of the molecules or atoms in the system. According to the **kinetic theory** of matter, molecules or atoms in fluids move chaotically in all directions, motion being restricted to the random vibration of particles within solids. As temperature decreases, molecular motion slows and it ceases completely at an **absolute temperature** of zero **kelvin**. As temperature increases, particles move more chaotically, increasing the internal energy of the substance. In general, we may classify heat as energy transferred through chaotic molecular motion.

KEY POINT

Heat is the flow of energy from one object or substance to another due to a difference in temperature. Objects are in thermal contact when they can exchange energy with each other through heat, which continues until they reach thermal equilibrium and are at the same temperature. This is an expression of the Zeroth Law of Thermodynamics. Heat is transferred through chaotic molecular motion.

Heat capacity

When a system absorbs heat from the surroundings, this will normally result in a rise in the temperature of the system. However, some materials will heat up more readily than others. This is dependent on the **heat capacity** of the material. Heat capacity at constant pressure has the symbol C_p and its value is affected by temperature. The heat capacity of a boundary will influence the flow of heat into and out of a system. It is often more useful to use molar heat capacity, being the amount of heat that one mole substance must absorb in order to increase in temperature by 1 K (Table 5.1). This has units of J $K^{-1}mol^{-1}$.

TABLE 5.1 Molar heat capacities of some selected materials at 298 K and 1 bar pressure

Substance	C_p/J $K^{-1}mol^{-1}$
Sucrose, $C_{12}H_{22}O_{11}$ (solid)	360.2
Benzene, C_6H_6 (liquid)	172.8
Water, H_2O (liquid)	75.3
Oxygen, O_2 (gas)	29.4

KEY POINT

Heat capacity, C_p, is a measure of how much heat a substance must absorb in order to bring about a temperature rise of 1 K at constant pressure.

Work

Heat will be transferred between two objects in thermal contact that are at different temperatures through the chaotic particle motion described earlier. However, if energy changes occur that cause or result in organized change in the direction of the molecular motion, then we say that **work** (w) is done.

Figure 5.3 shows a syringe full of gas. In Figure 5.3A, the gas fills the syringe and the molecules move randomly with a kinetic energy related to the temperature. If the plunger is moved down such that the volume of the gas decreases (Figure 5.3B), the molecules will be pushed into the lower regions of the syringe barrel. The pressure inside the syringe will increase and this is how, for example, a bicycle pump generates sufficient pressure to inflate a tyre.

The motion of particles during compression is no longer random, but is biased in the direction of the plunger movement. We say work has been done on the system. As the gas is compressed, the molecules have less space to move around in, and there are more collisions. This generates heat, which in turn increases the kinetic energy of the molecules and the internal energy

FIGURE 5.3 A syringe containing gas molecules. (A) The particles move randomly in all directions. (B) As the syringe plunger is depressed, the particles have net movement downwards

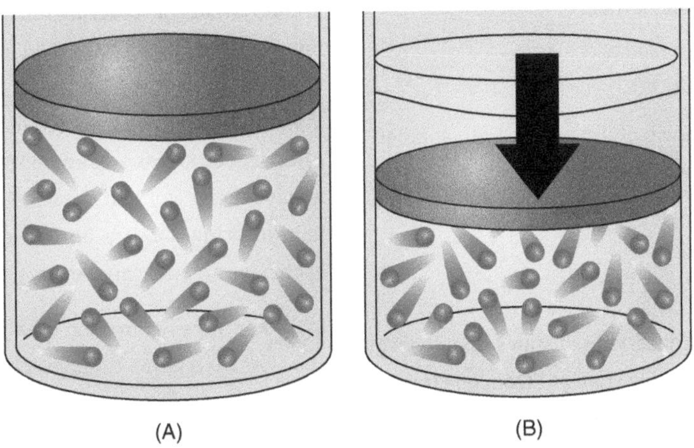

of the gas. If the compression takes place adiabatically, that is, with no heat either entering or leaving the system, then the temperature of the compressed gas will increase. This principle has practical applications. The fuel vapour in a diesel car engine, for example, is raised to the ignition temperature by compression, and not by the use of spark plugs as in a petrol engine.

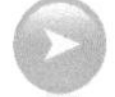
For more information on pressure, please refer to Section 4.1.

In Figure 5.3, the surroundings (including the plunger) did work on the system and the internal energy of the gas was raised. It is also possible for the system to do work on the surroundings. In Figure 5.4, a weight rests on a piston connected to a vessel in which a chemical reaction takes place that generates a gas. As the reaction proceeds, the weight is raised, work is done, and the potential energy of the weight will increase.

The particles that make up the weight, whilst continuing to vibrate randomly, will each move in an upwards direction. This uniform molecular motion is associated with work done on the system. Indeed, any system doing any type of work is capable of raising a weight. The energy associated with this process can be calculated using:

$$w = Fs \tag{5.1}$$

FIGURE 5.4 A chemical reaction generating a gas, pushing a piston that raises a weight and does work

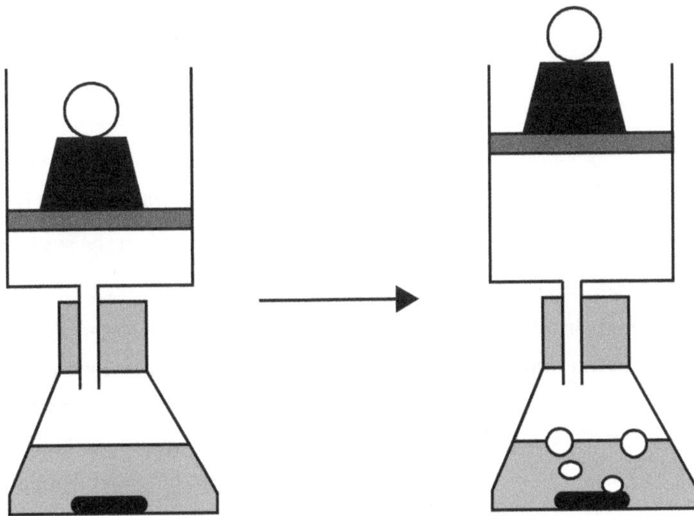

where w is the work done in joules, F is the force exerted by the weight in newtons, and s is the distance moved by the piston, in metres.

KEY POINT

Work is the flow of energy from one body to another through uniform molecular motion.

Conservation of energy

The law of energy conservation states that energy cannot be created, but only changed from one form to another. For example, when a candle is lit, the chemical energy contained within the wax is converted to heat and light; as a result, the candle is depleted and burns down. The battery that powers a torch contains chemical energy. As this energy is converted to light, the chemical energy is used up, until the battery is spent and must be replaced.

In the case of the gas syringe (Figure 5.3), work was done by the surroundings on the system and this led to an increase in the internal energy of the system. Thus, work energy was converted into internal (or 'chemical') energy. It follows that in the case of the chemical reaction and piston (Figure 5.4), work was done by the system on the surroundings and the internal energy of the system (the reacting mixture) decreased. Thus, internal energy was converted to work energy.

When substances such as pharmaceuticals are manufactured, they undergo many processes such as **milling**, **compression**, and **emulsification**. All these involve doing work on the system. All these processes help to bring about a desired change and they will each have an associated energy change.

For more information on milling and compression, please refer to 'Compressed and layered tablets' in Section 2.5 and for more information on emulsification, please refer to 'Stability of emulsions and nanoemulsions' in Section 10.6.

SELF CHECK 5.1

What is the difference between heat and temperature?

SELF CHECK 5.2

How can a temperature expressed in kelvin (K) be converted to degrees Celsius (°C)?

5.2 The First Law of Thermodynamics: what is possible?

We have seen that internal energy, U, is a state function and that changes in internal energy can be brought about by both heat and work, energy being conserved during these processes. We may use the symbol ΔU to represent this change. We will subsequently use the Greek letter Delta, Δ, alongside other state functions, again to represent changes in their value.

In general, the changes in internal energy can be calculated using:

$$\Delta U = q + w. \quad (5.2)$$

By convention:

- q is the energy transferred as heat from the surroundings to the system in joules.
- w is work done on the system by the surroundings in joules.

It follows that if the system does work on the surroundings, and heat energy flows from the system to the surroundings during that change, then both q and w will have negative values. Although internal energy is a state function, heat and work are **path functions**, as their value depends on the path taken to get between two states (see Box 5.1).

By application of equation 5.2, we can appreciate that, if the internal energy of a system increases by 5 J, this may have been by either of these two paths:

- $q = 2$ J, $w = 3$ J
- $q = 10$ J, $w = -5$ J.

Of course, innumerable other paths could also give rise to ΔU value of 5 J. The value of q and w between two states can have a variety of values depending on the path taken. Consequently, both heat and work cannot be described as state functions.

Although perhaps not immediately apparent, the principle that energy can be neither created nor destroyed, but must be conserved, is embodied within equation 5.2. This concept is more properly known as the First Law of Thermodynamics and states that the internal energy of an isolated system is constant. In an isolated system, no heat can be absorbed from the surroundings ($q = 0$ J) and no work can be done on the surroundings ($w = 0$ J). Thus, according to equation 5.2, $\Delta U = 0$ J, i.e. internal energy remains constant. If we consider the Universe to be a massive, isolated system, then the first law requires that the energy of the Universe is constant.

BOX 5.1

State functions and path functions

The fundamental difference between state and path functions can be understood by a simple example. Two towns, Churchtown and Hilltown, are connected by a ring road, shown in Figure 5.5. The distance between the two towns is 10 km but there is no road following a direct path. The ring road provides two possible routes of travel.

The distance between the towns is a state function and its value is 10 km. The distance travelled by a vehicle is a path function and depends on the route chosen. The distance travelled from Churchtown to Hilltown via the northern section is 12 km in a clockwise direction. The alternative route is 15 km in an anticlockwise direction. Variables such as fuel consumption of the vehicle depend on the path function, not the state function.

FIGURE 5.5 **The straight-line distance between the towns is a state function. The distance travelled on a journey between the towns is a path function and its value depends on the route taken**

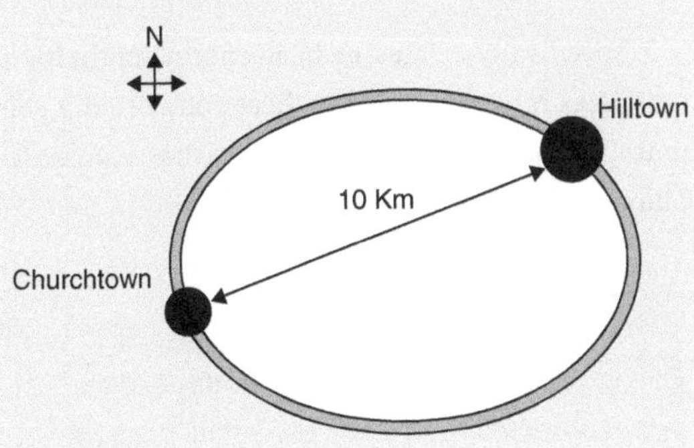

SELF CHECK 5.3

What is a path function?

KEY POINT

The First Law of Thermodynamics states that the internal energy of an isolated system is constant. It can be expressed as:

$$\Delta U = q + w$$

where ΔU is the change in internal energy, q is the energy transferred as heat from the surroundings to the system, and w is work done on the system by the surroundings.

Both heat and work are examples of path functions.

Calorimetry

The internal energy change, ΔU, for a chemical process can be determined by calorimetry. An adiabatic **calorimeter** is a vessel that is thermally insulated, restricting the transfer of heat to its surroundings. Any change in temperature that occurs as a result of the reaction within a calorimeter is proportional to the energy absorbed (or released) as heat. The ΔU for the reaction can then be calculated if the heat capacity of the material is known.

In differential scanning calorimetry (DSC), the amount of heat required to increase the temperature of a sample and reference material is measured over a range of temperatures. In this way, it is possible to determine the location of important transition temperatures, e.g. melting points. DSC is widely used in the pharmaceutical industry. For example, **amorphous** forms of APIs generally have superior bioavailabilities to the corresponding **crystalline** forms. DSC can be used to determine the temperature that must be maintained during processing to ensure crystallization does not occur.

For more information on amorphous and crystalline materials, please refer to Section 2.2.

KEY POINT

Calorimetry is an experimental technique that can be used to determine changes in both internal energy and enthalpy.

5.3 Enthalpy and Hess's Law

When chemical reactions take place, heat can flow in to or out of a system. If heat flows into the system when a change occurs, then that process is said to be **endothermic**. An example of an endothermic process is the evaporation of sweat from the skin. Vaporization of 1 mL of water requires that the liquid absorbs around 2 kJ of heat energy from the surroundings. Conversely, if heat flows out of the system when a process occurs, then that change is **exothermic**. The conversion of glucose to carbon dioxide and water during respiration is an exothermic reaction, releasing energy for use by the body.

Enthalpy, H, is a state function that is defined as the heat energy, q, absorbed by a system at fixed pressure. Many pharmaceutically relevant processes take place under constant atmospheric pressure, so this quantity is important. To mathematically define enthalpy, we must rearrange the first law of thermodynamics (equation 5.2), and express in terms of q:

$$q = \Delta U - w \tag{5.3}$$

If we only consider work done by the change in volume of a system, so-called 'expansion work', then it can be shown from equation 5.1 that:

$$w = -p\Delta V \tag{5.4}$$

where p is the external pressure that the system pushes against, and ΔV is the change in volume of the system, for example, due to the release of gas.

A minus sign is required so that when volume increases ($\Delta V > 0$), work has a negative sign, in accord with our convention: when w is less than zero, work is done by the system on the surroundings, in this case when the system expands in volume and pushes back the surroundings.

Substitution of equation 5.4 into 5.3 gives:

$$q = \Delta U + p\Delta V$$

As enthalpy is defined as the heat energy absorbed by a system at constant pressure, and all terms on the right-hand side of this equation are state functions, we may replace q with a new state function, H, and write:

$$\Delta H = \Delta U + p\Delta V \tag{5.5}$$

When a reaction takes place, we are concerned with changes in enthalpy, ΔH. To determine absolute values of H, it follows that we would use:

$$H = U + pV$$

As it specifically relates to heat energy, enthalpy is sometimes referred to as the 'heat content' of a substance, although we can see that it also has a pressure–volume component.

KEY POINT

Enthalpy, H, is a state function that is defined as the heat energy absorbed by a system at constant pressure.

Enthalpy changes associated with chemical reactions

When reactants combine to form products, the enthalpy of the system will normally increase or decrease. Figure 5.6A shows an exothermic reaction (i.e. one which releases heat). The enthalpy of the reactants is greater than the products, and the value of ΔH is negative. When the reaction is endothermic (i.e. absorbs heat), the enthalpy of the reactants is less than the enthalpy of the products and ΔH has a positive value, as shown in Figure 5.6B.

Standard enthalpy values

Values for the change in enthalpy when a chemical or physical process occurs are dependent on the conditions in which the process takes place. Generally, values are most useful if they relate to a standard set of conditions because this allows different processes to be compared directly. The standard conditions used in thermodynamic studies are 1 bar pressure and a specified temperature, normally 298 K. The standard state of a substance is its normal physical state under these conditions, e.g. the standard states of methane, water, and gold are gas, liquid, and solid, respectively.

FIGURE 5.6 Graphs of enthalpy, H, vs reaction path (the progress of a chemical reaction). (A) Shows the reaction path of an exothermic reaction. (B) Shows an endothermic reaction

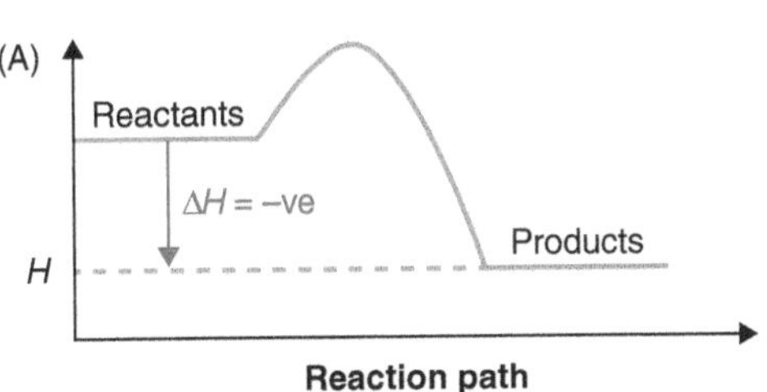

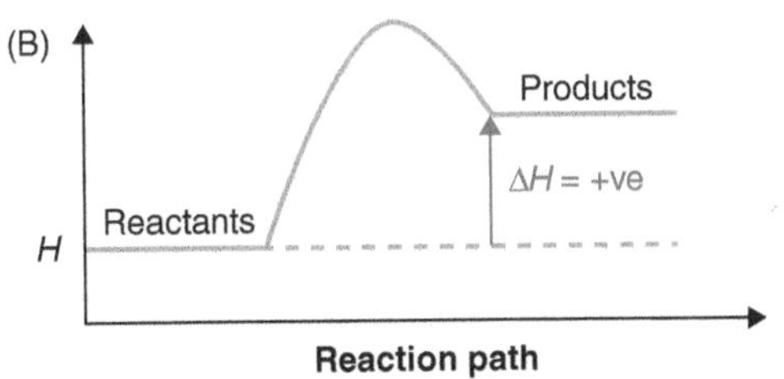

The standard enthalpy of a reaction, ΔH^{θ}, is equal to the enthalpy change when the reactants in their standard states react to give the products in their standard states, all under standard conditions. This can be written in the form of equation 5.6:

$$\Delta H^{\theta}_{\text{reaction}} = \Sigma H^{\theta}_{\text{(products)}} - \Sigma H^{\theta}_{\text{(reactants)}} \quad (5.6)$$

where Σ is standard mathematical notation meaning, 'the sum of...'

In practice, it is not possible to measure values of H^{θ} directly, although we can measure changes in its value. In a similar way, you may not know your exact altitude above sea-level. However, you do know that if you were to stand on your chair, you would be about 0.5 m higher than you were before. Thus, although you are able to determine altitude changes, you do not need you to know your absolute altitude in order to do this.

KEY POINT

Standard conditions for thermodynamic measurements are 1 bar pressure and a specified temperature.

Methane is the gas that fuels Bunsen burners or the gas ring in a kitchen. The chemical equation for the combustion of methane, CH_4 is:

$$CH_{4(g)} + 2O_{2(g)} \rightarrow CO_{2(g)} + 2H_2O_{(l)}$$

ΔH^{θ} (298 K) for this reaction is –890 kJ mol^{-1}. Notice that the energy change is stated for a specified temperature (298 K) and is measured per mole. Thus, the more material involved, the larger the release of heat. This ΔH^{θ} value has a negative sign, as the reaction is exothermic and releases heat. A negative sign indicates that the enthalpy of the products is less than the enthalpy of the reactants. Heat energy is transferred from the system to the surroundings during this reaction. The reverse reaction has the same enthalpy but the sign is reversed, thus:

$$\Delta H^{\theta}_{\text{forward}} = -\Delta H^{\theta}_{\text{reverse}}$$

Thus, a reaction that is exothermic in the forward direction will be endothermic in the reverse direction. Integration Box 5.1 discusses an exothermic reaction with which you might already be familiar.

KEY POINT

An exothermic reaction releases heat to the surroundings and has a negative value for ΔH. An endothermic reaction absorbs heat to the surroundings and has a positive value for ΔH.

Standard enthalpy of physical changes

We are often interested in the process of physical change and need to discuss the enthalpy changes that take place during changes of state, such as **vaporization**, **fusion** (melting), and **sublimation**. For example. Topical creams and gels often contain volatile solvents that evaporate from the skin. It helps to consider these enthalpy values under standard conditions so that we can compare values for different substances.

Enthalpy is a state function, so its value does not depend on the pathway by which a process occurs, only on the state of the system at the start, and at the end of the process. If you look at the graph shown in Figure 5.8, it shows how the **standard enthalpy** of fusion added to the **standard enthalpy** of vaporization will be the same as the **standard enthalpy** of sublimation. At a stated temperature, we can therefore calculate any of these values, as long as the other two are known. Here, it is important to use standard enthalpy values, i.e. values measured at standard pressure and fixed temperature, in order for the comparisons to be valid.

Hess's Law

Just as we used a mathematical approach to determine the enthalpy of physical changes, we can use a similar approach for chemical reactions. If a reaction takes place in a series of steps, the overall enthalpy change is the same as if it takes place in one chemical step. This principle, proposed by Germain Henri Hess (Box 5.2), is known as Hess's Law and it can be used to calculate

INTEGRATION BOX 5.1

Aspirin synthesis

Aspirin is manufactured by a synthesis reaction between salicylic acid and acetic anhydride. This is shown for you in Figure 5.7.

This reaction is exothermic. Because this energy release is per mole, if the reaction takes place on the scale of mass production, then a large release of energy takes place. A cooling system is needed to absorb the heat energy released.

For more information on aspirin synthesis, please refer to Chapter 1 'The importance of pharmaceutical chemistry' of the ***Pharmaceutical Chemistry*** book within this series.

FIGURE 5.7 Aspirin synthesis

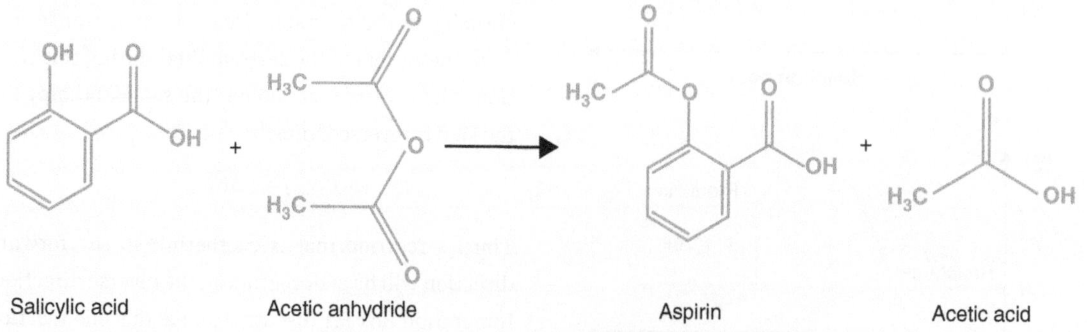

Salicylic acid + Acetic anhydride → Aspirin + Acetic acid

FIGURE 5.8 Enthalpy of sublimation can be calculated by the sum of the enthalpies of fusion and vaporization, measured under the same conditions: $\Delta H^{\theta}_{fus} + \Delta H^{\theta}_{vap} = \Delta H^{\theta}_{sub}$

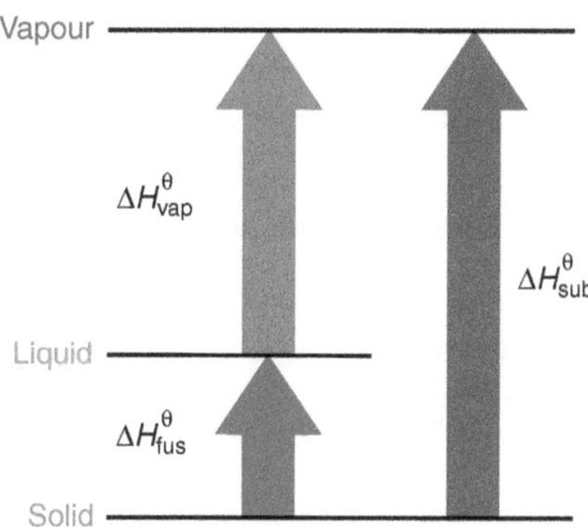

enthalpy changes that might be difficult or impossible to measure. Hess's Law states that the standard enthalpy change for any chemical or physical process at fixed temperature is independent of the number of steps taken to complete the process.

As an example of the application of Hess's law, consider aerobic respiration. We obtain energy from food by this exothermic process and the associated chemical equation may be written overall as:

$$C_6H_{12}O_6 + 6O_2 \rightarrow 6CO_2 + 6H_2O$$

This process releases energy, which is stored in the body as adenosine triphosphate (ATP). However, respiration is not a single chemical step, but takes place in a series of complex chemical steps outlined below:

1. Glycolysis, a reaction in which glucose is broken down to two molecules of pyruvate.
2. Pyruvate is oxidized by an enzymatic reaction to acetyl conzyme A (CoA).
3. Acetyl CoA enters a cycle of enzymatic chemical reactions known as the Krebs Cycle, which produces reduced nicotinamide adenine dinucleotide (NADH), which can donate electrons.
4. Electron transport takes place leading to the production of ATP.

Overall, these many steps produce the same output of energy as the overall process.

For more information on glycolysis and the Krebs cycle, please refer to Chapter 3 'The biochemistry of cells' of the *Therapeutics and Human Physiology* book within this series.

Enthalpy change can be measured for simple reactions; for example, the enthalpy of **dissolution** can be measured by recording the temperature change when a substance, such as paracetamol, is dissolved in water in an insulated vessel (an isolated system) such as a calorimeter.

For more information on dissolution, please refer to 'Pharmaceutically relevant phase transitions' in Section 7.1.

We can use Hess's Law to calculate the enthalpy of reactions, including those that cannot be measured directly, if we know the enthalpy of the intermediate reactions. See Box 5.3 for two examples.

BOX 5.2

Germain Henri Hess

Germain Henri Hess was a scientist who worked predominantly in Russia during the first-half of the nineteenth century. Having originally studied medicine, he also worked in the areas of geological science and chemistry. He is best remembered for his work on thermochemistry and his statement of Hess's 'Law of the constant summation of heat'. The principle of the law is a consequence of the First Law of Thermodynamics, which was discussed in Section 5.2. However, Hess published his work several years before the first law was stated.

KEY POINT

Hess's Law states that the standard enthalpy change for any chemical or physical process is independent of the number of steps taken to complete the process.

BOX 5.3

Practice calculation: finding the $\Delta H^{\theta}_{reaction}$

Example 1: Two-step reaction

Consider the oxidation of nitrogen at 298 K:

$$N_{2(g)} + 2O_{2(g)} \rightarrow 2NO_{2(g}$$

We can easily imagine this reaction taking place in two steps:

$$\text{Step1} \quad N_{2(g)} + O_{2(g)} \rightarrow 2NO_{(g)} \qquad \Delta H^{\theta} = 180\text{ kJ mol}^{-1}$$
$$\text{Step2} \quad 2NO_{(g)} + O_{2(g)} \rightarrow 2NO_{2(g)} \qquad \Delta H^{\theta} = -112\text{ kJ mol}^{-1}$$

This can be represented on an enthalpy diagram (Figure 5.9). As with convention, arrows pointing upwards represent endothermic processes, while downward arrows represent endothermic processes.

The reaction for the oxidation of nitrogen can be thought of as occurring in two steps. The total enthalpy change for the reaction, $\Delta H^{\theta}_{reaction}$, is the same as the sum of the enthalpies of the two intermediate steps 1 and 2.

$$\Delta H^{\theta}_{reaction} = \Delta H^{\theta}_{(step1)} + \Delta H^{\theta}_{(step2)}$$

FIGURE 5.9 **Enthalpy diagram for the oxidation of nitrogen**

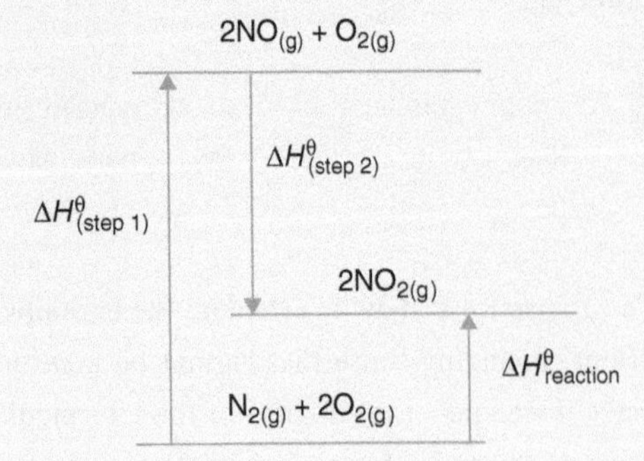

We can then calculate the $\Delta H^{\theta}_{reaction}$ as follows:

$$\Delta H^{\theta}_{reaction} = \Delta H^{\theta}_{(step1)} + \Delta H^{\theta}_{(step2)}$$
$$\Delta H^{\theta}_{reaction} = 180 + (-112)\text{ kJ mol}^{-1} = 68\text{ kJ mol}^{-1}$$

Example 2: Three-step reaction

The chemical equation for the combustion of the unsaturated hydrocarbon, ethene, C_2H_4, is written below:

$$C_2H_{4(g)} + 3O_{2(g)} \rightarrow 2CO_{2(g)} + 2H_2O_{(l)}$$

We can imagine this reaction taking place in a series of steps at 298 K:

$$\text{Step1} \quad C_2H_{4(g)} + H_{2(g)} \rightarrow C_2H_{6(g)} \qquad \Delta H^{\theta} = -136.7\text{ kJ mol}^{-1}$$
$$\text{Step2} \quad C_2H_{6(g)} + 3\tfrac{1}{2}O_{2(g)} \rightarrow 2CO_{2(g)} + 3H_2O_{(l)} \qquad \Delta H^{\theta} = -1556\text{ kJ mol}^{-1}$$
$$\text{Step3} \quad H_2O_{(l)} \rightarrow H_{2(g)} + \tfrac{1}{2}O_{2(g)} \qquad \Delta H^{\theta} = 285.5\text{ kJ mol}^{-1}$$

If we add these chemical equations together, in the same manner that we can add algebraic equations, then the sum will be the overall reaction equation:

$$C_2H_{4(g)} + H_{2(g)} \rightarrow C_2H_{6(g)}$$
$$C_2H_{6(g)} + 3\tfrac{1}{2}O_{2(g)} \rightarrow 2CO_{2(g)} + 3H_2O_{(l)}$$
$$H_2O_{(l)} \rightarrow H_{2(g)} + \tfrac{1}{2}O_{2(g)}$$
$$\overline{C_2H_{4(g)} + 3O_{2(g)} \rightarrow 2CO_{2(g)} + 2H_2O_{(l)}}$$

Any terms that appear on both sides of the equation will cancel. For example, $3\tfrac{1}{2}O_{2(g)}$ on the left in step 2 will cancel with $\tfrac{1}{2}O_{2(g)}$ on the right in step 3, to leave $3O_{2(g)}$, which is what we see in the overall equation.

We can arrive at the answer by adding the enthalpies of the individual steps:

$$\Delta H^{\theta}_{(r)} = \Delta H^{\theta}_{(step1)} + \Delta H^{\theta}_{(step\,2)} + \Delta H^{\theta}_{(step\,3)}$$
$$= (-136.7) + (-1556) + (285.5)$$
$$= -1407\text{ kJ mol}^{-1}$$

Calculating the enthalpy of combustion

We can use Hess's Law to determine values such as the **standard enthalpy of combustion, ΔH^{θ}_{c}**. Ethanol is a very widely used solvent, and is used in the formulation of medicines such as cough linctuses. We can use the principle of Hess's Law to determine the energy released when ethanol burns using **standard enthalpy of formation, ΔH^{θ}_{f}** data for the elements that make up ethanol (see Box 5.4).

BOX 5.4

Practice calculation: finding ΔH_c^θ

The reaction for the combustion of ethanol is:

$$C_2H_5OH_{(l)} + 3O_{2(g)} \rightarrow 2CO_{2(g)} + 3H_2O_{(l)}$$

The enthalpies of formation, ΔH_f^θ, for the substances involved at 298 K are:

$$\Delta H_f^\theta CO_{2(g)} = -393.0 \text{ kJ mol}^{-1}$$
$$\Delta H_f^\theta H_2O_{(l)} = -285.5 \text{ kJ mol}^{-1}$$
$$\Delta H_f^\theta C_2H_5OH_{(l)} = -273.1 \text{ kJ mol}^{-1}$$
$$\Delta H_f^\theta O_{2(g)} = 0 \text{ kJ mol}^{-1}$$

The enthalpy of formation of any element in its standard state, such as O_2(g), is always zero.

It follows from Hess's Law and equation 5.6 that ΔH_c^θ can be calculated using:

$$\Delta H_c^\theta = \Sigma H_{f(\text{combustion products})}^\theta - \Sigma \Delta H_{f(\text{reactants})}^\theta$$

Taking into account the chemical formula of ethanol, we may write:

$$\Delta H_c^\theta = (2 \times -393.0) + (3 \times -285.5) - (1 \times -273.1) - (0)$$
$$\Delta H_c^\theta = -1369 \text{ kJ mol}^{-1}$$

Dependence of enthalpy changes on temperature

The heat flowing into or out of a system during a chemical process is dependent on the heat capacity, C_p of the reactants and products. The heat capacity of a substance is a measure of how readily it absorbs heat. The value of C_p is dependent on temperature, so the value of the enthalpy change will be dependent on the temperature at which the reaction takes place.

For example, let us say that we know the value of the enthalpy change at one temperature, $\Delta H(T_1)$. We can then estimate its value if the same reaction takes place at another temperature, $\Delta H(T_2)$, using Kirchoff's Law:

$$\Delta H(T_2) = \Delta H(T_1) + \Delta C_p(T_2 - T_1)$$

where ΔC_p is the difference in heat capacities of the reactants and products, which can be assumed to be constant over small temperature changes, and $T_2 - T_1$ represents the change in temperature.

KEY POINT

Kirchoff's Law can be used to predict the enthalpy change at different temperatures if the heat capacities of the reactant and products are known.

SELF CHECK 5.4

How is standard enthalpy of fusion, ΔH_{fus}^θ, defined?

SELF CHECK 5.5

What is Hess's Law and what does it allow us to do?

5.4 Entropy and the Second Law of Thermodynamics: what is permissible?

We have learnt a lot about the energy changes that take place during a chemical reaction. However, thermodynamics can tell us much more than this about processes. We need to know, for example, why some reactions take place and some do not. This will help us to predict whether substances, such as medicines, are likely to degrade and whether materials used to store pharmaceutical formulations will be resistant to deterioration.

Of particular interest is whether reactions will occur spontaneously and, if so, whether or not they proceed to completion. By 'spontaneous' we mean a reaction that will occur naturally without needing to be forced. This includes, for example, combustion reactions that may require ignition, but then proceed unimpeded until all the fuel is spent. Knowing if a reaction will occur spontaneously does not tell us how fast it will occur. We can learn more about this by studying reaction kinetics. As well as change in enthalpy, ΔH, there are other changes that take place, which we need to think about in order to understand chemical processes more fully.

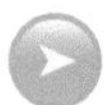

For more information on reaction kinetics, please refer to Chapter 12.

KEY POINT

A spontaneous process is one that will occur naturally without needing to be forced.

Entropy of a system

Entropy is a state function that measures the disorder in the system. You will know that in **gases**, particles are randomly arranged, and in **solids** they are arranged in regular patterns. Therefore, solids tend to have low entropy and gases have high entropy, with **liquids** somewhere in-between. Table 5.2 shows you some typical values for standard entropy. Entropy generally increases as molecules become more complex and ethanol, for example, has a greater entropy than water.

TABLE 5.2 Standard molar entropies of some selected materials at 298 K

Substance	S^θ/J K^{-1}mol^{-1}
Diamond, $C_{(s)}$	2.4
Water, $H_2O_{(l)}$	69.9
Ethanol, $C_2H_5OH_{(l)}$	160.7
Oxygen, $O_{2(g)}$	205.1

For more information on solids, liquids and gases, please refer to Chapter 2, Chapter 3, and Chapter 4.

The natural world tends to favour high entropy. This agrees with our everyday experience, as you can see by looking at Figure 5.10. In this example, the entropy of the system (the matches) increases during this naturally occurring change.

Entropy has the symbol, S, and it has units of J K^{-1}mol^{-1}. We can use ΔS^θ to represent the standard entropy change when a process such as a chemical reaction occurs:

$$\Delta S^\theta_{\text{reaction}} = \Sigma S^\theta_{\text{(products)}} - \Sigma S^\theta_{\text{(reactants)}} \qquad (5.7)$$

Processes that are spontaneous, that is, occurring without intervention or the need for work to be done on the system, are those that will increase the disorder or entropy of the Universe. This is the principle of the Second Law of Thermodynamics, which states that when an *isolated* system undergoes a *spontaneous* change, the entropy of the system will increase. Again, we can consider that the Universe is a special example of a very large, isolated system. Thus, the entropy of the Universe is continually increasing. Contrast this with the First Law of Thermodynamics, which states that the internal energy of the Universe is constant.

KEY POINT

Entropy is a state function that measures the disorder in the system. The Second Law of Thermodynamics states that the entropy of an isolated system increases during spontaneous change.

FIGURE 5.10 What happens when a box of matches is dropped? In (A) the matches are all facing the same direction, so the system has low disorder, which means low entropy. In (B), when the box is dropped, then the matches become jumbled and point in different directions. The pile of matches is now highly disordered: it has increased in entropy. Work would be needed to be done to reorder and lower the entropy of the pile of matches

(A)

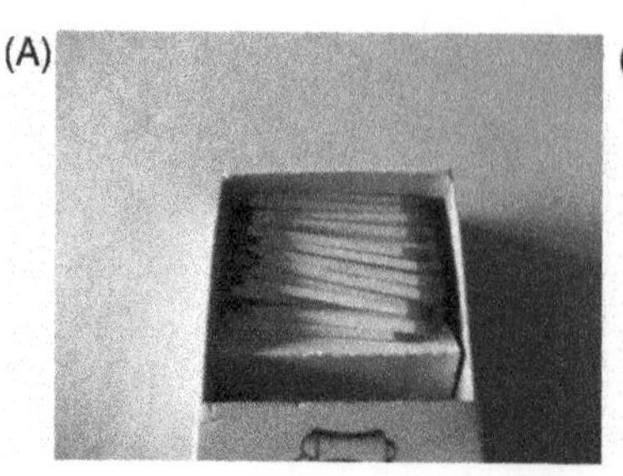

(B)

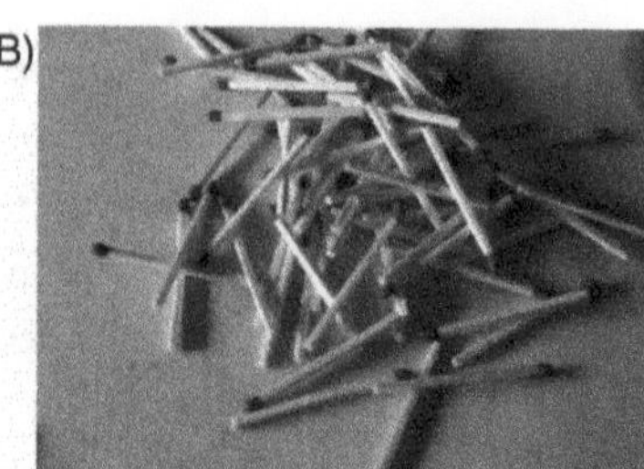

Remember that the Universe consists of both the system and the surroundings. The second law still allows for chemical and physical processes to lower the entropy of a system. Overall, we can conclude that the following types of process will generally be favoured:

- Those that result in an increase in the entropy of the system ($\Delta S^{\ominus}$=+ve).
- Those that result in an increase in an entropy of the surroundings. These will be those processes that release heat energy to the surroundings, making them more disordered (ΔH=–ve).

We can conclude that spontaneous processes are generally favoured when there is a release of dispersed matter (ΔS=+ve) and/or energy (ΔH=–ve).

Entropy is related to temperature. As temperature is increased, atoms have increased thermal motion and kinetic energy. As movements become more energetic, the entropy of the system increases. Therefore the temperature at which a reaction takes place will have an effect on $S^{\ominus}$ and by equation 5.7, $\Delta S^{\ominus}$.

At low temperatures, atoms are less energetic and their arrangements are more ordered. At absolute zero (0 kelvin), it is considered that the entropy of a perfect crystal is zero. This is a statement of the Third Law of Thermodynamics. Real substances do not exist as perfect crystals and, even at very low temperatures, will have some residual entropy.

KEY POINT

The Third Law of Thermodynamics states that for a perfect crystal, $S^{\ominus}=0\ J\ K^{-1}mol^{-1}$ when T=0 K.

Consider the following example of a spontaneous process. When coal (carbon) burns, it is converted into water vapour and carbon dioxide. $\Delta H^{\ominus}$ is negative (reaction is exothermic) and $\Delta S^{\ominus}$ is positive (solid converted to gas so entropy increases). The reaction is possible according to the first law because energy is conserved, the heat content of the reactants being released as heat energy. The reaction is permissible according to the second law because the entropy of both the system and surroundings increases.

KEY POINT

Spontaneous processes are generally favoured when there is a release of dispersed matter (ΔS=+ve) and/or energy (ΔH=–ve).

SELF CHECK 5.6

State the Second Law of Thermodynamics.

SELF CHECK 5.7

What is entropy?

5.5 Gibbs free energy

We can use the principles above to understand why processes accompanying the use of medicines occur spontaneously. For example, erythritol is a sugar alcohol that is used as an excipient to mask bitter flavours in oral care products, such as mouthwashes. Erythritol has an endothermic enthalpy of **dissolution** and gives a refreshing **mouth-feel** due to the associated cooling effect. As heat energy is absorbed from the oral cavity during dissolution, the entropy of the surroundings decreases. However, the entropy of the system increases as the erythritol dissolves. Overall, dissolution occurs spontaneously because the overall entropy of the Universe (system + surroundings) increases, in accord with the Second Law.

In order to know whether a reaction at constant pressure will occur spontaneously, we need to consider the balance of the quantities $\Delta H^{\ominus}$ and $\Delta S^{\ominus}$. To do this we relate enthalpy and entropy using a state function known as Gibbs free energy, also called the Gibbs energy or Gibbs function (after Josiah Willard Gibbs,

BOX 5.5

Josiah Willard Gibbs

Josiah Willard Gibbs was a theoretical physicist and chemist from the United States of America who worked during the nineteenth century. He graduated from Yale and was awarded the first engineering doctorate in the USA, in 1863. Following the loss of his parents, he spent several years in Europe, where he studied under some of the leading scientists of the time. Following his return to the USA, he was appointed professor of mathematical physics and it was during the 1870s that he published his major works on thermodynamic properties and equilibrium.

see Box 5.5). It relates enthalpy and entropy of a system at the reaction temperature according to equation 5.8:

$$G = H - TS \qquad (5.8)$$

where G is the Gibbs free energy. Throughout this chapter we will us the symbol ΔG^{θ}, to represent the standard change in Gibbs free energy associated with a reaction. Look at equation 5.9, which shows how we can calculate the standard Gibbs free energy change for a reaction. Compare it to equations 5.6 and 5.7:

$$\Delta G^{\theta}_{\text{reaction}} = \Sigma G^{\theta}_{\text{(products)}} - \Sigma G^{\theta}_{\text{(reactants)}} \qquad (5.9)$$

It can be shown that the **Gibbs free energy change** associated with a chemical or physical change is related to the maximum energy available to do work, hence the term 'free' energy. By the standard convention discussed previously, when ΔG^{θ} is negative, the system can do work on the surroundings. In this case, the accompanying change will always be spontaneous. Therefore, according to equation 5.9, for a reaction to occur spontaneously, the Gibbs free energy must be reduced as reactants are transformed into products.

An example of this type of process is the reaction of hydrogen gas with oxygen gas, where $\Delta G^{\theta} < 0$. This process can be harnessed to do work and this reaction has been used, for example, to power rocket engines. The reverse reaction, the conversion of water into its constituent elements, hydrogen and oxygen gas, is not spontaneous and $\Delta G^{\theta} > 0$. Although the decomposition of water does not naturally occur, it can be forced to happen by passing an electric current through the water. This is known as electrolysis, and in thermodynamic terms we would say that electrical work has been done on the system.

As discussed earlier, the definition of enthalpy takes into account any 'expansion work' that the system may do during a change of state, equation 5.4. As enthalpy is accounted for in the expression for G, equation 5.8, ΔG actually measures the remaining work available, the maximum 'non-expansion' work that a system can do.

'Non-expansion' work can include, for example, electrical work, **osmotic pressure** work, and energy changes associated with increases or decreases in **surface area**. Changes in volume and associated expansion work are quite common. Some types of non-expansion work are less common but are important in certain systems:

- Electrical work in an electrochemical cell that powers, say, a portable blood pressure monitor.
- Osmotic pressure work in drug-delivery systems that rely on **osmosis**.
- Surface area work in the formation of an **emulsion** from two **immiscible** liquids.

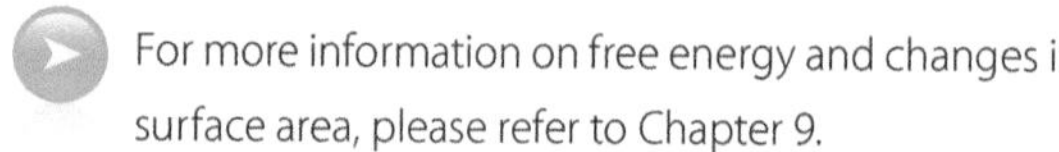
For more information on free energy and changes in surface area, please refer to Chapter 9.

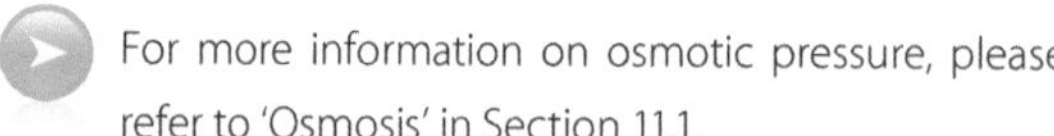
For more information on osmotic pressure, please refer to 'Osmosis' in Section 11.1.

KEY POINT

The Gibbs free energy change, ΔG, is the maximum amount of non-expansion work that can be done by a closed system undergoing a change of state.

Determination of temperature at which a reaction becomes spontaneous

Consider a sample of water in a pan. In order for it to boil, it must absorb energy from its surroundings, e.g. from a hotplate. This is an endothermic process and the **standard enthalpy of vaporization** has a positive value. During this process, liquid water (restricted movement of molecules) converts to gas (free movement of molecules). Therefore, the system increases in entropy and ΔS^{θ} for this process has a positive value. This increase in entropy is as a result of heat flow into the system (another name for enthalpy). Thus the surroundings have lost heat, and therefore the entropy of the surroundings has reduced. However, the temperature is very important: heating water gently from room temperature to 50 °C will increase its thermal energy and therefore increase its entropy, but will not bring about the spontaneous conversion to gas. We can say that at 50 °C and normal atmospheric pressure, the most thermodynamically stable state of water is liquid, a notion that can also be understood in terms of **chemical potential**.

For more information on chemical potential, please refer to Section 11.6.

We can conclude that whether a reaction or physical change will occur spontaneously will depend on temperature. Following on from equation 5.8, we can write an equation to describe how the standard enthalpy, entropy, and Gibbs free energy changes are connected, and this is written out for you in equation 5.10:

$$\Delta G^{\theta} = \Delta H^{\theta} - T\Delta S^{\theta} \qquad (5.10)$$

where T is the **absolute temperature** at which the process takes place (K).

It is apparent that the value of ΔG^{θ} depends on the value of T. When ΔH^{θ} is positive (as in an endothermic process), then ΔG^{θ} will be positive when T is low. When T is higher, the value for $T\Delta S^{\theta}$ will become larger than ΔH^{θ}, so that ΔG^{θ} becomes negative. So, when the temperature of water is below 100 °C, water exists as a liquid and the conversion to vapour does not occur. Above 100 °C, the conversion from liquid to vapour will be spontaneous and the water will boil.

We can apply the same approach to chemical reactions. If the change in Gibbs free energy is negative, then that process is predicted to occur spontaneously. This doesn't mean it will occur quickly. Some reactions are predicted to be spontaneous, but will occur very slowly or be disfavoured. For example, the process may have a large **activation energy** or reactant particles may be trapped in a solid lattice. Such a reaction mixture is said to be **metastable**. It is kinetically stable but thermodynamically unstable.

For more information on activation energy, please refer to Section 12.3.

The temperature at which reactions become spontaneous is of interest in pharmaceutics. For example, some solid APIs exhibit **polymorphism**. A **dosage form** may be formulated using a particular polymorph because it exhibits the greatest activity. In **enantiotropic** polymorphism, the different physical forms of the API each have a particular temperature range where they are most stable. If the most active polymorph is not the most stable at the storage temperature then it may spontaneously convert to a less active form, although this may be at a very low rate.

For more information on phase equilibrium, please refer to Chapter 7.

The temperature at which a reaction becomes spontaneous is the temperature at which ΔG^{θ} goes from a positive value (reaction will not occur) to a negative value (reaction will be spontaneous). This is the temperature at which ΔG^{θ} is equal to zero. Thus, at the standard boiling point of water the standard free energy of vaporization is zero. At this temperature, liquid water and water vapour are said to be in a phase equilibrium.

For more information on enantiotropic polymorphism, please refer to Section 2.3.

If we set $\Delta G^{\theta}=0$ in equation 5.10 then we can show that:

$$T = \left(\frac{\Delta H^{\theta}}{\Delta S^{\theta}}\right) \qquad (5.11)$$

We can use this to determine the temperature at which a reaction will occur spontaneously (see Box 5.6 for an example).

You should note that the processes we have considered here have been at standard pressure. Many real processes take place at pressures other than at 1 bar, and sometimes with changing pressure, such those within the lungs. Similarly, standard temperature is usually close to ambient, but biological process take place at body temperature, 37 °C.

BOX 5.6

Practice calculation: determining the temperature at which a reaction will occur spontaneously

Magnesium carbonate is an inorganic salt used in medicines and cosmetic products such as toothpaste. It decomposes by the following reaction:

$$MgCO_{3(s)} \rightarrow MgO_{(s)} + CO_{2(g)}$$

If the enthalpy (ΔH^θ) of the above reaction = +100.59 kJ mol^{-1} and the entropy (ΔS^θ) of the reaction = +174.98 J K^{-1} mol^{-1}, find the temperature at which magnesium carbonate will decompose spontaneously. Use equation 5.11:

$$T = \frac{\Delta H^\theta}{\Delta S^\theta}$$

$$T = \frac{(100.59 \times 1000)\,\text{J mol}^{-1}}{174.98\ \text{J K}^{-1}\,\text{mol}^{-1}} = 574.87\,\text{K}$$

This temperature is approximately equal to 300 °C, so below this temperature magnesium carbonate is thermodynamically stable.

KEY POINT

Standard free energy change is related to enthalpy and entropy change by:

$$\Delta G^\theta = \Delta H^\theta - T\Delta S^\theta$$

This equation can be used to predict the temperature at which a reaction will become spontaneous.

SELF CHECK 5.8

What is the value of ΔG^θ if a reaction occurs spontaneously?

SELF CHECK 5.9

Name four types of work that systems may do during a change of state.

SELF CHECK 5.10

How can we predict the temperature at which a reaction will occur spontaneously?

5.6 Reactions at equilibrium

We have seen how Gibbs energy can change with temperature. The Gibbs energy also varies with composition. A reaction mixture, for example, might start with a composition that is 100% reactants and finish with a composition that is 100% products. Equilibrium processes will have a final composition somewhere between these two extremes. A reaction has reached equilibrium when the concentrations of reactants and products have become constant. The forward and reverse reactions do not stop at equilibrium but effectively cancel each other out in a so-called **dynamic equilibrium**.

KEY POINT

A reaction has reached equilibrium when the concentrations of reactants and products have become constant. A reversible chemical reaction at equilibrium is an example of a dynamic equilibrium.

A system will always tend to the composition of reactants and products that has lowest Gibbs energy. When this is reached, the system is said to be at equilibrium and the Gibbs energy cannot decrease any further, $\Delta G = 0$. Notice that the standard symbol is missing from G here. This is because we are referring to a reaction mixture, rather than the reactants or products in their pure, standard states. Look at Figure 5.11 to see how a system at equilibrium has reached the lowest Gibbs energy available.

If the composition of a system at equilibrium is changed, e.g. if more reactant is added, then the system will spontaneously adjust by reacting to give more product and attain a new equilibrium composition, where the Gibbs energy again has its lowest value. This concept can be expressed in **Le Chatelier's principle** (Integration Box 5.2), which states that a system at equilibrium experiencing a change will respond to

FIGURE 5.11 At the equilibrium composition, the Gibbs energy is at a minimum

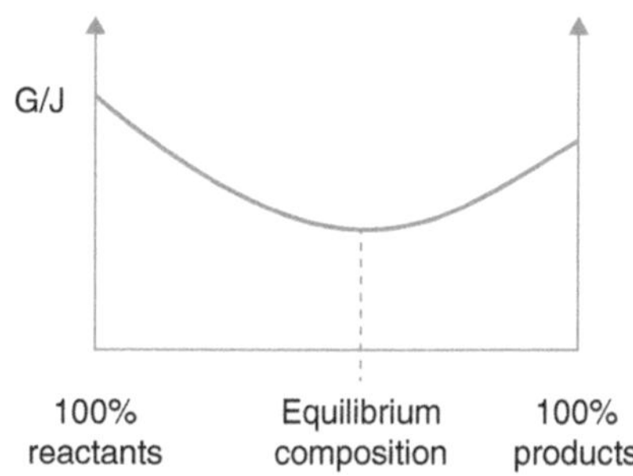

counteract the imposed change. The change may be caused by:

- The addition or removal of a reactant or product.
- A change of temperature.
- A change in volume or pressure.

According to Le Chatelier's principle, for example, adding extra reactant to a system at equilibrium will be counteracted by the system forming more product, shifting the equilibrium position to the right.

KEY POINT

A system will always tend to the composition of reactants and products that has lowest Gibbs energy. Le Chatelier's principle states that a system at equilibrium experiencing a change will respond to counteract the imposed change.

At equilibrium, the concentrations of reactants and products are constant, but this does not necessarily mean that the quantity of reactants and products are equal. The ratio of reactants to products is defined by the **equilibrium constant**. Consider the general reaction described below:

$$\alpha A + \beta B \rightleftharpoons \gamma C + \delta D$$

The equilibrium constant is calculated by:

$$K = \frac{[\text{products}]}{[\text{reactants}]} = \frac{[C]^\gamma [D]^\delta}{[A]^\alpha [B]^\beta} \quad (5.12)$$

So for a reaction such as:

$$N_2O_{4(g)} \rightleftharpoons 2NO_{2(g)}$$

$$K = \frac{[\text{products}]}{[\text{reactants}]} = \frac{[NO_2]^2}{[N_2O_4]}$$

The square brackets denote the molar concentration, or for gases we can use the partial pressure.

For more information on partial pressure, please refer to 'Partial pressure' in Section 4.2.

INTEGRATION BOX 5.2

Le Chatelier's principle in action

Respiratory alkalosis is a condition that occurs when a person hyperventilates or breathes in a rapid and shallow manner. This leads to too much carbon dioxide being expelled in the breath and alters the levels of CO_2 in the blood. Hydrogen ions and bicarbonate ions in the blood react to produce carbonic acid (H_2CO_3). H_2CO_3 in turn reacts with the enzyme carbonic anhydrase to produce CO_2, increasing the CO_2 level in the blood, bringing it closer to normal levels. These processes are shown in equation 5.13:

$$HCO_3^- + H^+ \rightleftharpoons H_2CO_3 \rightleftharpoons CO_2 + H_2O \quad (5.13)$$

Effect of temperature on equilibrium and reaction yield

The position of an equilibrium is affected by the conditions of the reaction. Look again at the graph shown in Figure 5.11. The equilibrium constant is a mathematical representation of where the position of lowest Gibbs energy lies. If the external conditions, such as temperature, change then the position of this minimum (and therefore the value of the equilibrium constant) also changes. The relationship between K and temperature is described by the van't Hoff equation, a version of which is written for you in equation 5.14:

$$\ln K = -\frac{\Delta H^\theta}{RT} + \frac{\Delta S^\theta}{R} \quad (5.14)$$

Over narrow temperature ranges, the standard enthalpy (ΔH^θ) and entropy (ΔS^θ) of reaction can be assumed to remain constant. For a reversible reaction that is exothermic in the forward direction, ΔH^θ has a negative value. Therefore K will decrease as the temperature increases, and the equilibrium will shift to the left, favouring reactants. This is consistent with Le Chatelier's principle: increasing temperature favours this reaction in the reverse, endothermic, direction as this absorbs heat energy and counteracts the imposed temperature change.

For an endothermic reaction, ΔH^{θ} is positive and, as the temperature increases, K increases. This means that the equilibrium will favour products and so the amount of products generated (known as yield of the reaction) will increase. When APIs are manufactured, the highest yield possible is desired and this must be considered alongside the kinetics of the reaction when choosing the reaction temperature.

It is helpful to be able to predict how much the position of equilibrium and therefore the reaction yield will change with changing temperature. By adapting the van't Hoff equation we can do this for equilibria where the standard enthalpy of reaction, ΔH^{θ} is known. Look at equation 5.15 to see how by knowing the value of K at one temperature, T_1, we can calculate the value of K at a different temperature, T_2. This tells us the position of the equilibrium at the new temperature and therefore the effect on reaction yield:

$$\ln K_2 - \ln K_1 = \frac{-\Delta H^{\theta}}{R}\left(\frac{1}{T_2} - \frac{1}{T_1}\right) \tag{5.15}$$

where K_1 is the value of K at T_1, K_2 is the value of K at T_2, and R is the gas constant

KEY POINT

The equilibrium constant, K, is a ratio that describes the composition of a system at equilibrium which undergoes a reversible reaction. The relationship between K and temperature is described by the van't Hoff equation.

SELF CHECK 5.11

What is the condition for free energy change, ΔG, for a system that has reached chemical equilibrium?

CHAPTER SUMMARY

- In order to study physical and chemical processes, we define the system as the region of interest and the surroundings as the rest of the Universe.
- The First Law of Thermodynamics states that the energy of the Universe is constant.
- The enthalpy of a substance is a state function that measures the heat content of a substance.
- Reactions can release heat energy (exothermic) or absorb heat energy (endothermic).
- We can calculate the enthalpy of reaction by the summation of the enthalpies of intermediate chemical steps and this is the principle of Hess's law.
- The Second Law of Thermodynamics states that a reaction will occur spontaneously if the entropy (or disorder) of the Universe increases as a result.
- The Gibbs energy relates enthalpy and entropy. If the Gibbs energy is lowered when a reaction takes place, that reaction will occur spontaneously. This does not necessarily mean that it will occur quickly.
- When the Gibbs energy change for a reaction is zero, then that reaction is said to be at equilibrium.
- The equilibrium constant for a reaction is dependent on temperature.
- We can predict the equilibrium constant, K for a given temperature if its value is known at another temperature. This can be used to predict decomposition and changes in yield with change in temperature.

FURTHER READING

Atkins, P. and de Paula, J. *Atkins' Physical Chemistry*, (9th edn) Oxford: Oxford University Press (2009).

An authoritative, rigorous coverage of the material with lots of worked examples to show the importance of thermodynamics to a variety of fields such as medicine, biochemistry and nanoscience.

Price, G. *Thermodynamics of Chemical Processes.* (Oxford Chemistry Primers), Oxford: Oxford University Press (1998).

This text covers the basic principles in a concise format. It covers any mathematical techniques needed to understand the material and doesn't assume too much prior knowledge.

6 Acids and bases

JUDITH MADDEN

Many chemical compounds can be characterized as either acids or bases. This information can be used to predict the properties of the compound, such as the way in which it reacts with other compounds and its solubility in particular solvents. Of the drugs currently available on the market, it is estimated that approximately 75% are basic in nature, and 20% are acidic. Thus, from a pharmaceutical perspective, acids and bases are of immense interest.

An ideal drug formulation is one in which the **active pharmaceutical ingredient (API)** is presented to the patient in an acceptable format. Medicines applied to sensitive areas such as the eye, for example, must not cause an irritant effect. This requires careful adjustment of the formulation to an appropriate **pH**. An understanding of acidic and basic behaviour is also essential in understanding how APIs will behave prior to, and following, administration to a patient. An ideal **dosage form** ensures that the API remains stable in storage for as long as reasonably practicable. The rate of degradation of a water-soluble API in a formulation is usually dependent on the pH of the environment. Of particular interest, therefore, is the pH at which the API is most stable.

In this chapter, key concepts relating to acid and base behaviour will be introduced. These will include:

- The behaviour of electrolytes and the difference between strong and weak electrolytes.
- The pH scale for measuring relative acidity and basicity (including the pH of various body fluids).
- Relative strengths of acids and bases.
- Ionization of acids and bases at different pHs.
- The ionization profile of zwitterionic compounds.
- Maintaining a specific pH using buffer systems, the buffering capacity and application of buffer systems.

These topics will be discussed in terms of their role in ensuring an appropriate formulation in terms of API stability and acceptability to the patient, as well as their influence on uptake and distribution of the drug in the body.

Learning objectives

Having read this chapter you are expected to be able to:

- Define the terms electrolyte, acid, base, conjugate pair, zwitterion, isoelectric point, buffer, and buffer capacity.
- Explain what is meant by the 'strength' of acids and bases, the scale by which these are recorded, and give several examples of factors that affect acid and base strength.
- Convert between hydrogen ion concentration and pH; K_a and pK_a; K_b and pK_b, appreciating the relationship

between the terms and the relevance of the ionic product of water.

- Calculate the extent to which particular APIs will be ionized or unionized at a given pH.
- Identify zwitterionic compounds (such as amino acids) and understand their behaviour in terms of ionization at different pHs.
- Determine the reagents required to produce a buffer of a particular pH and calculate the change in pH of that buffer when small amounts of acid or base are added.
- Give examples of how the principles of acid-base behaviour are incorporated into dosage form design.

6.1 Acidic and basic behaviour

When certain substances are added to water they produce ions; these substances are known as **electrolytes**. The name electrolyte is derived from the fact that these solutions are electrolytic, i.e. they contain charged ionic species that are capable of conducting electricity. Positively charged species are referred to as **cations** and negatively charged species as **anions**. We will see that all substances exhibiting acidic or basic behaviour can be classified as electrolytes.

Strong and weak electrolytes

When we talk about a substance being a strong or weak electrolyte, we are referring to the extent to which it ionizes when in a particular solution. A **strong electrolyte** is one that completely ionizes. An example of a strong electrolyte that you will be familiar with is table salt, sodium chloride, and this completely dissociates into its constituent ions when in aqueous solution:

$$NaCl_{(s)} \rightarrow Na^{+}{}_{(aq)} + Cl^{-}{}_{(aq)}$$

Other compounds that fully dissociate include hydroxides of group I and II elements in the periodic table, many salts, and some inorganic acids. In these examples, complete electrolytic dissociation occurs spontaneously as the **Gibbs free energy** of the system is significantly reduced when the solid breaks-up to yield solvated ions.

For more information on Gibbs free energy, please refer to Section 5.5.

Weak electrolytes are compounds that only partially ionize in solution. For example, household vinegar contains acetic acid and this is a weak electrolyte:

$$CH_3COOH_{(aq)} + H_2O_{(l)} \rightleftharpoons CH_3COO^{-}{}_{(aq)} + H_3O^{+}{}_{(aq)}$$

In this case the equilibrium lies to the left and only one molecule in around every 100 000 is in the ionized form. Other compounds that only partially ionize in aqueous solution include ammonia, organic bases, most organic acids, and some inorganic acids.

KEY POINTS

- A strong electrolyte completely ionizes when in solution.
- A weak electrolyte partially ionizes when in solution.

Brönsted and Lewis acids and bases

Acids and bases are substances that act as strong or weak electrolytes. There are different ways in which acids and bases can be defined. A definition that you may recognize from chemistry experiments is that an acid is a substance that reacts with a base to form a salt and water, for example:

$$H_2SO_{4(aq)} + 2NaOH_{(aq)} \rightarrow Na_2SO_{4(aq)} + 2H_2O_{(l)}$$

See also Case Study 6.1.

A stricter definition is that given by Brönsted–Lowry theory. In this, a **Brönsted acid** is defined as being a proton donor and a **Brönsted base** is defined as being a proton acceptor. For example, the chemical equation below shows hydrochloric acid donating its proton to water (which in this case acts as a base, accepting the proton):

$$HCl_{(aq)} + H_2O_{(l)} \rightarrow H_3O^+_{(aq)} + Cl^-_{(aq)}$$

Here, HCl behaves as a strong acid, a term clarified in Box 6.1. A proton may otherwise be known as a hydrogen ion (H^+). Thus, any substance that possesses ionizable hydrogen atoms would be characterized as a Brönsted acid. In some cases you may see protons in solution denoted as H^+ ions, however, in reality they exist as a species associated with water molecules and we may write this as H_3O^+ (hydroxonium) ions; both notations are often used.

Sodium hydroxide is a strong base, it fully dissociates in water and the OH^- ions formed then can act as a base, i.e. they are proton acceptors:

$$NaOH_{(aq)} \rightarrow OH^-_{(aq)} + Na^+_{(aq)}$$

Another definition of acids and bases is the Lewis definition. According to this classification, a **Lewis acid** is a substance that can accept an electron pair and a **Lewis base** can donate an electron pair. In Figure 6.1, ammonia (NH_3) acts as a Lewis base. It donates its lone pair of electrons to trifluoroboron (BF_3), which acts as the Lewis acid, forming a so-called Lewis adduct (Figure 6.1).

BOX 6.1

Acid and base strength

Imagine that you are in a laboratory looking at two solutions: one is labelled '1 M CH_3COOH' and the other is labelled '0.005 M HCl'. Which of these would you say is the stronger acid? One common misconception is that the 'strength' of an acid or base is related to its concentration – this is not true. The strength of an acid or base relates to the extent to which it dissociates. Hydrochloric acid is considered a strong acid as it fully dissociates in aqueous solution, hence in this case it is the hydrochloric acid that is the stronger acid. The acetic acid is a more concentrated solution, but acetic acid is the weaker acid in this example.

FIGURE 6.1 The Lewis adduct formed from NH_3 and BF_3

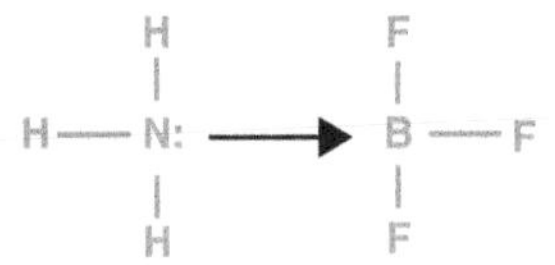

$$H-\ddot{N}(H)(H) \longrightarrow BF_3$$

Unless stated otherwise, the terms 'acid' and 'base' are routinely used to describe substances according to the Brönsted–Lowry definition. Lewis bases can often also be classified as Brönsted bases, given that a lone-pair is required to accept a proton. However, some Lewis acids (such as BF_3) cannot be Brönsted acids as they do not possess ionizable hydrogen atoms.

Conjugate pairs

Upon dissociation in solution, electrolytes yield 'conjugate pairs' that each consist of a neutral and an ionized species. Consider hydrochloric acid (HCl), which fully dissociates in aqueous solution:

$$HCl_{(aq)} + H_2O_{(l)} \rightarrow Cl^-_{(aq)} + H_3O^+_{(aq)}$$

Conjugate pair 1 (HCl / Cl^-)   Conjugate pair 2 (H_2O / H_3O^+)

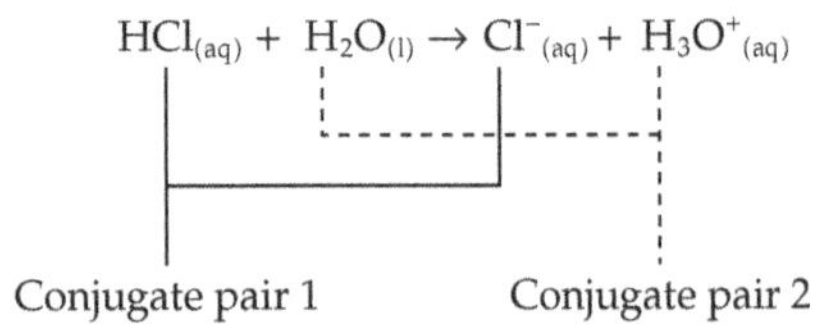

CASE STUDY 6.1

Following an evening of food-tasting with friends, Naina Patel awakes with indigestion.

REFLECTION QUESTION

What type of medicine might Naina take to alleviate this problem?

Answer

Indigestion is caused by a build-up of stomach acid. She could try taking one of many over-the-counter indigestion remedies that contain a basic compound, such as calcium carbonate ($CaCO_3$). This can react with the excess stomach acid (hydrochloric acid) forming a salt, water, and carbon dioxide:

$$2HCl_{(aq)} + CaCO_{3(s)} \rightarrow CaCl_{2(aq)} + H_2O_{(l)} + CO_{2(g)}$$

In this solution, the acid dissociates fully, i.e. the Cl^- ions do not readily accept protons to produce hydrochloric acid and the equilibrium position lies far to the right. We say that hydrochloric acid is a strong acid and that its conjugate ion (Cl^-) is a weak base. Together, HCl and Cl^- form a conjugate pair, as do H_2O and H_3O^+.

Conversely, if you consider a weak acid such as acetic acid, this will have a correspondingly strong conjugate base. In solution, more of the acid exists in the undissociated form than the dissociated form:

$$CH_3COOH_{(aq)} + H_2O_{(l)} \rightleftharpoons CH_3COO^-_{(aq)} + H_3O^+_{(aq)}$$

Conjugate pair 1 Conjugate pair 2

The CH_3COO^- ion readily accepts a proton to form CH_3COOH and the equilibrium lies to the left.

SELF CHECK 6.1

When a strong electrolyte enters solution, does the equilibrium position for the dissociation reaction lie to the left or to the right?

SELF CHECK 6.2

Why does the strength of an acid not increase as the concentration of the acid in an aqueous solution increases?

KEY POINTS

- Acids and bases are always electrolytes and they may fully or partially ionize in solution.
- According to the Brönsted–Lowry definitions, an acid is a proton donor and a base is a proton acceptor.
- According to the Lewis definitions, an acid is an electron pair acceptor and a base is an electron pair donor.
- Acid or base strength is not related to its concentration but to the equilibrium position of electrolytic dissociation.
- When a compound dissociates in solution, a conjugate pair is formed by the dissociated and undissociated species.
- A strong acid forms a conjugate pair that includes a weak conjugate base; a weak acid forms a conjugate pair that includes a strong conjugate base.

6.2 Factors affecting acid and base strength

The pharmaceutical activity of APIs is often reliant on their acidic or basic strength. The strength of acids and bases is determined by:

- Structural features of the undissociated molecule.
- The stability of the charged species that forms when the molecule ionizes.
- The solvent environment into which the acid or base is placed.

These principles can be applied in designing APIs, so that they have appropriate acid/base characteristics.

Structural features of the undissociated molecule

In order for an acid to lose a proton, the bond that connects the proton to the remainder of the molecule must be broken. Hence structural features that weaken the bond to the proton increase acid strength, i.e. make the proton more likely to be lost. If electron-withdrawing groups are present on the molecule, these can reduce the electron density of this bond and weaken it. Similarly, structural features, such as electron-donating groups that strengthen the bond to the proton, result in a weaker acid. Consider the three acids below:

- Cl_3CCOOH (trichloroacetic acid).
- CH_3COOH (acetic acid).
- $CH_3CH_2CH_2CH_2COOH$ (pentanoic acid).

Trichloroacetic acid is the strongest acid, as it possesses three chlorine atoms that exert an electron withdrawing effect. This is known as an **inductive effect** and it operates mainly through the σ bond framework of the molecule. Pentanoic acid is the weakest as the electron releasing inductive effect of small alkyl groups generally increases with alkyl chain length. The converse applies to bases; the strength of a base is related to its electron pair availability. Hence aminoethane ($CH_3CH_2NH_2$) is a stronger base than ammonia (NH_3), as the electron-releasing inductive effect of the alkyl chain increases electron pair availability and consequently base strength.

For more information on inductive and mesomeric effects, please refer to Chapter 7 'Introduction to aromatic chemistry' of the ***Pharmaceutical Chemistry*** book within this series.

The stability of the ionized molecule

The stability of the ion that forms following dissociation will, in part, determine the equilibrium position of electrolytic dissociation, i.e. the extent to which the molecule dissociates. Resonance stabilization of the resulting ion, for example, will favour the dissociation of the parent molecule. This is an example of a **mesomeric effect** and these are distinct from inductive effects because they operate through the conjugated π bond framework of a molecule.

Due to mesomeric effects, phenol (C_6H_5OH) is more likely to dissociate and form the $C_6H_5O^-$ ion than ethanol (CH_3CH_2OH) is to dissociate and form the $CH_3CH_2O^-$ anion. This is because the ion formed from the phenol is more stable. The resonance forms of the phenoxide ion ($C_6H_5O^-$) are shown in Figure 6.2.

For more information on the resonance forms of the phenoxide ion, please refer to Chapter 5 'Alcohols, phenols, ethers, organic halogen compounds, and amines' of the ***Pharmaceutical Chemistry*** book within this series.

The stabilizing of charge need not always be due to mesomeric effects. Thus, aminomethane (CH_3NH_2) is a stronger base than ammonia as the positive charge of the quaternary ammonium ion ($CH_3NH_3^+$) is stabilized by the electron donating inductive effect of the methyl group.

Choice of solvent

The environment in which an acidic or basic substance is placed will affect the degree of dissociation. The behaviour of acids or bases in a particular medium will depend on the classification of that solvent. Four different types of solvent may be identified:

- **Protogenic** solvents are those that donate protons, e.g. liquid hydrogen chloride (HCl).
- **Protophilic** solvents are those that accept protons, e.g. liquid ammonia (NH_3).
- **Amphiprotic** solvents are those that can both accept or donate protons, e.g. water.
- **Aprotic** solvents neither accept nor donate protons, e.g. dimethylsulphoxide (DMSO).

Liquid acetic acid is generally classified as a protogenic solvent, but can act as an extremely weak base, so it is technically an amphiprotic solvent. When hydrogen chloride dissolves in liquid acetic acid, it is not able to fully ionize as it does in water. The dissociation equilibrium lies well to the left:

$$HCl + CH_3CO_2H \rightleftharpoons Cl^- + CH_3C(OH)_2^+$$

Thus, HCl is only a weak acid when dissolved in acetic acid as this solvent has a very poor proton-accepting ability when compared to water.

In some instances, the choice of solvent can enhance acidic and basic behaviour. Acetic acid is a weak acid in water, but is a strong acid when dissolved in a protophilic solvent, such as liquid ammonia:

$$CH_3CO_2H + NH_3 \rightarrow CH_3CO_2^- + NH_4^+$$

The basic solvent accepts protons so that acetic acid can then lose protons more easily.

Solvents may also be characterized as being polar or non-polar. Water and DMSO are polar solvents, as the

FIGURE 6.2 The resonance forms of the phenoxide ion

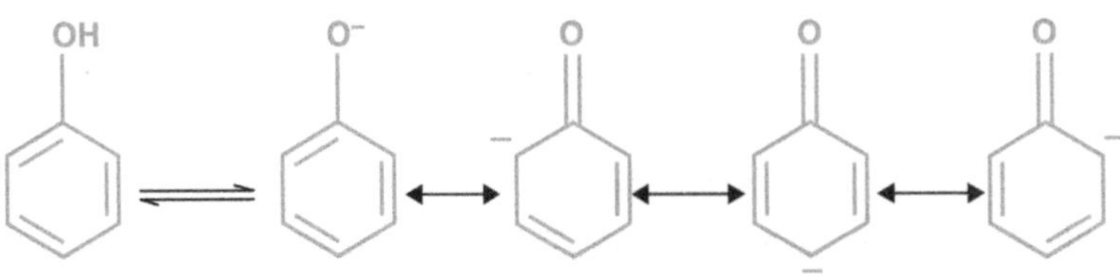

molecules bear partial positive and negative charges. In DMSO, this is due to the differing electronegativities of the sulphur and oxygen atoms that form the S=O bond. Polar aprotic solvents, such as DMSO, are not able to accept or donate protons. Consequently, acids and bases are generally weaker in these types of media. DMSO is a particularly important solvent in pharmaceutics as it can dissolve a wide range of compounds. As a skin-penetration enhancer it is useful in increasing the absorption of pharmaceuticals that are applied to the skin.

KEY POINT

The strength of acids and bases is determined by structural features that increase or decrease the likelihood of dissociation, the stability of the charged species that results from ionization, and the solvent environment into which the acid or base is placed.

SELF CHECK 6.3

Which is the stronger acid: acetic acid or trifluoroacetic acid?

6.3 The ionic product of water and the pH scale

The **pH** scale is used to indicate the relative acidity or basicity (alkalinity) of solutions. The majority of solutions fall in the pH range of 1 to 14, but how can a pH value be interpreted and what is meant by a **neutral solution**? Consider the equilibrium constant for the dissociation of water. The reaction is:

$$2H_2O \rightleftharpoons H_3O^+ + OH^-$$

This process is referred to as **autoprotolysis** and the **equilibrium constant** is related to the free energy change that accompanies the process. The equilibrium constant (K) for the reaction is:

$$K = \frac{[H_3O^+][OH^-]}{[H_2O]^2} \qquad (6.1)$$

For more information on the equilibrium constant, please refer to Chapter 5.

The hydroxonium ion (H_3O^+) is a very strong acid and the hydroxide ion (OH^-) is a very strong base. Thus, they react together very quickly to reform the water. This means that very few OH^- and H_3O^+ ions exist in solution at equilibrium. As the concentration of water remains effectively unchanged as a result of autoprotolysis, we can discount the expression $[H_2O]^2$ in the denominator of equation 6.1. This gives a new expression, where the equilibrium constant 'K' is replaced with 'K_w', which is referred to as the **ionic product of water** (equation 6.2).

$$K_w = [H_3O^+][OH^-] \qquad (6.2)$$

At a temperature of 25 °C it has been experimentally determined that K_w has a value of 1.0×10^{-14} mol^2 dm^{-6}. In pure water, the amount of H_3O^+ ions equals the amount of OH^- ions. This means that the concentration of H_3O^+ ions equals 1.0×10^{-7} mol dm^{-3} and the concentration of OH^- ions also equals 1.0×10^{-7} mol dm^{-3}.

As only a small amount of water dissociates it is more convenient to convert the K_w value to a more user-friendly value that avoids negative indices (see Box 6.2). For this reason we use the pK_w value:

$$pK_w = -\log_{10}K_w \qquad (6.3)$$

$$pK_w = -\log_{10}(1.0 \times 10^{-14})$$

Thus, pK_w = 14 at a temperature of 25 °C.

Neutral pH refers to conditions where the concentration of OH^- ions equals the concentration of H_3O^+ ions. At 25 °C, the concentration of both OH^- ions and H_3O^+ ions is the same and equal to 1.0×10^{-7} mol dm^{-3}. Again, to avoid the use of negative indices, this is more conveniently expressed by the pH scale:

$$pH = -\log_{10}[H_3O^+] \qquad (6.4)$$

where $[H_3O^+]$ is the value of the molar concentration of hydrogen ions in solution.

Note that this square bracket notation is always used to indicate molar concentration in mol dm^{-3} and should not be used for quantities with other concentration

BOX 6.2

pH measurement and activity

It is convenient to express hydrogen ion concentration in logarithmic form as we then avoid the need to express [H^+] as a very small number. It is also useful to use pH as some experimentally measurable quantities that depend on hydrogen ion concentration are found to be proportional to the logarithm of [H^+]. An example is the electrode potential of a glass electrode. In dilute acid solution, this electrode potential is found to be dependent on log [H^+] (so-called ideal behaviour) and a glass electrode is the main component of a pH meter. At low pH, it is found that the recorded pHs are often different than those predicted by equation 6.4 (so-called non-ideal behaviour). In concentrated acid, the distance between ions in solution is relatively small. Under these conditions, interactions between charged species are significant. The pH of a solution is more properly expressed as:

$$pH = -\log_{10} a_{H_3O^+} \quad (6.5)$$

where $a_{H_3O^+}$ is the **activity** of hydrogen ions in solution.

Thus, a pH meter actually measures the activity of hydrogen ions in solution. This will only be equal to the molar concentration under conditions where ionic concentrations are at their lowest (close to pH 7). Activity is the 'effective concentration' of a species in solution and takes into account the fact that solutions do not always behave as **ideal solutions**. Although equation 6.5 should be used in place of equation 6.4 for accurate work, in dilute solutions it is assumed that:

$$a_{H_3O^+} = [H_3O^+] \quad (6.6)$$

In introductory texts, this assumption is often extended to cover concentrated solution, although it is understood that these behave non-ideally. Thus, any calculation of pH using −log [H^+] can only be considered to be approximate.

units, e.g. $g\,m^{-3}$. For neutral pH, we know the concentration of H_3O^+ ions (at 25 °C) = 1.0×10^{-7} mol dm^{-3}. Hence if we substitute this value for H_3O^+ ion concentration into equation 6.4, this gives us a value of pH = 7. This is neutral pH at 25 °C.

The dissociation of water into ions is an **endothermic** process, i.e. a process that absorbs heat from the surroundings. This energy is needed to break the single covalent bond between the oxygen atom and a hydrogen atom in water. According to **Le Chatelier's principle**, if a change is made to a system that is in dynamic equilibrium, then the position of the equilibrium will move to counteract the change. From this we can predict that if the temperature of the water is increased, then more ions will be formed, as the ionization process absorbs the heat. At 100 °C, the ionic product of water is 51.3×10^{-14} mol^2 dm^{-6}. Hence from equation 6.2, the molar concentration of H_3O^+ (and OH^-) ions in a neutral solution at this temperature is 7.2×10^{-7} mol^2 dm^{-3}. Using equation 6.4 it follows that the pH of a neutral solution at 100 °C is therefore 6.1. It follows that a solution with a pH of 7 would be described as basic at this temperature.

For more information on Le Chatelier's principle, please refer to Section 5.6.

The pH scale (Figure 6.3) is used to indicate the relative acidity or basicity (alkalinity) of solutions. Solutions can be tested using universal indicator and this is red in acidic conditions, green at neutral pH, and blue in alkaline conditions. Alternatively, litmus paper may be used: blue litmus turns red in acidic

FIGURE 6.3 The pH scale for acidity and alkalinity

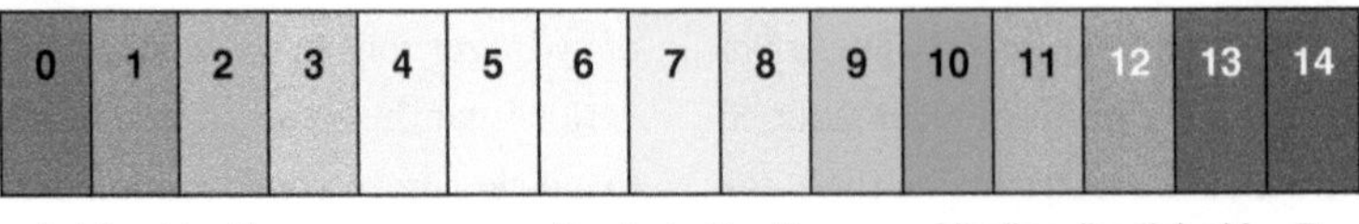

conditions and red litmus turns blue in alkaline conditions.

We have already determined that a neutral solution (pH=7 at 25 °C) contains 1.0×10^{-7} mol dm^{-3} of H_3O^+ ions. An acidic solution will always contain more H_3O^+ ions than are present in a neutral solution. For example, consider an acidic solution where the concentration of H_3O^+ ions is 6.0×10^{-6} mol dm^{-3}. By substitution into equation 6.4 we have:

$$pH = -\log_{10} 6.0\times10^{-6}$$

$$pH = 5.2$$

Now consider a basic solution where the concentration of $[H_3O^+]$ is less than 1.0×10^{-7} mol dm^{-3}. For example, the pH of a solution that contains 6.0×10^{-8} mol dm^{-3} H_3O^+ ions is given by:

$$pH = -\log_{10} 6.0\times10^{-8}$$

$$pH = 7.2$$

pH calculations for strong acids

We can use equation 6.4 to calculate the pH of solutions of strong acids that fully dissociate in water. Thus, a 0.050 M solution of HCl will contain 0.050 M of hydrogen ions. This gives:

$$pH = -\log_{10}(0.050)$$

$$pH = 1.3$$

Of course, the converse calculation is also useful. For example, if a sample is found to have a pH of 4.62, we can determine the concentration of the H_3O^+ ions in that solution. Substituting the given value into equation 6.4 we have:

$$4.62 = -\log_{10}[H_3O^+]$$

Taking the antilog of each side gives:

$$[H_3O^+] = \text{Antilog}(-4.62)$$

Therefore:

$$[H_3O^+] = 2.40\times10^{-5}\,\text{mol dm}^{-3}$$

If the sample was HCl, then we could conclude that the concentration of the acid must also be 2.40×10^{-5} mol dm^{-3}. If the sample were H_2SO_4, then the concentration of acid would be 1.20×10^{-5} mol dm^{-3}, given that each molecule of sulphuric acid has two ionizable hydrogen atoms. Both HCl and H_2SO_4 are strong acids, and we can assume that they are fully dissociated in solution. To determine the concentration of a weak acid in a solution of known pH, we require a quantitative understanding of the degree to which it dissociates; this is discussed in Section 6.4.

pH calculations for strong bases

We have shown in equation 6.4 that pH=$-\log_{10}[H_3O^+]$. An analogous expression can be derived for pOH:

$$pOH = -\log_{10}[OH^-] \qquad (6.7)$$

From the ionic product of water, that was derived previously, we can determine that:

$$pK_w = pOH + pH \qquad (6.8)$$

We may use this principle to determine the pH of strong bases, such as a 0.1 M solution of $Ba(OH)_2$. As mentioned previously, hydroxide ions of group II elements tend to be strong bases, i.e. they fully dissociate:

$$Ba(OH)_2 \rightarrow Ba^+ + 2OH^-$$

If the concentration of $Ba(OH)_2$=0.1 M, then the concentration of OH^-=0.2 M (according to the stoichiometric ratio):

If

$$pOH = -\log_{10}[OH^-]$$

then

$$pOH = -\log(0.2)$$

$$pOH = 0.7$$

Rearranging equation 6.8 above gives:

$$pH = pK_w - pOH$$

$$\text{i.e. } pH = 14 - 0.7 = 13.3$$

KEY POINTS

- The pH scale is used to indicate the relative acidity or basicity (alkalinity) of solutions where pH=$-\log_{10}[H_3O^+]$.
- The ionic product of water, K_w, is given by $K_w=[H_3O^+][OH^-]$ and $pK_w=-\log K_w$.

- The pH of neutral solutions depends on temperature.
- $pOH = -\log_{10} [OH^-]$ and $pK_w = pH + pOH$.
- For strong acids and bases, the concentration of the dissolved species can be calculated if the stoichiometry of the ionization equilibrium and the pH or pOH are known.

SELF CHECK 6.4

At 0 °C the ionic product of water is 0.114×10^{-14} mol^2 dm^{-6}. What is neutral pH at 0 °C?

SELF CHECK 6.5

Nitric acid is a strong acid; what is the pH of a 0.02 M solution of nitric acid (HNO_3)?

SELF CHECK 6.6

A solution of nitric acid (HNO_3) has a pH of 3.8. What is the concentration of H_3O^+ ions in this solution?

6.4 Measuring the strengths of acids and bases

Earlier, we determined that the strength of an acid or base was related to the extent to which it dissociates. The equilibrium constant (K) for a reaction is a measure of how far it proceeds towards completion. We can develop specific equilibrium constants that may be used to quantify the strength of weak acids and bases.

Acid dissociation constant

Consider the equilibrium constant for a typical acid, HA, in water:

$$HA + H_2O \rightleftharpoons A^- + H_3O^+$$

$$K = \frac{[A^-][H_3O^+]}{[HA][H_2O]} \quad (6.9)$$

Again, the change in concentration of water as the equilibrium is established is negligible. Hence, as we did when deriving K_w, we can discount the expression $[H_2O]$ in the denominator. This gives us the acid dissociation constant (K_a), which is derived from the equilibrium constant K:

$$K_a = \frac{[A^-][H_3O^+]}{[HA]} \quad (6.10)$$

For weak acids, only a relatively small amount of HA dissociates. To avoid the use of negative indices (similar to the derivation of pH) we convert the K_a value to a pK_a value:

$$pK_a = -\log_{10} K_a \quad (6.11)$$

As can be seen from equation 6.11, the further the dissociation reaction goes towards completion, the higher the K_a will be (and the lower the lower pK_a will be). In general, strong acids have high K_a values and low pK_a values, while weak acids have low K_a values and high pK_a values.

From equation 6.11, it can be seen that when half of the acid is dissociated then the concentrations of the dissociated and undissociated species are equal, i.e,. $[A^-] = [HA]$. This requires that $K_a = [H_3O^+]$. Thus, the pK_a of an acid is the pH at which 50% of it is dissociated. Table 6.1 shows the pK_a values of some common acids, in particular note the pK_a values for the examples given above where we discussed factors affecting acid strength.

pH of weak acids

When determining the pH of a solution of a strong acid we can assume that all of the acid dissociates and it is

TABLE 6.1 pK_a values for example compounds

Compound	pK_a value
Trichloroacetic acid	0.77
Methanoic acid	3.75
Pentanoic acid	4.84
Hexanoic acid	4.88
Phenol	9.95
Ethanol	15.9

relatively straightforward to calculate the concentration of H_3O^+ ions. However, if we want to determine the pH of a weak acid solution, then we need to know the K_a value of the acid in order to determine the pH. If the starting concentration of a weak acid HA is C, and the concentration of HA that dissociates is x then we can determine the concentration of each species involved at equilibrium:

$$\begin{array}{ccc} HA + H_2O & \rightleftharpoons A^- & + H_3O^+ \\ C - x & x & x \end{array}$$

Which gives:

$$K_a = \frac{x^2}{C - x} \tag{6.12}$$

We know that only a very small amount of HA has dissociated, therefore we can assume that the equilibrium concentration of HA is almost the same as the initial concentration i.e. $C - x \approx C$. We can also deduce from the equilibrium that $x = [H_3O^+]$. Substituting these equalities gives:

$$K_a = \frac{[H_3O^+]^2}{C} \tag{6.13}$$

Which upon rearrangement yields:

$$[H_3O^+] = \sqrt{K_a C} \tag{6.14}$$

We can use this expression to calculate the pH of a 0.01 M solution of the weak acid phenol (C_6H_5OH); for example, given that its $K_a = 1.1 \times 10^{-10}$ mol dm^{-3}. From equation 6.14:

$$[H_3O^+] = \sqrt{1.1 \times 10^{-10} \cdot 0.01} = 1.0 \times 10^{-6} \text{M}$$

It follows that:

$$pH = -\log_{10}(1.0 \times 10^{-6})$$

$$pH = 6.0$$

Base dissociation constant

In the same way that a pK_a scale can be devised to indicate relative strengths of acids, a pK_b scale can be devised to show the relative strengths of bases.

For a generic base B, the ionization reaction takes the form:

$$B + H_2O \rightleftharpoons BH^+ + OH^-$$

The equilibrium constant (K) for the reaction would be:

$$K = \frac{[BH^+][OH^-]}{[B][H_2O]} \tag{6.15}$$

To calculate the base dissociation constant (K_b), we discount the expression $[H_2O]$ in the denominator (as we did for the calculation of K_a) and we are left with:

$$K_b = \frac{[BH^+][OH^-]}{[B]} \tag{6.16}$$

To convert K_b values to more manageable figures we use the conversion:

$$pK_b = -\log_{10} K_b \tag{6.17}$$

The stronger the base the more it will dissociate, i.e. strong bases have high values of K_b and a low value of pK_b.

Relationship between K_a and K_b

For a particular acid, HA, we can define a K_a value. The acid anion, A^-, is the conjugate base of this acid and we can define a K_b value for this species. By consideration of the expressions for K_a, K_b and K_w we can then show that:

$$K_a \times K_b = K_w \tag{6.18}$$

Taking logs of this expression gives:

$$pK_a + pK_b = pK_w \tag{6.19}$$

We know that pK_w has a value of 14 at 25 °C. Therefore, if we know the pK_a for an acid then we can calculate the corresponding pK_b value for its conjugate base. The reverse also applies: if we know the pK_b for a base, then we can calculate the corresponding pK_a value for its conjugate acid. For example, as the pK_b of ammonia is 4.7, it follows that the pK_a of the ammonium ion, NH_4^+, will be 9.3.

SELF CHECK 6.7

The weak acid HCN has a K_a value of 4.9×10^{-10}. What is the pH of a 0.01 M solution of this acid?

KEY POINTS

- The acid dissociation constant, K_a, is a modified equilibrium constant for acid ionization equilibria. Strong acids have high K_a and low pK_a, where p$K_a = -\log_{10} K_a$.
- For the general weak acid HA, the hydrogen ion concentration may be determined using $[H_3O^+] = \sqrt{K_aC}$. where C is the molar concentration of acid.
- The base dissociation constant, K_b, is a modified equilibrium constant for the base ionization equilibrium. Strong bases have high K_b and low pK_b, where p$K_b = -\log_{10} K_b$.
- pK_a+pK_b=pK_w.

6.5 Ionization of acidic and basic APIs

The vast majority of APIs are weak acids or weak bases, and they may exist in both neutral and ionized forms, both in solution and in the body. Ionized compounds are more soluble in aqueous phases, whilst neutral molecules are more soluble in lipid phases. This differential solubility of ionized and neutral forms must be taken into consideration in the production of the dosage form; for example, in determining the solubility of an API in creams, gels, or ointments for topical preparations, and in the preparation of injections. It also has implications for orally administered tablets that undergo **dissolution** in the liquid of the gastrointestinal tract (GIT). We would predict that APIs that remain largely unionized in the low pH conditions of the stomach will be absorbed more readily into the lipid membranes of the stomach lining, in accordance with the **pH-partition hypothesis**.

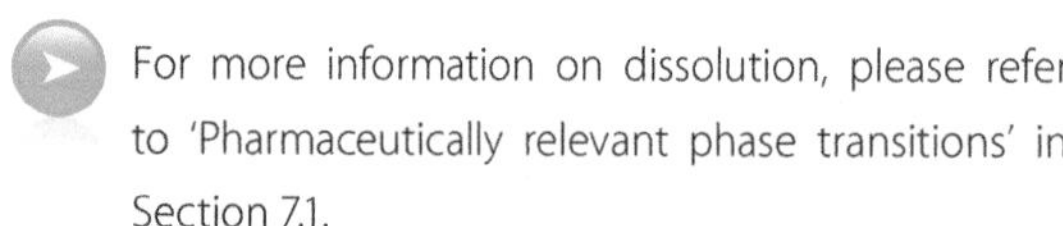
For more information on dissolution, please refer to 'Pharmaceutically relevant phase transitions' in Section 7.1.

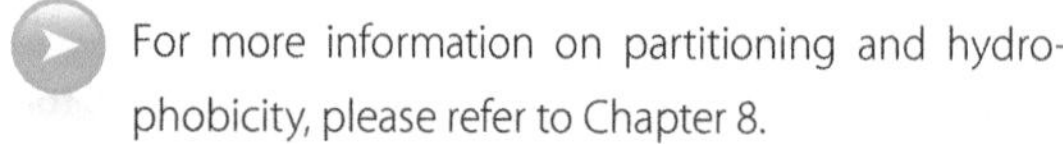
For more information on partitioning and hydrophobicity, please refer to Chapter 8.

In order for the API to interact with its biological target, it needs to possess specific functional groups that are associated with a particular activity. Many of these functional groups are ionizable, and binding to a target often requires the API to be in an ionized form.

All of the principles above can be used to rationalize the observed behaviour of some specific APIs:

- Anionic and cationic antibacterial and antiprotozoal agents are more active when they are ionized.
- Antibacterial sulphonamide APIs can be active in both ionized and unionized forms.
- General anaesthetic drugs that need to cross the blood–brain barrier and interact with cell membranes are more active when neutral.

Another important way in which acid and base behaviour influences drug formulation is in the enteric coating of tablets. An enteric coating provides a protective layer covering an orally administered medicine. The coating is designed to be resistant to the acidic environment of the stomach so that the API is not released. However, when the enteric coating encounters the more basic conditions in the intestine, the coating breaks down to release the API.

For more information on tablet coatings, please refer to 'Coated tablets' in Section 2.5.

Degree of ionization of APIs

The extent to which an API is ionized *in vivo* will depend upon:

- The pK_a or pK_b of the API.
- The pH of the physiological fluid that contains the API.

As an example of a common API possessing an acidic functionality, let us consider the non-steroidal anti-inflammatory drug (NSAID) naproxen (Figure 6.4). Naproxen is used for the treatment of pain and

FIGURE 6.4 The structure of naproxen

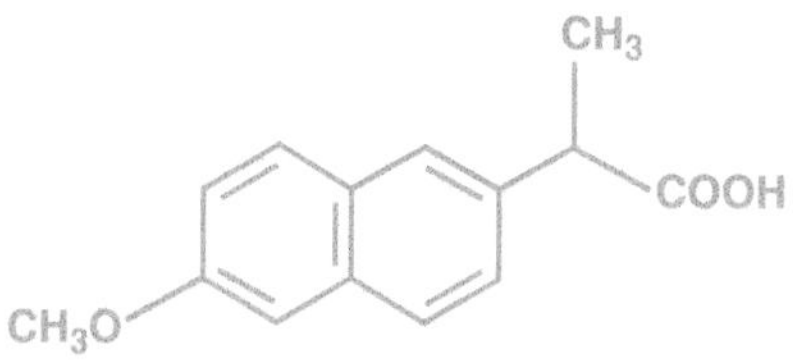

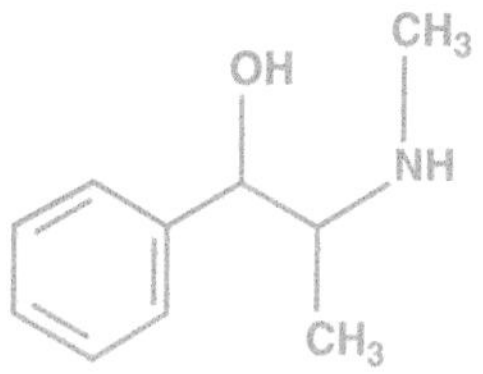

inflammation and like many NSAIDs, this compound contains a carboxylic acid (COOH) function.

The carboxylic acid group present on naproxen can be ionized as follows:

$$\mathrm{RCOOH} \rightleftharpoons \mathrm{RCOO^-} + \mathrm{H^+}$$

A carboxylic acid functionality means naproxen can exist as the more lipid-soluble neutral form or as the more aqueous-soluble ionized form according to the equilibrium reaction shown above.

At any given pH, the extent to which a weakly acidic API will be ionized is given by the equation:

$$\%\ \text{ionization} = \frac{100}{1 + \text{antilog}(\mathrm{p}K_\mathrm{a} - \mathrm{pH})} \qquad (6.20)$$

The pK_a of naproxen is 4.2 and it is therefore a weak acid. We can predict that in more basic conditions (i.e. higher pH) it should be more ionized than at conditions of lower pH. We can confirm this by considering the extent of ionization at (i) pH 3.5 and (ii) pH 7.4. Substituting the known values of pK_a and pH into equation 6.20, we can calculate that:

(i) at pH 3.5 the % ionization of naproxen = 16.6% and

(ii) at pH 7.4 the % ionization of naproxen = 99.9%.

Thus, as expected, more naproxen is ionized at higher pH.

Whilst many APIs are weak acids, the majority of APIs are weak bases. This includes, for example, some APIs that act as mimics of neurotransmitters involved in signalling pathways. Like the neurotransmitters themselves, the APIs contain an amine functional group. This gives the API the properties of a weak base that may exist in the ionized or unionized form. Figure 6.5 shows the structure of ephedrine, an amine-containing adrenergic **agonist** that is used as a stimulant and appetite suppressant.

FIGURE 6.5 Structure of ephedrine

For more information on agonists, please refer to Chapter 4 'An introduction to drug action' of the *Therapeutics and Human Physiology* book within this series.

Amine functional groups can be ionized according to the scheme below:

$$\mathrm{RNH_2} + \mathrm{H^+} \rightleftharpoons \mathrm{RNH_3^+}$$

At any given pH, the extent to which a weakly basic API will be ionized is given by the equation:

$$\%\ \text{ionization} = \frac{100}{1 + \text{antilog}\,(\mathrm{pH} - \mathrm{p}K_\mathrm{w} + \mathrm{p}K_\mathrm{b})} \qquad (6.21)$$

Now let us consider the ionization of ephedrine, which is weakly basic and has a pK_b of 4.64. We can calculate the percentage of ephedrine that will remain unionized in solutions of pH 5.5 and pH 9.0. First, we need to use equation 6.21 to find the percentage that is ionized at these given pHs. We have previously shown that pK_w = 14, therefore we need to substitute in the given values for pK_b and pH. This will give us the percentage of the API that is ionized. The percentage that remains unionized is 100 − percentage ionized. Therefore, at pH 5.5 we can show that the percentage ionization of ephedrine = 99.99%, so the percentage unionized = 0.01%. At pH 9.0, the percentage ionization of ephedrine = 69.61%, so the percentage unionized = 30.39%.

SELF CHECK 6.8

What percentage of aspirin (pK_a = 3.5) would be ionized in the stomach, given the pH of the stomach is 1.4?

SELF CHECK 6.9

The pH of a solution containing morphine is adjusted to pH 6. How much of the API remains unionized at this pH, given the pK_b for morphine is 6.1?

Diprotic and polyprotic acids

Acids such as HCl or CH_3COOH each possess only one proton that can dissociate from the molecule. These are referred to as **monoprotic** acids. **Diprotic acids** are compounds that possess two protons that may dissociate and **polyprotic acids** may lose more protons. In the case of a monoprotic acid, the pK_a of the acid equals the pH at which half of the acid exists in its ionized form. Where two or more protons may be lost, each dissociation has a specific acid dissociation constant K_a (and hence pK_a) value.

An example of a diprotic acid is carbonic acid (H_2CO_3). This can dissociate as:

$$H_2CO_3 \rightleftharpoons H^+ + HCO_3^- \quad K_{a1} = 4.2 \times 10^{-7} \quad pK_{a1} = 6.38$$

$$HCO_3^- \rightleftharpoons H^+ + CO_3^{2-} \quad K_{a2} = 4.8 \times 10^{-11} \quad pK_{a2} = 10.32$$

Another example is the polyprotic acid phosphoric acid, H_3PO_4, and this has three ionizable hydrogen atoms:

$$H_3PO_4 \rightleftharpoons H^+ + H_2PO_4^- \quad K_{a1} = 7.4 \times 10^{-3} \quad pK_{a1} = 2.13$$
$$H_2PO_4^- \rightleftharpoons H^+ + HPO_4^{2-} \quad K_{a2} = 6.2 \times 10^{-8} \quad pK_{a2} = 7.21$$
$$HPO_4^{2-} \rightleftharpoons H^+ + PO_4^{3-} \quad K_{a3} = 4.8 \times 10^{-13} \quad pK_{a3} = 12.32$$

Together, HCO_3^-, H_2CO_3, $H_2PO_4^-$, and HPO_4^{2-} play an important role in forming part of the buffering systems that maintain physiological pH. Buffer systems are discussed later in this chapter.

Zwitterions

Proteins are essential to life and they are built up in the body from linear chains of amino acids. There are 20 amino acids used to build these chains and they can be represented by the general formula $H_2NCHRCOOH$, where R represents the side-chain, which is specific to an individual amino acid. Figure 6.6 shows the generic structure for amino acids.

FIGURE 6.6 The generic structure for an amino acid

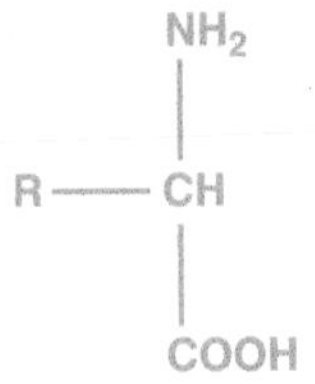

NH_2
R — CH
COOH

Amino acids contain both an acidic carboxylic acid group (COOH) and a basic amine group (NH_2). Amino acids therefore exhibit **amphiprotic** behaviour, i.e. they can behave as both acids and bases, and may therefore be described as ampholytes. At low pH, amino acids predominantly act as bases, i.e. the amine functional group will accept a proton to become ionized and the cationic form dominates. At high pH, amino acids act mainly as acids, i.e. the carboxylic acid function will donate a proton and become ionized and the majority of molecules are in the anionic form. At intermediate pH, both the amine and carboxylic acid groups will be ionized at the same time. If two opposite charges are present within one molecule, then the molecule is referred to as a hybrid ion or **zwitterion**.

An amino acid can exist as the neutral molecule or the zwitterion if the pH of the solution is above the pK_a of the acid and below pK_a of the base (typically in the range of pH 2–9). In this range, cationic or anionic forms of the molecule can also exist so that the amino acid will bear a net positive or negative charge. At a specific pH, however, the concentrations of the positive and negative species will be same and the net charge on the molecules will be zero. This is referred to as the isoelectric point. Figure 6.7 shows the amino

FIGURE 6.7 The structure of alanine showing the different ionization states

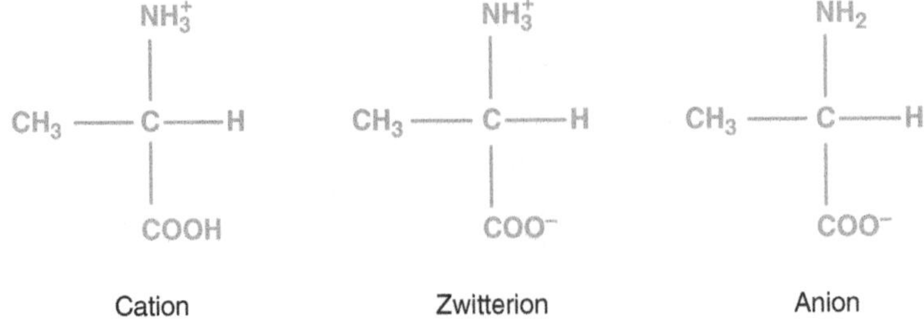

FIGURE 6.8 The structure of cetirizine

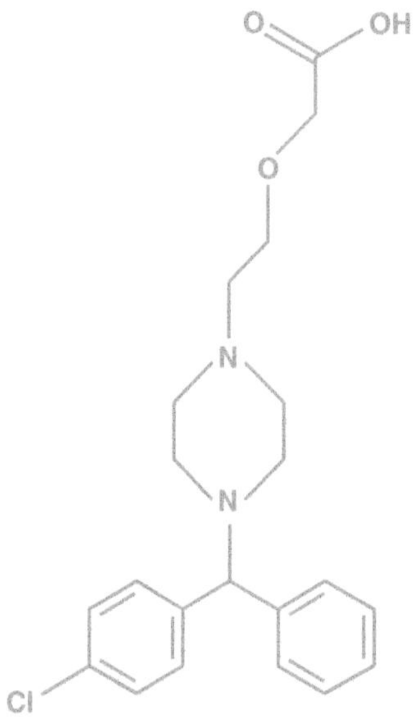

acid, alanine, in its positive, negative, and zwitterionic forms. For alanine the side-chain group R is CH_3.

The isoelectric point is midway between the two pK_a values for the acid dissociation constants of the acidic and basic groups. For example, consider the amino acid alanine, where the pK_a of the COOH group is 2.35 and the pK_a for the NH_3^+ group is 9.69. Hence, the isoelectric point for alanine is given as:

$$\frac{2.35+9.69}{2}=6.02$$

Certain APIs also exist as zwitterions; for example, L-DOPA (3,4-dihydroxylphenylalanine), which is used in the treatment of Parkinson's disease and cetirizine, an anti-histamine, the structure of which is shown in Figure 6.8.

KEY POINTS

- Many APIs are weak organic acids or bases; these APIs can ionize in solution.
- Whether an API exists predominantly in an ionized or unionized form will determine its solubility, absorption, distribution around the body, and interactions with biological targets.
- The degree of ionization of an API depends on the surrounding pH and the pK_a (or pK_b) of the API.
- Monoprotic acids possess only one ionizable hydrogen atom per molecule, whereas polyprotic acids are able to donate more than one proton per molecule.
- A zwitterion is a molecule that bears both negative and positive charges.
- Ampholytes exhibit amphiprotic behaviour and will form zwitterions at specific pH ranges.

SELF CHECK 6.10

Find the isolelectric point for leucine given the pK_a for the COOH group is 2.36 and the NH_3^+ group is 9.60.

6.6 Buffers

Changes to pH can have a significant impact on chemical and biological systems, so it is important that pH can be maintained within a narrow range. **Buffers** play an important role both in physiological systems and in chemical applications (including drug formulation), as they enable pH to be maintained around at the required value. Within defined limits, a buffer can resist changes to pH, even when acids or bases are added to the system. In this section we will consider the role of buffers in both physiology and drug formulation.

Maintaining the pH of body fluids

Biologically, maintaining the correct pH of different regions of the body is essential to ensure normal functioning of the organs and tissues. For example, biological enzymes perform efficiently within narrowly defined pH ranges. Each region of the body has a specific pH for optimum function, examples of which are shown in Table 6.2; this table also indicates the mechanisms responsible for the pH associated with specific physiological fluids.

TABLE 6.2 **Example pH values for different physiological fluids and factors responsible for maintaining the pH**

Physiological fluid	Approximate pH	Factors responsible for pH
Blood	7.4	Buffering action of haemoglobin, plasma proteins, carbonic acid, bicarbonate, and phosphate
Urine	5–8	Main constituents are water, urea, chloride, sodium, potassium, creatinine, dissolved organics, and inorganics. pH can be significantly altered by diet and drugs
Cerebrospinal fluid (CSF)	7.4	Physiological buffers maintain pH. The buffering capacity of CSF is lower than that of blood
Sweat	5	Main constituents are water, mineral ions, lactate, and urea. Sebum and sweat combine to form a protective layer on the skin
Lachrymal fluid	7.4	Complex fluid acting to protect and lubricate the eye, contains physiological buffers to maintain pH
Saliva	6.5	Comprises water, electrolytes, mucus, enzymes, and glycoproteins; maintains acidic environment to reduce infection
GIT fluid (stomach)	1–3	Hydrochloric acid secretion gives low pH
GIT fluid (small intestine)	8	Bicarbonate is released into small intestine, neutralizes stomach acid and raises pH; bile salts also released to aid digestion
GIT fluid (colon)	7.0–7.5	Short chain fatty acids formed from fermentation of carbohydrates in gut lowers pH

Disruption of physiological pH

If the correct pH for a given region of the body is not maintained, then the consequences can vary from mild irritation of the affected area to a potentially fatal outcome. You may be familiar with the burning sensation that you can feel in your muscles after excessive physical activity. Under normal conditions, glycolysis in muscles produces pyruvic acid, which is oxidized in the mitochondria to release the energy required for muscle contraction. If strenuous exercise is undertaken for an extended period of time, the muscles cannot be supplied with sufficient oxygen. Under these circumstances, the pyruvic acid formed is converted to lactic acid. When lactic acid is produced more rapidly than it can be removed, the build-up of acid lowers pH, irritating the muscle and producing a 'burning' sensation.

Vaginal pH is normally maintained between 3.8 and 4.2, i.e. it is an acidic environment. This acidic pH is essential as it limits the growth of bacteria preventing infection. Factors that affect vaginal pH, such as the use of some soaps or body washes, menopause, or the use of certain antibiotics (that disrupt the normal balance of bacteria), can reduce acidity and make women susceptible to infection.

More serious effects can occur when the systemic acid–base balance is disrupted. The normal pH range of arterial blood is 7.35–7.45; this is predominantly maintained by the carbonic acid: bicarbonate buffer system. This balance can be disrupted leading to metabolic acidosis or metabolic alkalosis. Acidosis can be caused by malfunction of the kidneys (which leads to insufficient hydrogen ions being excreted or too many carbonate ions being excreted) or by severe diarrhoea, which can also result in a loss of carbonate ions. Alkalosis can result from excessive vomiting (resulting in a significant loss of hydrochloric acid from the stomach) or by excessive intake of alkaline drugs. Systemic acidosis results in depression of the nervous system by reducing synaptic transmission of nerve impulses. This can lead to disorientation, coma, and, if untreated, eventually death. Conversely, systemic alkalosis leads to over-excitation of peripheral and central nerves, which can lead to muscle spasm, convulsions, and, in extreme cases, death.

Buffering in pharmaceutical formulations

In terms of pharmaceutical formulation, buffers are essential to the production of effective, stable, dosage forms. As discussed previously, the extent to which an API is ionized will depend upon the pH of the environment and this will govern the extent to which it is absorbed into, and subsequently distributed around, the body.

The rate of breakdown of an API can also be dependent upon the pH of the formulation. Determining the pH at which water soluble APIs within liquid dosage forms will show the slowest rate of degradation is critical if the shelf life is to be optimized.

For more information on the effect of pH on rates of degradation, please refer to Section 12.1.

It may be necessary to select a pH that provides the best compromise between extended shelf life and other factors, such as solubility. Acidic compounds dissolve more readily in basic solution, while basic compounds are more soluble in acidic media. Another important consideration is the sensitivity of the body to acidic and basic solutions where dosage forms for topical delivery are required; for example, in the formulation of eye drops. Extremes of pH would have a highly irritant effect on the eye, overwhelming the intrinsic buffering ability of lachrymal fluids. Buffer solutions can be used to maintain a suitable pH and avoid discomfort to the patient. Similarly, injections must be formulated between pH 3 and pH 9 to avoid causing pain and swelling at the site of administration. Care must be taken to ensure that the concentration of dissolved species, including buffers, gives a liquid dosage form of appropriate **tonicity**.

For more information on tonicity, please refer to Section 11.3.

Acidic buffers

Acidic buffers are made up of a mixture of an acid and a salt of that acid. The acid is usually selected such that the pK_a of the acid is within +/−1 pH unit of the required pH of the buffer. An example of such a buffer system is a mixture of acetic acid and sodium acetate. The pK_a of acetic acid is 4.8, therefore it is useful for producing buffers in the pH range of 3.8 to 5.8.

The components of this buffer react according to the following two equations:

1. $CH_3COOH + H_2O \rightleftharpoons CH_3COO^- + H_3O^+$
2. $CH_3COONa \rightarrow CH_3COO^- + Na^+$

Overall, this leads to an excess of acetate ions (CH_3COO^-) being present in the solution. If a small amount of acid is added to this system, the excess H_3O^+ will react with the CH_3COO^- ions, i.e. the equilibrium (1) moves to the left and the overall concentration of H_3O^+ ions remains roughly constant. As pH is related to the concentration of H_3O^+ ions, then the pH remains approximately constant. Similarly, if a base is added to this system, this will react with the H_3O^+ ions and the equilibrium (1) will shift to the right to replace the H_3O^+ ions. Again the concentration of H_3O^+ ions is maintained and the pH remains approximately constant.

As different formulations require specific pH values to be maintained, we need to be able to calculate the correct amount of acid and salt to add to a system to create a buffer for the desired pH. The choice of which acid would be most suitable is also important and this will be discussed later. To calculate the amount of acid and salt required for the buffer, we need to be able to relate the acid strength (pK_a), the pH of the system, and the amounts of salt and acid. This is provided by the Henderson–Hasselbalch equation, which is derived from the definition of K_a and is written as:

$$\mathrm{pH} = \mathrm{p}K_\mathrm{a} + \log\frac{[\mathrm{A}^-]}{[\mathrm{AH}]} \qquad (6.22)$$

This can be written in the following form in the case of acidic buffers:

$$\mathrm{pH} = \mathrm{p}K_\mathrm{a} + \log\frac{[\mathrm{salt}]}{[\mathrm{acid}]} \qquad (6.23)$$

As the volume of a buffer solution is the same for both the acid and salt components, we can replace molar concentration with number of moles, n:

$$\mathrm{pH} = \mathrm{p}K_\mathrm{a} + \log\frac{n(\mathrm{salt})}{n(\mathrm{acid})} \qquad (6.24)$$

Let us assume that we have found that a pH of 5.0 gives the optimum stability for a particular API in a liquid dosage form. As the pK_a for acetic acid is 4.76, the sodium acetate and acetic acid buffer system could be used. What mass of sodium acetate (relative molecular mass=82) should be added to 1 L of 0.100 M acetic acid to produce a buffer at the required pH?

Substituting this information into the Henderson–Hasselbalch equation we have:

$$5.0 = 4.76 + \log\frac{[\text{salt}]}{0.100}$$

Re-arranging the equation and taking the antilog of both sides gives:

$$\text{antilog}\,(5.0 - 4.76) = \frac{[\text{salt}]}{0.100}$$

From this we have:

$$[\text{salt}] = 1.74 \times 0.100 = 0.174\,\text{M}$$

Hence, 0.174 mol of salt is required to prepare 1 L of this buffer. Remember that:

$$\text{number of mols} = \frac{\text{mass}}{\text{relative molecular mass}}$$

Thus, 14.3 g of sodium acetate is required.

Basic buffers

A basic buffer can be made up from a mixture of a weak base and the salt of the weak base, for example, ammonia and ammonium chloride:

1. $NH_3 + H_2O \rightleftharpoons NH_4^+ + OH^-$
2. $NH_4Cl \rightarrow NH_4^+ + Cl^-$

In this system, the NH_4^+ ions exist in excess. If acid (H_3O^+) is added to the system, this will react with the OH^- ions and the equilibrium (1) will shift to the right to replace any OH^- ions that have been used up. In this way, the concentration of H_3O^+ ions (and hence the pH) will remain roughly constant. If a base (OH^-) is added to the system, then this can react with the NH_4^+ ions and the equilibrium (1) will shift to the left. Again, the pH of the system is maintained.

Calculating the pH of a buffer upon addition of acid or base

We know how to make up an appropriate buffer, but how effective are buffers at resisting changes to pH when acid or base is added? Consider the example of the acetic acid and sodium acetate buffer, earlier. If 10 mL of a 0.8 M hydrochloric acid (HCl) solution were added to this pH 5 buffer, we can calculate how much the pH will change. From the Henderson–Hasselbalch equation we know that the pH is related to the amounts of acid and salt present.

If acid is added to the system then this will react with the excess CH_3COO^- ions to form CH_3COOH. HCl will react in a 1:1 ratio with the acetate ions. We have added 10 mL of 0.8 M HCl, i.e. 0.008 mol of HCl. Remember that HCl is a strong acid that fully dissociates in solution so 0.008 mol of HCl will form 0.008 mol of H^+ ions. The buffer solution will then 'mop-up' the added H^+ according to the following reaction:

$$\begin{array}{ccccc} CH_3COO^- & + & H^+ & \rightarrow & CH_3COOH \\ 0.008\,\text{mol} & & 0.008\,\text{mol} & & 0.008\,\text{mol} \end{array}$$

We showed previously that 1 litre of our pH 5 buffer would have 0.100 mol of acetic acid and 0.174 mol of acetate ions. The 0.008 mol of HCl added will react with 0.008 mol acetate ions, leaving us with 0.174 − 0.008=0.166 mol of acetate ions remaining. Similarly, the amount of undissociated acid present is now the initial 0.100 mol plus the 0.008 mol formed from the reaction between the acetate ions and the H^+, i.e. 0.108 mol.

If we substitute these new values for the amount of acid and salt into the Henderson–Hasselbalch equation, we can calculate the new pH of the system:

$$\text{pH} = 4.76 + \log\frac{0.166}{0.108}$$

$$\text{pH} = 4.95$$

This value is only 0.05 units from the original buffer pH and demonstrates that when acid is added to a buffer system, the change in pH is much less than if, for example, it were added to water.

Buffer capacity

The ability to resist changes to pH is quantified as the buffer capacity of the system. **Buffer capacity, β,** is defined as the amount of acid or base that must be added to a buffer so that the pH changes by 1 unit. One way to determine the buffer capacity of a system is to use van Slyke's equation:

$$\beta = \frac{2.303 \cdot C \cdot K_a \cdot [H_3O^+]}{(K_a + [H_3O^+])^2} \quad (6.25)$$

where C = total buffer concentration, being the sum of the molar concentrations of the acid and the salt.

Buffer capacity is therefore raised as the amount of the acid and salt used in preparing the buffer is increased. The presence of the $[H_3O^+]$ terms in the equation shows that buffer capacity also depends on pH. Acidic buffers are most effective when the required pH of the buffer is equal to the pK_a of the acid. As stated previously, the acid should be chosen to have a pK_a within +/–1 pH unit of the desired pH. Diprotic and polyprotic acids can be used to buffer over a broader range of pH values, as they possess multiple pK_a values, one value for the dissociation of each ionizable hydrogen atom.

Continuing our example of an API that was most stable when stored at pH 5.0, we designed a buffer that was 0.174 M in sodium acetate and 0.100 M in acetic acid. We know that the pK_a of acetic acid is 4.76 so the buffer capacity can be calculated:

$$C = 0.174 + 0.100 = 0.274 \text{ M}$$

We know that:

$$pH = -\log_{10}[H_3O^+]$$

hence if:

$$pH = 5$$

then:

$$[H_3O]^+ = 1 \times 10^{-5} \text{ M}$$

Similarly:

$$pK_a = -\log_{10} K_a$$

hence if:

$$pK_a = 4.76$$

then:

$$K_a = 1.74 \times 10^{-5} \text{ M}$$

Substituting into the van Slyke equation, we obtain:

$$\beta = \frac{2.303 \times 0.274 \times 1.74 \times 10^{-5} \times 1 \times 10^{-5}}{(1.74 \times 10^{-5} + 1 \times 10^{-5})^2}$$

$$\beta = 0.146 \text{ mol L}^{-1} \text{ pH unit}^{-1}$$

The units of buffer capacity are mol per litre per pH unit.

Maximum buffer capacity (β_{max})

If buffers are most effective when the pH required is equal to the pK_a of the acid, we can derive an equation for maximum buffer capacity (β_{max}). If the pH of the system equals the pK_a of the acid, then $[H_3O^+]$ is equal to K_a. Substituting these terms into the van Slyke equation gives us a much simpler expression for the calculation of maximum buffer capacity, i.e:

$$\beta_{max} = 0.576\, C \quad (6.26)$$

Whilst buffers play a vital role in formulation, it is important to realize that buffer capacity is finite. Once this buffer capacity is used up, by the addition of large quantities of acid or base, then the system will behave as any ordinary solution.

KEY POINTS

- Buffers play an important role in maintaining the pH of both physiological systems and pharmaceutical formulations.
- A number of different buffer systems in different regions of the body maintain physiological pH.
- In pharmaceutical formulations, a buffer may be used to confer stability, aid API solubility, or ensure that the medicine does not irritate the body.
- Acidic (and basic) buffers may be made by combining a weak acid (or weak base) with an associated salt.
- The pH of acidic buffers, and the change in pH on adding acid or base, may be determined using the Henderson–Hasselbalch equation.

SELF CHECK 6.11

If 0.008 mol HCl were added to 1 L of water at pH 7 what would be the change in pH? Assume that the addition of the HCl has a negligible effect on the volume of the liquid.

SELF CHECK 6.12

What is the maximum buffer capacity of a buffer comprising 0.015 mol of sodium acetate in 100 mL of 0.100 M acetic acid?

CHAPTER SUMMARY

- The vast majority or APIs are either weak acids or weak bases, and understanding of this behaviour is key to developing appropriate dosage forms.
- According to the Brönsted–Lowry definitions, an acid is a proton donor and a base is a proton acceptor.
- The strength of acids and bases is determined by their structure and the solvent environment.
- The pH scale is used to indicate the relative acidity or basicity (alkalinity) of solutions where $pH = -\log_{10} [H_3O^+]$.
- The acid dissociation constant, K_a, is a modified equilibrium constant for acid ionization equilibria. Strong acids have high K_a and low pK_a.
- Whether an API exists predominantly in an ionized or unionized form will determine its solubility, absorption, distribution around the body, and interactions with biological targets.
- In pharmaceutical formulations, a buffer may be used to confer stability, aid API solubility, or ensure the medicine does not irritate the body.

FURTHER READING

Cairns, D. Chemistry of acids and bases. Chapter 1 in *Essentials of Pharmaceutical Chemistry*, (4th edn). London: Pharmaceutical Press, (2012), pp 1–28.

Introduces the concepts of acids, bases and buffers including useful question and answer sections.

Florence, T. and Attwood, D. Physicochemical properties of drugs in solution. Chapter 2 in *Physicochemical Principles of Pharmacy*, (5th edn). London: Pharmaceutical Press, (2011), pp 43–88.

Introduces acid and base chemistry, buffers and zwitterions as applicable to drugs and their properties.

Moynihan, H.A. and Crean, A.M. Pharmaceutical solutions. Chapter 2 in *The Physicochemical Basis of Pharmaceuticals*. Oxford: Oxford University Press, (2009), pp 22–55.

Provides a simple introduction to acidity and basicity and the relevance to the behaviour of drugs in solution.

7

Phase equilibria and transitions

STEVE ENOCH

The aim of this chapter is to introduce the concepts of phase, phase equilibria, and phase transitions. It will be shown how these ideas are used in the pharmaceutical sciences, particularly in relation to how medicines are formulated and delivered. The chapter is split into two parts, the first of which deals with some important definitions, concepts, including the introduction of the phase rule. The second part builds upon these concepts and will cover phase diagrams for pure compounds and mixtures. This discussion is placed in terms of how such data help pharmaceutical scientists to make decisions about the formulation of medicines to be administered to patients.

Learning objectives

Having read this chapter you are expected to be able to:

- Define the terms phase, phase transition, and phase equilibria.
- Recognize some pharmaceutically relevant phase transitions.
- Use phase diagrams to understand the behaviour of one-, two-, and three-component systems.
- Give examples of how phase diagrams are used to assist in the formulation of dosage forms.

7.1 Phases, phase transitions, and phase equilibria

Any substance can exist as a solid, liquid, or gas. These three physical states each represent a different **phase** of matter. Changes of phase, called **phase transitions**, can occur at specific temperatures and pressures. As the temperature of a solid system at constant pressure is increased, for example, it will melt to become liquid. Upon continuation of heating, the substance will vaporize from the surface of the liquid. In an **open system**, further heating will result in boiling. This is where the liquid changes to a gas and vaporization occurs not just at the surface, but throughout the bulk of the liquid. The opposite phase transitions occur when a system is cooled. Thus, a gas will condense to become a liquid and then, upon continued cooling, will freeze to become a solid.

Some solid substances convert directly to a gas upon heating, without going through a liquid phase. This is known as sublimation and occurs for some materials, e.g. carbon dioxide, at normal atmospheric pressure. The reverse of sublimation, deposition, occurs when a gas is cooled and converts directly into a solid. These transitions are summarized in Figure 7.1.

For more information on open systems, please refer to 'System and surroundings' in Section 5.1.

Phase changes and the temperatures at which transitions occur can be illustrated by considering water and its common physical states of solid, liquid, and vapour. At atmospheric pressure (1 atm), the solid phase of water (ice) exists at and below 0 °C. As the temperature is raised a little above 0 °C, water is most thermodynamically stable as a liquid and, finally, at temperatures above 100 °C, as a vapour. The two important temperatures in this discussion are the **melting point** and the **boiling point**, which occur at 0 °C and 100 °C, respectively (see Box 7.1). These are the phase transition temperatures for water at atmospheric pressure and these terms are generally preferred when a substance is being heated. For a substance that is being cooled, the terms **condensation point** and **freezing point** may be used. Of course, the transition temperatures are unchanged and, for example, the melting and freezing points are equal to each other.

A phase equilibrium exists at each of the phase transition temperatures. Thus, at 0 °C and atmospheric pressure, solid and liquid water are in thermodynamic equilibrium. The associated free energy change between the phases, ΔG, is equal to zero and this is the general condition for equilibrium. This makes sense because at temperatures that are a fraction of a degree below 0 °C, the conversion of ice to water is not spontaneous and $\Delta G > 0$. At temperatures that are a fraction above 0 °C, the conversion of ice to water is spontaneous and $\Delta G < 0$. At 0 °C precisely, $\Delta G = 0$.

In advanced work, it is preferable to use the **chemical potential** to represent the free energy of each chemical species involved in a chemical or physical process. This would be necessary, for example, when considering the thermodynamics of systems that are not pure. As $\Delta G = 0$ at equilibrium, we may say that the chemical potential of water molecules in the solid and liquid phases is the same at 0 °C and 1 atm.

If the system at equilibrium is in **thermal equilibrium**, then it will have a uniform temperature throughout its composition. In this case, the temperature of the system will remain at the phase transition temperature until the one phase has been completely converted to the second. For example, upon heating water from the solid phase (ice) to the liquid phase, the system remains at 0 °C until all of the ice has melted (Figure 7.2).

FIGURE 7.1 **Outline of the three phases of matter and the transitions between them**

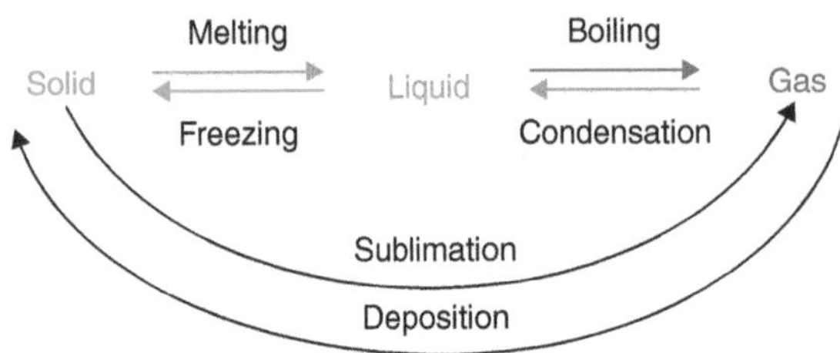

BOX 7.1

Standard melting and boiling points

A pure substance under atmospheric pressure (1 atm) has defined transition temperatures known as the normal melting and boiling points. For water, these values are 0 °C and 100 °C, respectively. If not stated otherwise, we can assume that quoted transition temperatures for a substance are the 'normal' values recorded at 1 atm. In modern thermodynamic studies, however, standard pressure is 1 bar (= 0.987 atm). The transition temperatures recorded at this pressure are known as the standard melting and boiling points, and they differ slightly from the normal transition temperatures. For example, the standard boiling point of water is 99.6 °C.

For more information on free energy change, please refer to Section 5.5.

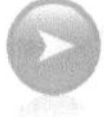

For more information on chemical potential and transition temperatures, please refer to 'Chemical potential and transition temperatures' in Section 11.6.

FIGURE 7.2 The phase transition between a solid and a liquid showing the phases present and how the temperature varies with time. T_m = normal melting point

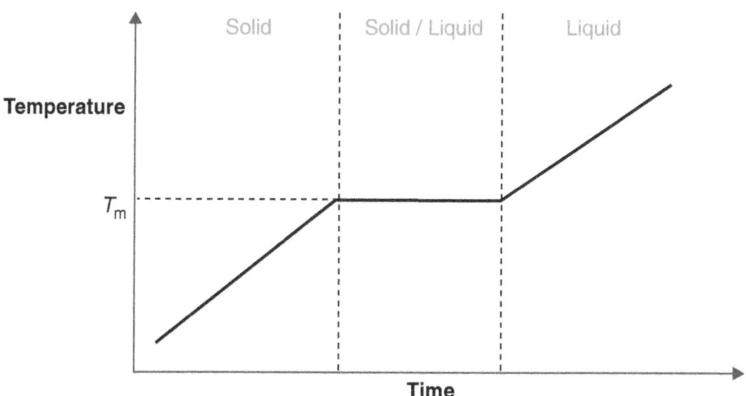

Until now, we have only considered the various phases of water, a pure substance. These types of substances may also be referred to as unitary systems, as they contain only one **component**. Almost all pharmaceutically relevant materials are mixtures, however, and we need to broaden our understanding of both phases and phase transitions. By definition, a phase is a form of matter that is uniform throughout in both its physical state and chemical composition.

A mixture of two **immiscible** liquids, such as oil and water, for example, consists of two layers. Each layer represents a distinct phase, as each layer has a different chemical composition. This would, therefore, be described as a two-phase system, even though it is entirely liquid. A solid containing a mixture of two different forms of the same compound (**polymorphism**) would also be described as a two-phase system, given that each polymorph represents a different physical state.

For more information on polymorphs, please refer to Section 2.3.

Melting and boiling are examples of phase transitions as they involve changes in physical state. However, phase transitions can also occur through changes in chemical composition. Thus, when ethanol and water are mixed we obtain an homogeneous system as these two liquids are miscible. Although the system remains liquid throughout, this process would also be described as a phase transition, as the chemical composition of final liquid is different from the starting liquids.

Pharmaceutically relevant phase transitions

There are a number of key phase transitions that are associated with the delivery of an **active pharmaceutical ingredient (API)** to the site of action. These are as follows:

- **Dissolution**: This is a phase transition in which an API, typically as a solid, dissolves in the biological aqueous environment. This a key process for medicines formulated as tablets or suspensions. It is also an important phase change for liquid droplets and solid particles delivered via an inhaler.

For more information on tablets, please refer to 'Compressed and layered tablets' in Section 2.5.

For more information on suspensions, please refer to 'Suspensions and nanosuspensions' in Section 10.2.

For more information on inhalers, please refer to 'Pressurized aerosols' in Section 4.5.

- **Vaporization**: This phase transition involves a solid formulation undergoing a phase transition to a vapour. This is important in the formulation of medicines, such as chest rubs, that release vapour for the patient to inhale. The composition of the rub needs to be such that the active ingredient is released as a vapour at around body temperature. However, the formulation must be such that the active ingredient remains in the formulation at room temperature.

For more information on chest rubs, please refer to 'Non-prescription inhalations' in Section 4.4.

- Melting: The solid to liquid phase transition of medicines that are applied topically to the skin or that are taken as suppositories needs to be considered during their formulation. In these cases the melting point of the formulation must be such that the API is released at around body temperature.

For more information on suppositories, please refer to Section 2.6.

- Precipitation: An API formulated as a liquid may well precipitate out within the body and this is most commonly due to changes in pH. An orally delivered, weakly acidic drug that is only soluble in the ionized form, for example, will precipitate out in the acidic environment of the stomach as the unionized form. In order to be absorbed by the body, dissolution of the precipitate must then occur.

For more information on percentage ionization, please refer to 'Degree of ionization of APIs' in Section 6.5.

- Gas absorption: This is an important phase change associated with gaseous APIs administered via the airways. The absorption of these APIs into the blood represents a gas to liquid phase change.

For more information on medical gases, please refer to 'Medical gases' in Section 4.4.

- Partitioning. This phase change has particular relevance to liquid and semi-solid formulations applied topically to the skin. The transfer of the API from the medicine to the skin is an example of partitioning. This same type of phase transition is also relevant for APIs dissolved in the fluid of the gastrointestinal tract (GIT), perhaps following dissolution. In order to be absorbed, the API must partition into the walls of the GIT.

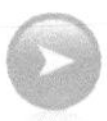

For more information on partitioning, please refer to Chapter 8.

Dissolution and the Noyes–Whitney equation

Dissolution is one of the most commonly encountered phase changes associated with drug delivery. When a solid particle composed of a soluble API is placed in a liquid medium, a diffusion layer will be established around the particle. This region contains dissolved API that has not yet entered the bulk of the dissolution medium (Figure 7.3). The concentration of the API within this layer will equal the maximum **solubility** of the API in the chosen solvent (the saturation solubility). The diffusion layer is separated from the bulk solution by a boundary region of intermediate concentration.

The rate of dissolution can then be measured as the mass, m, of solid entering the liquid phase per unit time, t. This can be calculated using the Noyes–Whitney equation:

$$\frac{dm}{dt} = -\frac{DA(C_S - C_B)}{L} \tag{7.1}$$

FIGURE 7.3 The diffusion layer surrounding a solid particle and the associated concentration profile

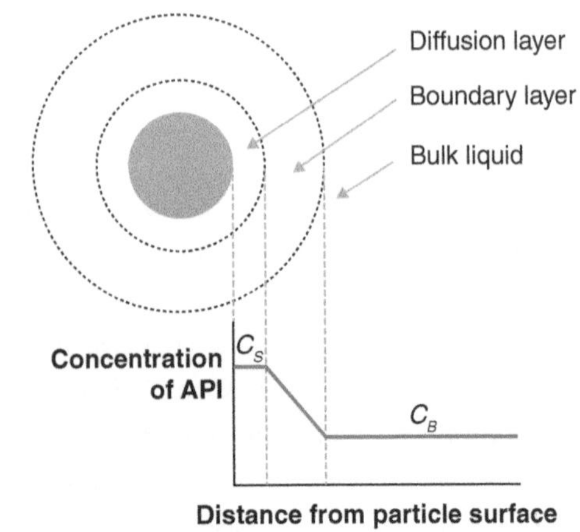

where:

$\frac{dm}{dt}$ = rate of dissolution of the solid,

A = solid/liquid interfacial area,

C_S = concentration of the solid in the diffusion layer surrounding the solid,

C_B = concentration of the solid in the bulk dissolution medium,

D = the diffusion coefficient,

L = thickness of the diffusion layer.

The negative sign in equation 7.1 indicates that the mass of the solid will continue to decrease with time as long as C_S is larger than C_B, the rate being greatest when the difference between C_S and C_B is at its greatest.

The Noyes–Whitney equation shows that a primary driver for the rate of dissolution is the surface area of the solid in contact with the liquid, A. In pharmaceutical applications this can involve increasing a tablet size to increase dissolution. This would result in an increase in the onset of action of the drug, as its dissolution rate would be increased. Conversely, decreasing a tablet size would slow the onset of action by decreasing the dissolution rate. It is also possible to alter the dissolution rate by altering the crystalline form of the API, as certain polymorphs will undergo dissolution more rapidly than others. The required rate of dissolution depends on the intended use of the drug in question.

For more information on polymorphism, please refer to Section 2.3.

KEY POINTS

- A phase is a form of matter that is uniform throughout in both its physical state and chemical composition.
- For pure substances, phase transitions from one phase to a second phase occur at specific temperatures and pressures. At these conditions, a phase equilibrium exists.
- Phase changes include changes in physical state and/or chemical composition.
- A number of pharmaceutically relevant phenomena involve phase changes.
- The Noyes–Whitney equation can be used to predict the rate of dissolution of a soluble solid in a liquid medium.

SELF CHECK 7.1

Define the terms phase and phase transition.

SELF CHECK 7.2

Briefly define vaporization and melting. In each case, give one example of a dosage form that relies on these phase transitions.

7.2 Phase diagrams for pure substances

The above discussion regarding the phase transitions of water considered the effect of varying temperature at fixed (atmospheric) pressure. However, the observed phase transitions of substances depend on both temperature and pressure. For pure substances, a convenient way to display the relationship between the preferred phase and the conditions of a closed system is to plot a single-**component** phase diagram (Figure 7.4).

The phase diagram in Figure 7.4 has the following key features:

- The lines represent phase boundaries where the phases shown on either side are at equilibrium, i.e:
  - solid–liquid equilibrium.
  - liquid–vapour equilibrium.
  - solid–vapour equilibrium.

FIGURE 7.4 Example phase diagram for a pure substance. T_m = normal melting point, T_b = normal boiling point, T_c = critical temperature, p_c = critical pressure and T_3 = triple point

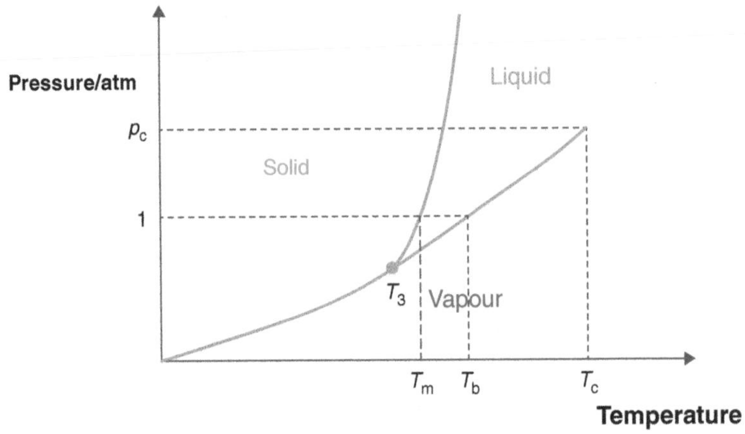

- The normal melting and boiling points for atmospheric conditions (1 atm) are shown by the symbols T_m and T_b.
- Where the three phase boundaries intersect, all three phases can co-exist in equilibrium and this is known as the **triple point**, indicated by T_3 in Figure 7.4.
- The phase diagram can be used to predict what phase a substance will be in at a given temperature and pressure. At equilibrium, this will always be the phase that is the most thermodynamically stable.

It is possible to lower the temperature of a liquid or gas below the normal freezing point without it becoming a solid. This is discussed further in Box 7.2.

Vapour pressure

The **vapour pressure** is the pressure of a vapour that is in thermodynamic equilibrium with its condensed phase in a closed system, the term condensed phase referring to either a liquid or a solid. **Vapour pressure** can be understood by considering a liquid that partly occupies a sealed container of fixed volume at constant temperature. In this closed system, some of the liquid molecules will have sufficient energy to leave the surface of the liquid phase. The vapour that is released by this evaporation will exert a pressure within the container. At equilibrium, the rate of vaporization will equal the rate of condensation and a constant pressure is attained. This pressure is the vapour pressure (Figure 7.5).

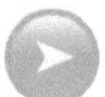

For more information on vapour pressure, please refer to 'Vapour pressure' in Section 4.2 and Section 11.1.

Once a system reaches equilibrium, the vapour pressure remains constant, if the temperature of the system remains constant. As the temperature of the system is increased, the density of the gas begins to rise as more molecules enter the vapour phase. There is a corresponding fall in the density of the liquid due

BOX 7.2

Supercooling

Supercooling is defined as the process of lowering the temperature of a liquid or gas below the normal freezing point without it becoming a solid. Crystallization requires a nucleation site, and this is normally a seed crystal or tiny fleck of solid material, e.g. dust. Supercooling occurs when the temperature is lowered in a purified liquid system where potential nucleation sites have been removed. The process of supercooling a liquid is pressure dependant. For example, at atmospheric pressure water can be supercooled to around −48 °C. A supercooled liquid is **metastable** i.e. it is thermodynamically unstable but kinetically stable, i.e. the rate of crystallization is effectively zero.

FIGURE 7.5 Schematic diagram illustrating the origin of vapour pressure in a closed system. The blue spheres represent molecules in the liquid phase and the red spheres represent molecules in the vapour phase. The phases are in equilibrium

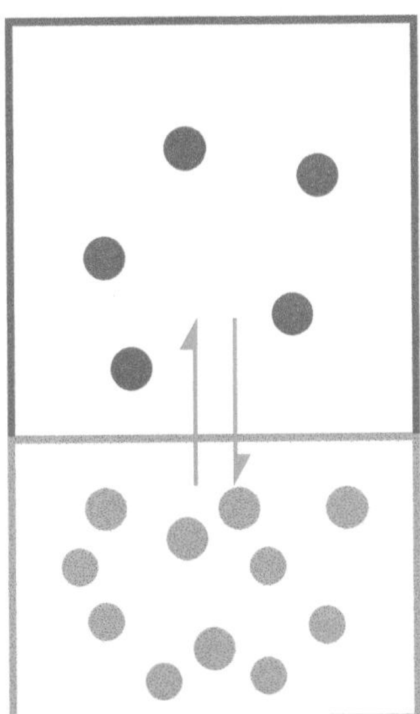

to the increase in volume caused by the rise in temperature, so-called thermal expansion. The change in density of the two phases continues until the so-called **critical temperature (T_C)** is reached (Figure 7.4). At this point, the density of the liquid and the density of the vapour are equal to one another and the liquid–vapour surface between the two phases disappears (Figure 7.6). The pressure at which the critical temperature is reached is known as the **critical pressure (p_C)**. Above the critical temperature and pressure, the system is described as a supercritical fluid (SCF), having properties intermediate between those of a gas and liquid (see Box 7.3).

We can now clarify the distinction between the terms 'gas' and 'vapour'. A vapour is a gas that is at a temperature below the critical temperature of the substance. For example, the critical temperature of water is 374 °C. Below this temperature, water vapour can be converted to liquid by increasing the pressure. Pressurized medicinal gases, such as entonox, may require careful storage to avoid liquefaction.

For more information on entonox, please refer to 'Medical gases' in Section 4.4.

BOX 7.3

Uses of supercritical fluids (SCF)

Supercritical fluids have flow properties similar to a gas and solvating properties that are comparable to a liquid. Consequently, they have applications in manufacturing and processing, where a soluble species needs to be removed from a raw material, e.g. the extraction of caffeine from coffee beans. In other applications, SCF chromatography can be used to separate compounds with very similar structures, such as polyunsaturated fatty acids. The excellent flow and solvent properties of SCFs also mean they have potential applications in impregnating porous matrixes, such as transdermal patches, with an API.

FIGURE 7.6 The effect of increasing the temperature on liquid-vapour phase equilibrium. At and above the critical temperature, T_C, the system is a homogenous supercritical fluid.

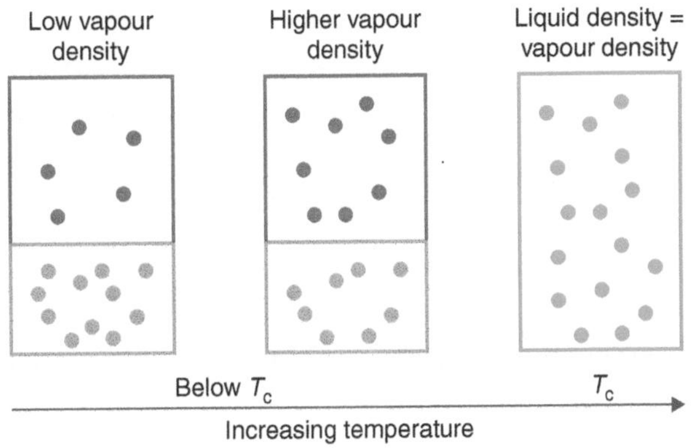

The phase rule

The closed systems shown in Figure 7.6 are all in equilibrium and can therefore be described mathematically using Gibbs' phase rule. This is expressed as:

$$F = C - P + 2 \tag{7.2}$$

where:

F = the number of degrees of freedom in the system (see Box 7.4),

C = the number of chemical components in the system,

P = the number of phases in the system.

When considering the number of phases in a system the following rules apply:

- Two (or more) gases are always miscible. Therefore, a gaseous system can only contain a single phase.
- Two (or more) liquids can either be miscible or immiscible. Therefore, a wholly liquid system can contain multiple phases.
- Two (or more) solids can either be miscible or immiscible. Therefore, an entirely solid system can contain multiple phases.

We may apply the phase rule to a pure substance that is homogenous throughout, e.g. ice, water, or water vapour:

- The system only has a single phase, so $P = 1$.
- The number of chemical components is one: $C = 1$.

Therefore, the number of degrees of freedom, F can be calculated:

$$F = C - P + 2$$
$$F = 1 - 1 + 2$$
$$F = 2$$

This can be interpreted by examining Figure 7.4. This figure shows that for a single-component system, the state of the system (in terms of which phase is present) varies with both temperature and pressure. Thus, in order to define the exact phase of a single-component system, one requires knowledge of both temperature and pressure, i.e. two independent factors (or degrees of freedom).

At the phase boundaries, represented by the lines in Figure 7.4, there is an equilibrium between two phases. By application of the phase rule, we may calculate that the degrees of freedom, $F = 1 - 2 + 2 = 1$. Thus, if we have a pure substance and a phase equilibrium between two phases, we need only state the value of one variable in order to fully characterize the system. For example, if ice and water are at equilibrium at a pressure of 1 atm, we know that the temperature must be 0 °C. Conversely, if ice and water are at equilibrium at a temperature of 0 °C, we know that the pressure must be 1 atm.

BOX 7.4

Degrees of freedom (F)

The 'degrees of freedom' of a system is the number of independent factors that are required in order to be able to characterize the state of a system. Typically, these factors are temperature and pressure.

For example, consider water at its triple point. This system contains a pure substance, so we may conclude that $C = 1$. At the triple point, solid, liquid, and vapour co-exist, so $P = 3$. According to the phase rule (equation 7.2), we can calculate the degrees of freedom of this system:

$$F = C - P + 2$$
$$F = 1 - 3 + 2$$
$$F = 0$$

Thus, a pure substance at the triple point has zero degrees of freedom. In practice, this means that there is only one unique temperature and pressure that define the triple point of water. Any deviation from these values means we are no longer at the triple point. As 'zero' deviation is allowed in order to remain at the triple point, we say that the system has zero degrees of freedom.

SELF CHECK 7.3

State the phase rule, clearly outlining the meaning of each term.

KEY POINTS

- A single-component phase diagram shows which phase(s) will exist at specific temperatures and pressures for a pure substance within a closed system.
- The vapour pressure is the pressure of a vapour that is in thermodynamic equilibrium with its condensed phase in a closed system.
- Above the critical temperature and pressure, a pure substance is described as a supercritical fluid.
- The phase rule relates the number of degrees of freedom to chemical components and phases in a system.

SELF CHECK 7.4

Define the terms critical temperature and critical pressure.

SELF CHECK 7.5

Define the term triple point. How many degrees of freedom are there at the triple point for water and what does this mean in terms of the allowed temperature and pressure values at which the triple point can exist?

7.3 Solid–liquid phase diagrams for two-component systems

Phase diagrams can also be used to illustrate the most thermodynamically stable phase(s) of a two-component system at a given temperature. In a solid–liquid phase diagram, solid and/or liquid phases are present over the range of temperatures investigated. The behaviour of the system is generally shown at constant pressure and this is usually atmospheric pressure (1 atm) in pharmaceutical applications. The phase diagram itself is normally constructed by mixing together the two constituents and recording the composition of this mixture as % (w/w) or mole fraction of each component. The mixture is then heated and the temperatures at which there is sharp change in the physical appearance of the sample are recorded. This includes the **thaw point**, where the sample first starts to melt, and the **melting point**, where melting is complete.

For more information on % (w/w) and mole fraction, please refer to Section 3.4.

Binary systems consist of two components and if they:

- do not react with each other to form a complex,
- have liquid forms that are miscible,
- are immiscible as solids,

then the resulting phase diagram has a characteristic appearance (Figure 7.7) with a number of important features:

- The melting points of the pure compounds are shown by the values T_A (for compound A) and T_B (for compound B).
- Increasing the ratio of compound B to compound A results in a decrease in the melting point of the system.
- This decrease in the melting point continues as the ratio of compound B to compound A is increased until the **eutectic point** is reached. This point represents the lowest possible melting point for the system. It is not necessarily at the point where the ratio of compound A to compound B is equal. Two-component phase diagrams can have more than one eutectic point (see Section 7.4).
- Continuing to increase the ratio of compound B to compound A after the eutectic point causes the melting point to start increasing again. This continues until system is 100% (w/w) compound B.

Three distinct regions are evident for the system shown in Figure 7.7:

FIGURE 7.7 Solid-liquid phase diagram for a binary system of A and B. T_A and T_B are the melting points for pure compound A and B, respectively. 'e' represents the eutectic point

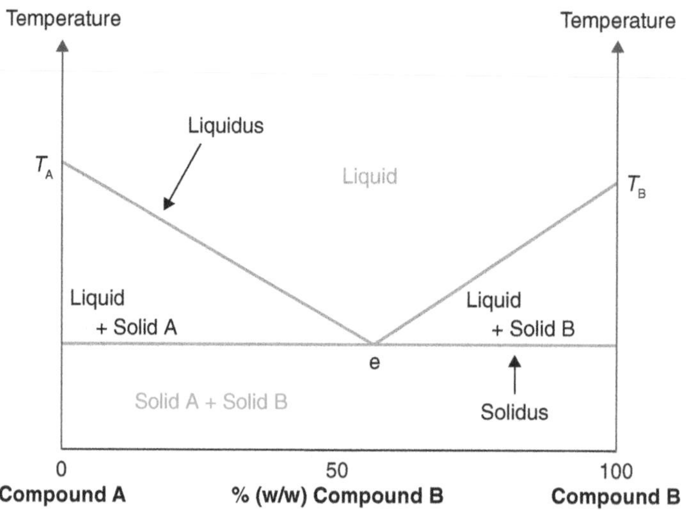

- Both compounds are in the liquid phase at all temperatures above the **liquidus**. This line is formed by plotting the recorded melting temperatures.
- Both compounds are in the solid phase at all temperatures below the **solidus**. This line is formed by plotting the recorded thaw points.

Two-phase mixtures exist at temperatures above the solidus and below the liquidus. These are regions where the liquid and solid phases co-exist.

Phase diagrams for pharmaceutical formulations may be constructed through thermal analysis. Differential scanning calorimetry (DSC), for example, may be used to study the melting behaviour of mixtures of an API and an excipient at various ratios. Using this technique, it has been found that mixtures of diacetylmorphine and caffeine within pharmaceutical heroin for inhalation exhibit the general behaviour described in Figure 7.7, the eutectic point being observed in mixtures containing around 92% (w/w) diacetylmorphine (Klous *et al.*, 2005).

For more information on calorimetry, please refer to Section 5.2.

Eutectic point

This is the point on the phase diagram at which the mixture solidifies (or melts) at a temperature lower than that of any other composition. This temperature is known as the eutectic melting point. If we consider a mixture of compounds A and B held at this temperature, then we can see from Figure 7.7 that a fractional increase in temperature will result in liquid formation. However, only a mixture with the eutectic composition will change entirely to liquid. As mixtures with the eutectic composition will revert to liquid most readily, they are described as having the maximum solubility (see Integration Box 7.1 for a clinical example).

INTEGRATION BOX 7.1

Eutectic formulation

The dermal anaesthetic Emla is a eutectic formulation of two poorly water-soluble anaesthetics, procaine and lignocaine. These are solid bases that, when mixed together in equal weight quantities, form a eutectic mixture. This mixture is an oil with a melting point of 18 °C. This is considerably lower than either procaine or lignocaine, which have melting points of 155 °C and 66 °C, respectively. The low melting point oil is formulated as an oil-in-water emulsion that can be applied topically to the skin. Emla is widely used to numb the skin for minor skin operations, such as superficial surgery.

For more information on oil-in-water emulsions, please refer to 'Emulsions' in Section 10.2.

A system with the eutectic composition that is cooled results in the two compounds crystallizing simultaneously. This is in contrast to cooling from any other point on the phase diagram in which one of the compounds would begin to crystallize before the other. The result of simultaneous crystallization is the production of small crystals. The resulting small crystals have high rates of dissolution and this is often desirable within solid formulations.

SELF CHECK 7.6

Define the term liquidus and solidus.

SELF CHECK 7.7

What phases are present in the region of the phase diagram above the solidus but below the liquidus?

SELF CHECK 7.8

What is the eutectic point and how are the properties of a mixture of eutectic composition useful in the formulation of medicines?

Tie lines and the lever rule

A two-component phase diagram can be used to answer a number of key questions with regard to the phase composition of a mixture. Consider the example phase diagram shown in Figure 7.8. Using this diagram, there are four questions that can be addressed:

1. What is the bulk composition at points 1 and 2?

   The bulk composition is simply the ratio of compound A to compound B at any given point on the phase diagram. This includes the total amount of each component, regardless of the physical form (solid or liquid). This ratio does not change with temperature and can be understood on the phase diagram by drawing a vertical line connecting point 1 and point 2 to the horizontal axis. This line is known as an **isopleth**.

   The bulk composition is given by noting the intersection of the isopleth and the horizontal axis (Figure 7.8). Thus, we can see that the bulk composition of the mixture at points 1 and 2, in terms of the % (w/w) compound B, is equal to Z. It follows that the bulk composition in terms of % (w/w) compound A is equal to 100 – Z.

2. What phases are present at points 1 and 2?

   To answer this question, we can inspect the two regions on Figure 7.8 in which points 1 and 2 are located. Point 1 is above the liquidus and thus both compounds exist entirely as liquids. In contrast, point 2 lies below the liquidus and above the

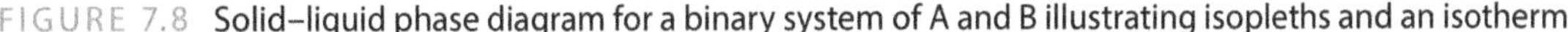

FIGURE 7.8 Solid–liquid phase diagram for a binary system of A and B illustrating isopleths and an isotherm

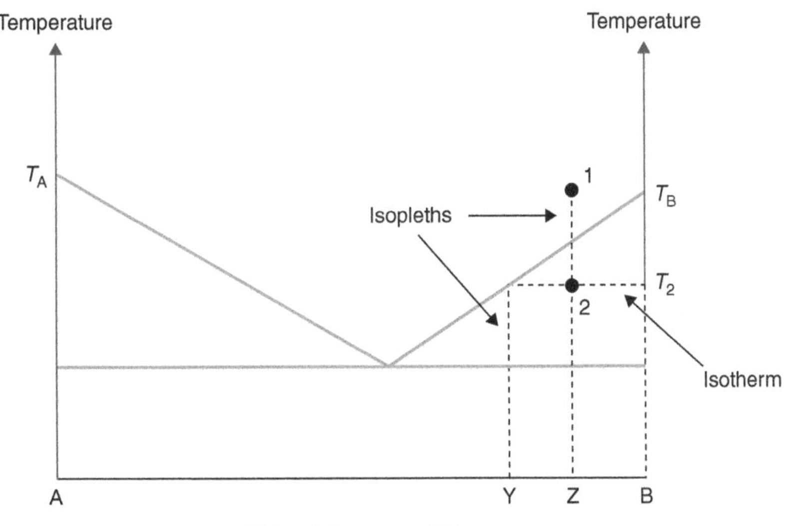

solidus, in a region of the phase diagram where both solid (compound B) and liquid (mixture of compound A and B) phases exist. This can be easily rationalized by considering that, to get from point 1 to point 2 on the phase diagram, the system has to be cooled. We can see that at this composition, the first solid to fall out of solution during cooling is compound B.

3. What are the compositions of the phases present at points 1 and 2?

In contrast to the bulk composition, the composition of each phase does vary with temperature. At point 1 on Figure 7.8, the system consists of a liquid phase only. Whenever the system exists as a single phase, the composition of this phase will be equivalent to the bulk composition.

At point 2, the composition of each phase can be determined using the following procedure.

- A horizontal line is drawn from point 2 in both directions until a boundary is reached. This line is known as an **isotherm** (or tie line), given that it indicates a region of the phase diagram in which the temperature is constant. In the phase diagram shown in Figure 7.8, the tie line is drawn at temperature T_2 and reaches the liquidus when extending to the left of point 2, and to the phase diagram boundary to the right of point 2.
- Isopleths are drawn where the isotherm intersects these boundaries. When extended down to the horizontal axis, these then give the composition of each phase that is present.

The isopleth drawn at the intersect of the tie line with the liquidus represents the composition of the liquid phase. In terms of the % (w/w) compound B, this is equal to Y in Figure 7.8. The isopleth drawn at the intersect of the tie line and the phase diagram boundary gives the composition of the solid phase. This is equal to B in Figure 7.8 and this represents a mixture with a composition of 100% (w/w) compound B, i.e. pure compound B.

4. What are the proportions of the phases present at point 2?

We have established that only one phase is present at point 1 on Figure 7.8. When two phases are present, we can use the phase diagram to determine the proportion of each phase. At point 2, we have established that both solid and liquid phases exist. To calculate the proportion of each phase, the lever rule is employed. We may use the tie line and isopleths that were drawn to determine the composition of the each phase in the previous question. If YZ, YB, and ZB measure the separation between the labels indicated, then the lever rule requires that:

$$\%\,\text{solid B} \times \text{ZB} = \%\,\text{liquid} \times \text{YZ}$$

As YZ + ZB = YB, and the % proportion of the two components will always add up to 100%, it can be shown that:

$$\%\,\text{Solid B} = \text{YZ/YB} \times 100$$

$$\%\,\text{Liquid} = \text{ZB/YB} \times 100$$

The units of YZ, YB, and ZB are not critical, as long as they are consistent. Thus, we may use millimetres or the same units as the horizontal axis.

KEY POINTS

- A solid–liquid phase diagram for a two-component system shows the most thermodynamically stable phase(s) at a given temperature and fixed pressure.
- Solid–liquid phase diagrams for two-component systems often exhibit a eutectic point that represents the lowest possible melting point of the system.
- The liquidus and the solidus are lines on phase diagrams that bound the areas of the diagram where the mixture is wholly liquid and wholly solid, respectively.
- A phase diagram for a two-component system can be used to determine the phases present, their compositions, and proportions using the lever rule.

SELF CHECK 7.9

Determine phases present and their composition at Point 2 in Figure 7.8 if Z = 93% and Y = 82%. What is the proportion of each phase?

7.4 Solid–liquid phase diagrams for two-component systems with complex formation

Consider the behaviour shown in Figure 7.7 in which the melting points of compounds A and B are affected by the percentage composition of the mixture. In this type of phase diagram the two compounds mix but there is no formation of any third chemical species. More complicated, if less common, phase diagrams can be obtained for two-component systems that involve the formation of a molecular complex. This has a dramatic effect on the resulting phase diagram, as shown in Figure 7.9. As before, the liquid forms of A and B are miscible. This phase diagram has the following key features:

- It has the appearance of two conventional phase diagrams placed side by side and contains two eutectic points (denoted by 'e').
- The formation of the complex between components A and B is denoted by presence of solid C in the phase diagram. Each of these three compounds is immiscible in the solid form.
- Frequently, the formation of this complex occurs at a stoichiometry of 1:1, i.e. when the percentage of compound B is 50 % (w/w), as in Figure 7.9. However, it is possible for other stoichiometric complexes to exist, for example, 2:1.
- Above the liquidus there is a single homogenous liquid phase. Complex C may or may not be stable in the liquid phase.
- There are two distinct solid phase regions, containing a mixture of solids. It should be noted that there is no region in the phase diagram where Solid A and Solid B coexist.
- Finally, there are three distinct regions containing a solid and a liquid phase. In each of these regions; the solid phase is made up completely of a single compound or complex.

Despite the additional complexity of this type of phase diagram, we can still use the same techniques that we considered in the previous Section. Again, we will look at two specific points on the phase diagram labelled 1 and 2 (Figure 7.10).

1. What is the bulk composition at points 1 and 2?

FIGURE 7.9 Solid–liquid phase diagram for a binary system of A and B where compound formation occurs. 'e' represents a eutectic point

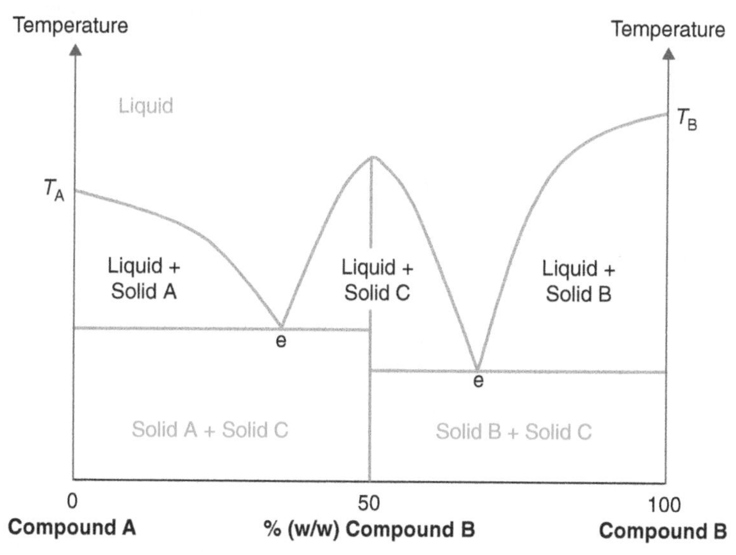

FIGURE 7.10 Solid–liquid phase diagram for a binary system of A and B where complex formation occurs

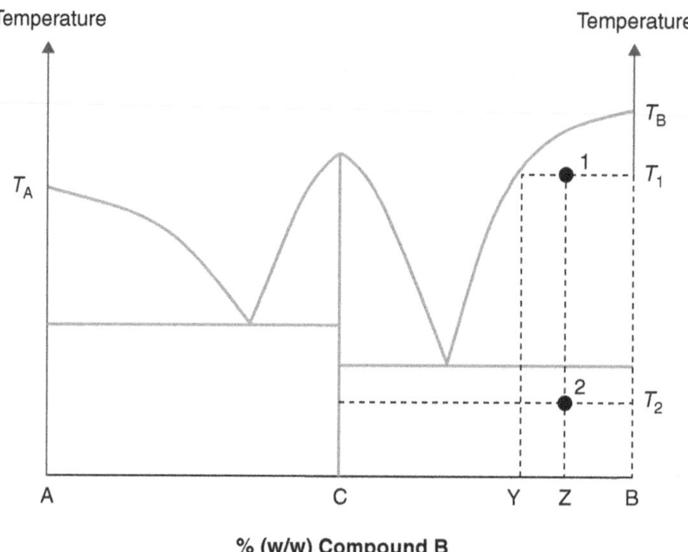

As points 1 and 2 are on the same isopleth, we can see that the bulk composition, in terms of the % (w/w) compound B, is equal to Z.

2. What are the phases present at points 1 and 2?

   Point 1 is below the liquidus and above the solidus. The diagram tells us that two phases are present: liquid and solid B. Point 2 is below the solidus and here the mixture is wholly solid, being a two-phase system consisting of solid B and solid C.

3. What is the composition of the phases present at point 1 and point 2?

   By drawing the tie line at temperature T_1 and the isopleths shown in Figure 7.10, we can determine that the compositions of the two phases present at point 1, in terms of the % (w/w) compound B, are Y and B. As before, the liquidus gives the composition of the liquid phase (Y), while the phase diagram boundary gives the composition of the solid phase (B, i.e. pure compound B).

   At point 2, the tie line is drawn at temperature T_2 and the associated isopleths reveal that the composition of the two solid phases present are C and B. The former is equivalent to 50% (w/w) compound B and this represents pure compound C. The latter is equivalent to 100% (w/w) compound B and this represents pure compound B.

4. What is the proportion of phases present at point 1 and point 2?

   Again, we will use YZ, YB, ZB, CZ, CB, and ZB to represent the separation between the pair of labels indicated. At point 1, application of the lever rule gives:

$$\%\,\text{Solid B} = \text{YZ} / \text{YB} \times 100$$

$$\%\,\text{Liquid} = \text{ZB} / \text{YB} \times 100$$

   At point 2, application of the lever rule gives:

$$\%\,\text{Solid B} = \text{CZ} / \text{CB} \times 100$$

$$\%\,\text{Solid C} = \text{ZB} / \text{CB} \times 100$$

The calculations shown above, and in the previous section, provide us with a means to obtain the wealth of information that is contained on a phase diagram. In doing so, we obtain a thorough understanding of the thermal behaviour of solid mixtures. It is not uncommon, therefore, for solid–liquid phase diagrams to be examined when deciding upon the most appropriate method for manufacturing a particular medicine. This may include considerations of complex formation and Integration Box 7.2 presents an example.

INTEGRATION BOX 7.2

Stearic acid and ibuprofen

Stearic acid is a waxy solid made up of long chain carboxylic acid molecules and it is used in the formulation of suppositories. Ibuprofen is an over the counter (OTC) analgesic that belongs to the class of non-steroidal anti-inflammatory drugs (NSAIDs). Mixtures of stearic acid and ibuprofen, analysed via DSC, have been found to show the general behaviour shown in Figure 7.9. Two eutectic melt temperatures at 62 °C and 63 °C have been recorded for the ibuprofen-stearic acid system, at 42% and 65% (w/w) ibuprofen, respectively (Lerdkanchanaporn *et al.*, 2001). It has been concluded that the complex is composed of two molecules of stearic acid for each molecule of ibuprofen.

KEY POINTS

- Some binary mixtures have components that combine together to produce a molecular complex.
- This behaviour is often characterized by the appearance of two eutectic points on the solid–liquid phase diagram for the system.
- We may use isopleths, tie lines and the lever rule to analyse these types of diagrams.

7.5 Liquid–vapour phase diagrams for two-component systems

Phase diagrams can also be constructed for two-component systems where the individual components are either a vapour or a liquid over the temperature range investigated. Again, the pressure of the system is kept constant. This type of phase diagram is constructed by measuring the **bubble point** and **dew point** for a two-component mixture at a range of mole fractions or percentage weights.

Components in a binary gas phase mixture are always miscible. If the liquids are miscible in the liquid phase then liquid–vapour diagrams have the general form shown in Figure 7.11. This has a number of key features, these being:

- The vaporus shows the dew point at each molar combination of the two compounds.
- The liquidus shows the bubble point at each ratio of the two compounds.
- The area below the liquidus is a single-phase liquid system consisting of the two miscible components.

FIGURE 7.11 Liquid–vapour phase diagram for a binary system of A and B. T_A and T_B are the boiling points for pure compound A and B, respectively

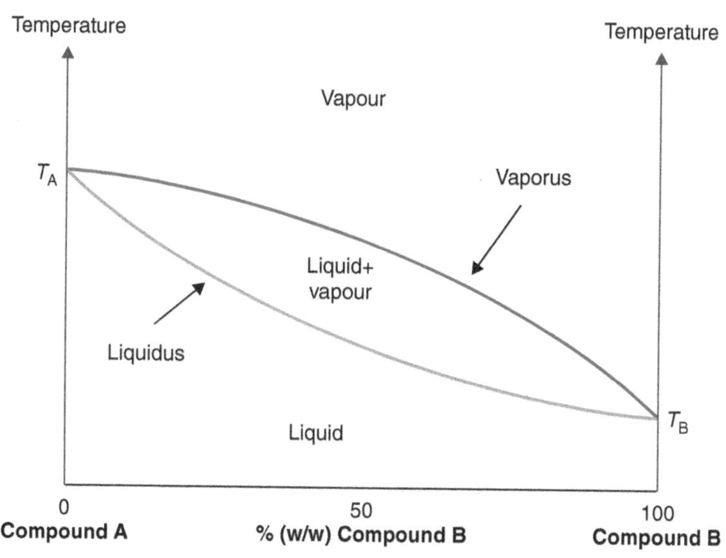

- The area above the vaporus is a single-phase system where both compounds are in the vapour phase.
- The temperatures T_A and T_B are the boiling (or condensation) points of pure compounds A and B, respectively.

As for solid–liquid phase diagrams, both the phase and lever rules are applicable to a two-component liquid-vapour phase diagram. Figure 7.12 shows the analysis required to calculate the mole fractions of liquid and vapour for each compound at point 1. This analysis consists of drawing an isotherm at the temperature of interest, T_1. An isopleth is then drawn at the point where the isotherm meets the liquidus and vaporus. The following questions can be answered for this type of phase diagram using the lever rule:

1. What is the bulk composition at point 1 on the phase diagram?

   As before, we can obtain this information by noting where the isopleth from point 1 intersects the horizontal axis in Figure 7.12:

$$\%\text{Composition B} = \text{Z}$$

$$\%\text{Composition A} = 100 - \text{Z}$$

2. What phases are present at point 1?

   There are two phases present: liquid and vapour. Pure liquid and pure vapour phases are only observed at the edges of the phase diagram where the bulk composition is either 100% A or 100% B. In between these extremes, the liquid and vapour phases will each contain both compound A and compound B.

3. What are the compositions of the phases present at point 1?

   The intersect of the isotherm at T_1 and the liquidus gives the composition of the liquid phase. The intersect of the isotherm and the vaporus gives the composition of the vapour phase. By drawing isopleths to the horizontal axis from these intersects (Figure 7.12), the compositions can be recorded. We can see that at point 1, the composition in terms of %(w/w) compound B for the liquid phase is equal to X, while that for the vapour phase is Y.

Consider an increase in temperature for a mixture with bulk composition Z by following the isopleth upwards from point 1 in Figure 7.12. If tie lines were added, they would show that the composition of the vapour phase becomes closer to the bulk composition, Z, with increasing temperature. This occurs as the composition of the liquid phase becomes closer to that of pure compound A. This makes sense because we can see that as $T_A > T_B$. Therefore, compound A is less volatile than compound B and would be expected to be more reluctant to enter the vapour phase.

FIGURE 7.12 Liquid–vapour phase diagram for a binary system of A and B illustrating isopleths and an isotherm

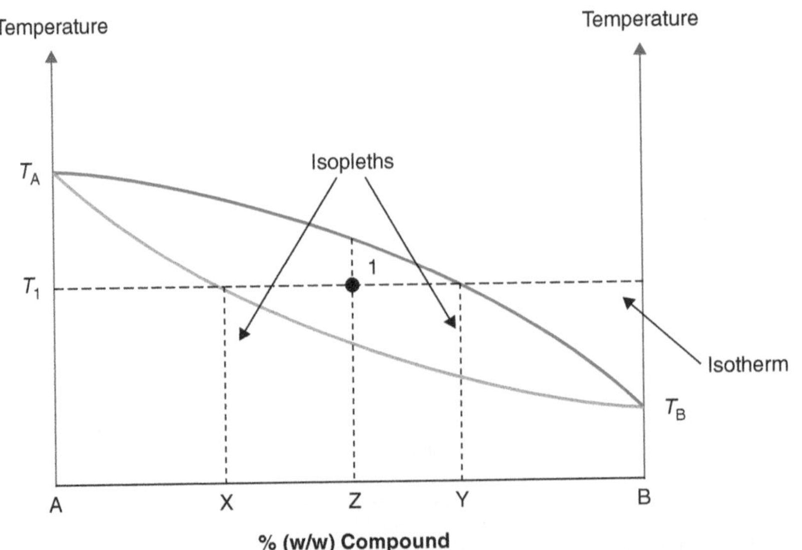

4. What are the proportions of the phases present at point 1?

By application of the lever rule, as before, we obtain:

$$\% \text{Vapour} \times \text{ZY} = \% \text{Liquid} \times \text{XZ}$$

It then follows that:

$$\% \text{Liquid} = \text{ZY} / \text{XY} \times 100$$

$$\% \text{Vapour} = \text{XZ} / \text{XY} \times 100$$

An increase in temperature of this system corresponds to following the isopleth upwards from point 1 in Figure 7.12. We can see that if tie lines were added, the lever rule would predict that the percentage of liquid in the mixture will decline, whereas the percentage of vapour would increase. This is in accord with expectation and is one way to confirm that the lever rule has been applied correctly.

The behaviour represented in Figure 7.11 is demonstrated by a number of mixtures and is that expected for an **ideal solution**. Here, the strength of the intermolecular forces between molecules of A and A is comparable to those between molecules of B and B, which in turn are of a similar magnitude to the forces those between molecules of A and B.

In non-ideal mixtures, molecules of A and B may have favourable interactions actions that stabilize the liquid phase. Alternatively, molecules of A and B may interact unfavourably and destabilize the liquid. In each case, an azeotrope may be observed. At the azeotropic composition, the liquid will convert directly into a vapour without an intermediate two-phase liquid–vapour system, as in Figure 7.11. This behaviour can be compared to the eutectic composition, where a solid melts to yield a liquid without an intermediate two-phase solid–liquid system.

Azeotropic systems have consequences for pharmaceutical manufacturing because they can result in liquid mixtures that cannot be separated by distillation. This is of particular importance for companies attempting to recycle solvents used during manufacture e.g. during large-scale chromatography. Acetonitrile (CH_3CN), for example, is a common solvent in pharmaceutical manufacturing and forms an azeotrope with water. Attempts to separate this mixture by distillation always result in a distillate that is impure and has the azeotropic composition (of around 85% (w/w) acetonitrile).

KEY POINTS

- Liquid–vapour phase diagrams for two-component systems show which phases will be present at various temperatures and fixed pressure.
- These diagrams are composed of liquidus and vaporus curves that bound an area where liquid and vapour coexist.
- In the region of the phase diagram where two phases are present, the proportion and composition of each phase can be determined by the use of isotherms, isopleths, and by application of the lever rule.
- In ideal behaviour, a mixture of A and B will always convert from liquid to vapour via an intermediate two-phase liquid–vapour system upon heating.
- In non-ideal behaviour, an azeotrope may be observed where the system converts directly from a liquid to a vapour at a specific composition upon heating.

7.6 Liquid–liquid phase diagrams for two component systems

Until now, we have only considered mixtures that are **miscible** when liquid. Some mixtures of liquids are **immiscible**, however, regardless of the experimental conditions. In a number of systems, temperature-dependent miscibility is observed and this can be represented on a temperature-composition phase diagram. Liquid systems exhibit an upper critical solution temperature (T_{UC}) when the components remain immiscible until a maximum temperature is attained (Figure 7.13). This phenomenon can be attributed to interactions between the two components that disfavour mixing at lower temperatures. As the temperature is increased, these interactions are overcome due to the increased thermal motion of molecules and the liquids become more miscible.

This behaviour is shown by mixtures of phenol and water and the T_{UC} is around 70 °C. Above this temperature, mixtures of phenol and water are always miscible, regardless of the composition.

Although less common, it is also possible for a lower critical solution temperature (T_{LC}) to be observed. The T_{LC} is the minimum temperature at which two components will exist as two distinct liquid phases (Figure 7.14). This phenomenon normally arises due to strong interactions between the two components, typically the presence of polar interactions or hydrogen bonds. At low temperatures, these forces result in the formation of complexes of the two components and the

FIGURE 7.13 Temperature–composition diagram for a binary system of A and B. The upper critical temperature, T_{UC}, is highlighted

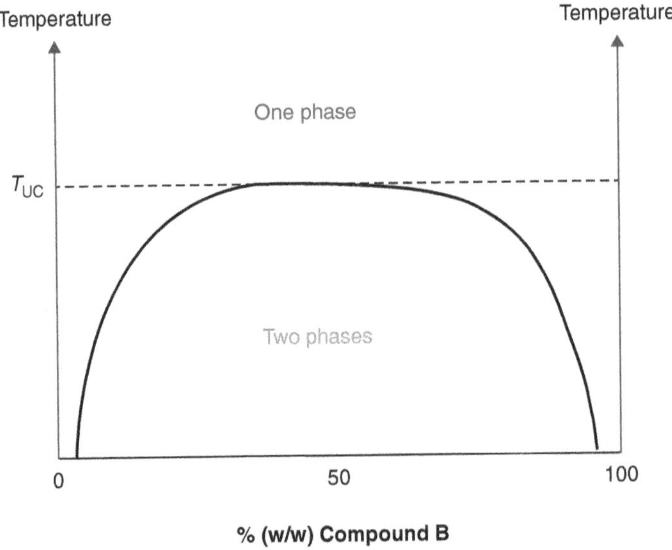

FIGURE 7.14 Temperature–composition diagram for a binary system of A and B. The lower critical temperature, T_{LC}, is highlighted

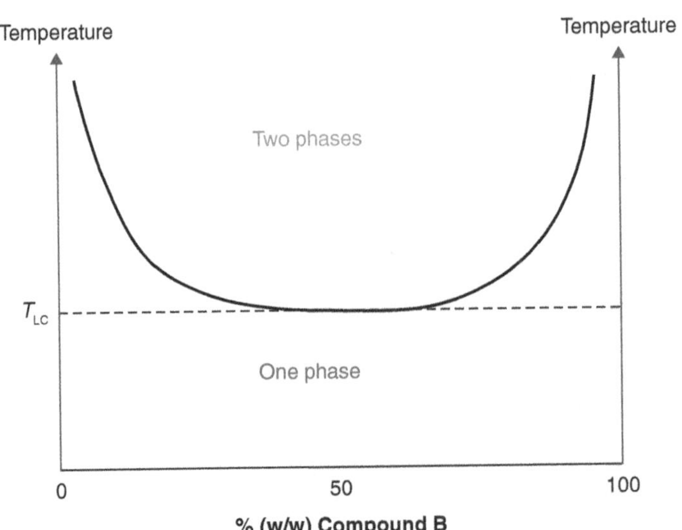

FIGURE 7.15 Temperature–composition diagram for a binary system of A and B. Both the upper and critical solution temperatures are highlighted

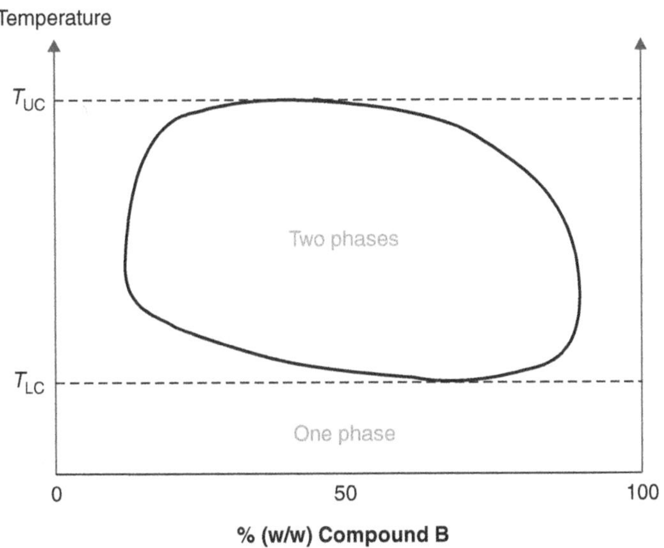

liquids are miscible. At higher temperatures, these complexes break up due to increased thermal motion and the liquids are less miscible.

Systems can also exist that exhibit both an upper and a lower critical solution temperature (Figure 7.15). The most commonly studied is the nicotine–water system in which the T_{LC} is 61 °C and the T_{UC} is 210 °C. Once again, complexes form between the two components at low temperatures and the liquids are miscible. As temperature is increased, the complexes break down and a two-phase system results. As the temperature is increased still further, the thermal motion of the molecules becomes sufficient to mix the two components together and miscibility returns.

The transition of a liquid system from one to two phases as a result of a change in temperature has biomedical applications. Thermoresponsive polymers are examples of 'smart' materials that can response to external stimuli (in this case, heat). They have applications in novel drug delivery and can be used in controlled release formulations. Preloaded polymer networks can be designed to release an API at body temperature over extended periods, the polymer structure being chosen so the lower critical solution temperature of the material in water is close to body temperature.

7.7 Phase diagrams for three-component systems

Phase diagrams can be extended to understand the behaviour of three-component, or ternary, systems. Three-component phase diagrams are triangular, in which both temperature and pressure are kept constant. In this type of phase diagram, the pure components are represented by the each of the corners. In a ternary phase diagram, the number and types of phases are experimentally determined for a range of composition ratios (component A: component B: component C). This allows for the prediction of the phase composition of the mixture at a given component ratio.

An example of the triangular axes used to plot this type of phase diagram is shown in Figure 7.16. Point 1 on the diagram represents a system with a composition that is 20% (w/w) compound A, 30% (w/w) compound B, and 50% (w/w) compound C.

FIGURE 7.16 Three-component phase diagram axes for a ternary system of A, B, and C

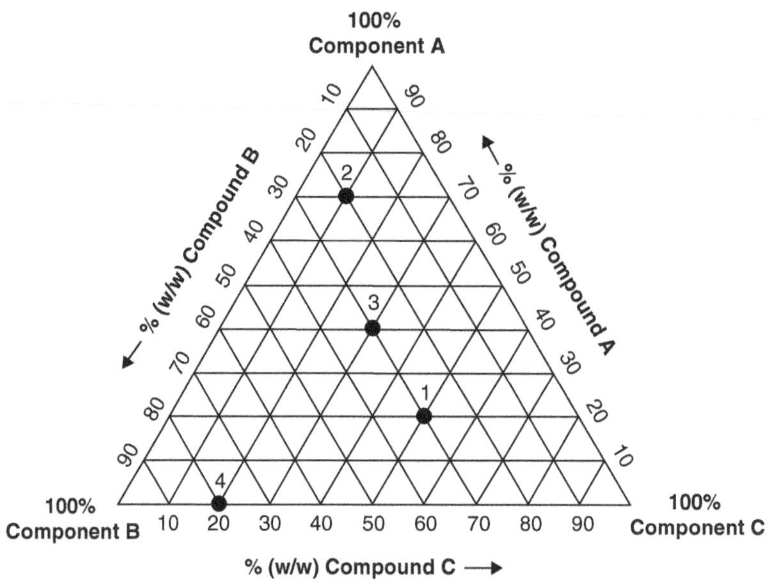

Three-component phase diagrams are widely used to assist in the formulation of medicines that contain a poorly soluble API. These **dosage forms** may be composed of emulsions within which the poorly soluble API is stabilized. The creation of an emulsion involves mixing water, emulsifier and oil in the correct combination to create oil-in-water (o/w) or water-in-oil (w/o) emulsions. In this use of a phase diagram there is no API component, however, the diagram can be used to determine the optimum ratios of water, emulsifier and oil. In terms of stabilizing a poorly soluble API, o/w emulsions are desirable. The precise amounts of each component will also determine the class of emulsion that can form.

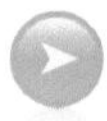
For more information on emulsions, please refer to 'Emulsions' in Section 10.2.

Three-component phase diagrams can also be used in the design of formulations that are resistant to the acidic environment of the stomach. This is extremely useful if the API is susceptible to acid degradation or if it is irritating to the stomach. These types of formulation are generally designed to deliver the API to the more basic environment of the small intestine. One such formulation method is to create microparticles coated by enteric polymers such as cellulose acetate trimellitate (CAT). As in the case of emulsion formation, the three components (for example CAT, oil, and acetone/ethanol) need to be mixed in the correct combination for microparticles to form. The compositions that correspond to the formation of microparticles are then displayed on a phase diagram (Figure 7.17). See Integration Box 7.3 for another example.

INTEGRATION BOX 7.3

Formulation of oral non-steroid anti-inflammatory drugs

NSAID drugs, such as ibuprofen, are insoluble in water. Ibuprofen is commonly available as both a tablet and a liquid capsule with the latter offering improved release of the API and thus quicker pain relief. NSAIDs formulated as a capsule are liquid aqueous suspensions in which the insoluble API is formulated as microparticles. Here, fine particles of solid API are coated by a polymer, such as cellulose acetate phthalate and gelatin. The precise amount of each constituent required for this microparticle formation is guided by the use of a three-component phase diagram.

FIGURE 7.17 **Example three-component phase diagram showing microparticle formation**

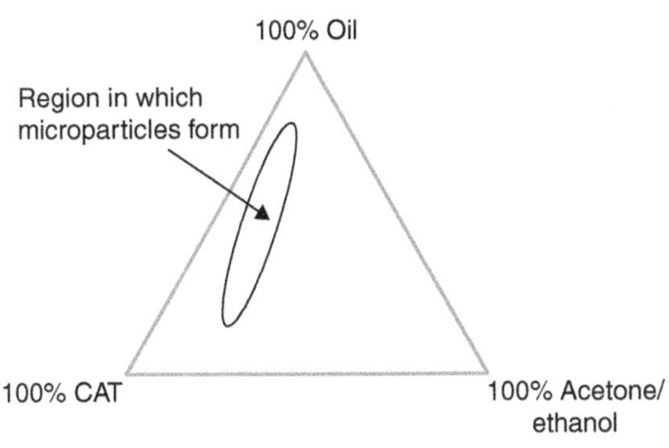

KEY POINTS

- Three-component phase diagrams show the most stable phases present for a ternary system at constant temperature and pressure.
- Ternary phase diagrams are triangular, the composition of a particular point on the diagram being determined by examination of the horizontal and diagonal axes.
- Three-component phase diagrams are widely used to assist in the formulation of medicines that contain a poorly soluble API.

SELF CHECK 7.10

State the composition of the mixtures represented by points 2, 3 and 4 in Figure 7.16.

CHAPTER SUMMARY

- A phase is a form of matter that is uniform throughout in both its physical state and chemical composition.
- A phase transition occurs when one or more phases change physically and/or chemically to produce a new phase or phases.
- Phase transitions occur at a specific temperature and pressure and, at these conditions, the phases involved are at equilibrium.
- Vaporization, melting, dissolution, precipitation, gas absorption, and partitioning are pharmaceutically-relevant phase transitions.
- The Noyes–Whitney equation can be used to calculate the rate of dissolution for a solid particle within a solvent.
- A single-component phase diagram shows the most thermodynamically stable phases at various temperatures and pressures for a pure substance.
- The triple point is the specific temperature and pressure at which all three phases; solid, liquid, and gas, can coexist in equilibrium.
- The Gibbs' phase rule establishes the relationship between the number of chemical components, the number of degrees of freedom, and the number of phases in an enclosed system.
- Phase diagrams for two-component systems illustrate the preferred phase/phases at a given temperature, pressure being kept constant.
- The eutectic point on a solid–liquid phase diagram represents a mixture with a composition that yields the lowest melting point.
- The composition of the solid, liquid, and vapour phases can be determined on an appropriate phase diagram from the intersection of an isotherm with the solidus, liquidus, or vaporus, respectively.
- The lever rule enables information about the proportion of two phases at any point on a two component phase diagram to be calculated.
- A temperature–composition diagram can be used to show whether two liquids will be miscible or immiscible over the temperature range represented.
- Three-component phase diagrams are used to illustrate the preferred phase/phases of a system containing three substances at constant temperature and pressure.

FURTHER READING

Atkins, P.W. and de Paula, J. *Physical Chemistry.* (9th edn). Oxford: Oxford University Press (2009).

This textbook goes into the chemistry associated with phase transitions and diagrams in more detail. It is also an excellent general physical chemistry textbook.

REFERENCES

Klous, M.G., Bronner, G.M., Nuijen, B., van Ree, J.M. and Beijnen, J.H. Pharmaceutical heroin for inhalation: thermal analysis and recovery experiments after volatilisation. *Journal of Pharmaceutical and Biomedical Analysis* (2005). 39: 944–50.

Lerdkanchanaporn, S., Dollimore, D. and Evans, S.J. Phase diagram for the mixtures of ibuprofen and stearic acid. *Thermochimica Acta* (2001). 367: 1–8.

8

Hydrophobicity and partitioning

WILLIAM McAULEY

Understanding, or having a measure of, the **hydrophobicity** of a drug molecule is important for a wide range of situations when considering pharmaceutical products. These range from the biological activity and **pharmacokinetics** associated with a particular **active pharmaceutical ingredient (API)**, through to issues associated with formulating and packaging.

Partitioning is an example of a **phase transition** and it occurs when an API distributes itself, or 'partitions', between two immiscible liquids. The effect is also evident when other types of solutes, such as dyes, are added to two-phase liquid systems. In Figure 8.1, phenol red tends to concentrate in the aqueous phase after partitioning, a relatively smaller amount being present in the organic layer, n-butanol. The concentration of the solute in each phase can be experimentally measured and, at equilibrium it is found to be constant. This information can be used to quantify the hydrophobicity of the solute, including APIs.

Learning objectives

Having read this chapter you are expected to be able to:

- Define hydrophobicity and explain its relevance for pharmaceuticals.
- Describe what partition and distribution coefficients are and how they can be measured.
- Understand how partitioning equilibria can be understood from considerations of solute chemical potential.
- Explain why octanol is the most widely used lipophilic phase when determining log P for APIs.
- Explain drug absorption in terms of the partitioning of an API into and out of a lipophilic biological membrane.
- Account for the origin of optimum log P values among a series of APIs that yields maximum biological activity.
- State and apply the pH-partition hypothesis and understand some of its limitations.
- Give examples of how partitioning can be used to aid the selection of preservatives and dosage form containers.

8.1 Hydrophobicity

The word 'hydrophobicity' comes from the Greek *hydro* (water) and *phobos* (fear) and characterizes the preference of a substance for a non-aqueous solvent over water. Its antonym, **hydrophilic**, literally

FIGURE 8.1 (A) The dye phenol red is added dropwise to a two-phase system of water (lower layer) and n-butanol (upper layer). (B) After shaking and standing for 15 minutes, the preference of the dye for the aqueous phase is apparent (photos courtesy Phil Denton)

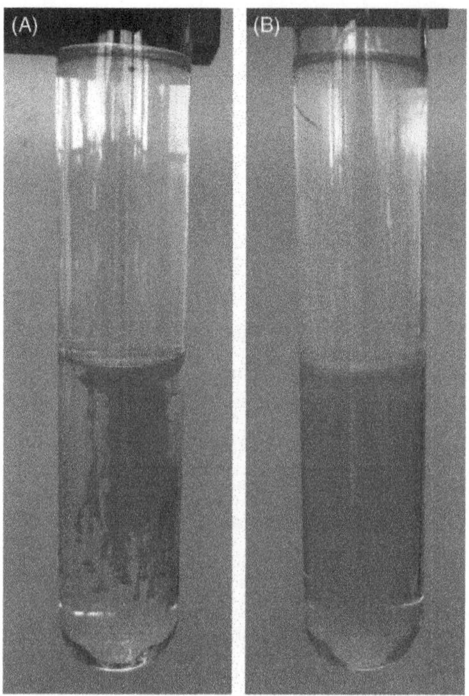

means 'water loving'. Many new drugs are highly hydrophobic and, in recent years, much work has been done to develop **dosage forms** that enable the delivery of poorly water-soluble APIs. This might lead to the assumption that hydrophobic APIs present a problem; however, hydrophobic character is extremely important for drug molecules affecting, for example:

- Binding to target **receptors**.
- Absorption across biological membranes.
- Their interaction with some types of pharmaceutical packaging.

Thus, an understanding of the hydrophobicity of an API is essential to understand its role as a medicine.

Hydrophobicity is associated with non-polar portions of molecules, such as hydrocarbon chains, that limit the ability of the molecule to interact with water. The hydrophobic effect arises from the comparatively low **entropy** associated with the relatively ordered structuring of water molecules around hydrophobic solutes. This is necessary so that hydrogen bonds between water molecules are preserved. This explains why globules of oil in water have a tendency to spontaneously **coalesce**. This process reduces the overall interfacial area of hydrophobic globules and this liberates water molecules in an entropically favoured process.

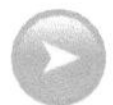
For more information on entropy, please refer to Section 5.4.

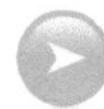
For more information on coalescence, please refer to 'Coalescence/aggregation' in Section 10.5.

KEY POINTS

- A hydrophobic substance prefers non-aqueous solvents over water.
- A hydrophilic substance prefers water over non-aqueous solvents.
- The hydrophobicity of APIs has an influence on various pharmaceutically relevant phenomena, including solubility, interaction with packaging, absorption across biological membranes, and binding to target receptors.

SELF CHECK 8.1

Why is the coalescence of two globules of oil suspended in water an entropically favourable process?

8.2 Partition coefficient

If an API is added to a system of two immiscible liquids, then the drug will partition between the two phases until a constant ratio is reached at equilibrium. The **partition coefficient** measures the relative affinity of the API for the two liquids; for example, water and an organic **lipophilic** solvent. Dilute solutions can be assumed to behave as **ideal solutions** and the concentration of the API in the two phases can be used to calculate the **partition coefficient**, *P*:

$$P = Co/Cw \qquad (8.1)$$

where *P* is the partition coefficient, *Co* (*o*=organic) is the concentration of the API in the lipophilic phase and *Cw* (*w*=water) is the concentration in the aqueous phase.

P remains constant at fixed temperature and pressure and is not dependent on **pH**. When calculating the partition coefficient of any chemical between an aqueous and a non-aqueous phase, the concentration of solute in the aqueous phase is always in the denominator (i.e. below the dividing line in equation 8.1).

For more information on pH, please refer to Section 6.3.

Critically, equation 8.1 expresses the concentrations of *exactly* the same species in the two media. Thus, when acetic acid is added to water, the partition coefficient would be calculated by dividing the concentration of CH_3COOH in the lipophilic solvent by the concentration of CH_3COOH in the aqueous medium. This solute is an acid and will ionize to yield CH_3COO^-. However, the concentration of this species is not directly included in the expression for partition coefficient, as it is not exactly the same as CH_3COOH.

For more information on acids, please refer to Chapter 6.

The partition coefficient is often converted to a logarithmic value, log *P*, because of the large range of values obtained for different compounds:

- When *P*=1, there are equal concentrations of API in both phases and log *P*=0.
- When *P*=100, there is a one-hundred-fold greater concentration of the API in the non-aqueous phase than the aqueous phase and log *P*=2. As the drug has a greater affinity for the organic phase, the API can then be considered to be hydrophobic.
- When *P*=0.1 there is a ten-fold greater concentration of the drug in the aqueous phase than the non-aqueous phase and log *P*=−1. As the drug has a greater affinity for the aqueous phase, it can be considered hydrophilic.

Thus log *P* provides a convenient measure of an API's behaviour, hydrophobic APIs having positive log *P* values and hydrophilic APIs having negative log *P* values. Some example values for log *P* at 298 K are shown in Table 8.1.

According to the International Union of Pure and Applied Chemistry (IUPAC) nomenclature for liquid-liquid distribution, the term 'partition ratio' is preferable to partition coefficient and is defined as:

> The ratio of the concentration of a substance in a single definite form, in one phase to its concentration in the same form in the other phase at equilibrium, e.g. for an aqueous-organic system.

The term 'partition coefficient' can also be defined in this way and, as it continues to be the predominantly used term, it will be used here.

TABLE 8.1 **Values of log *P* for selected APIs measured for the octanol–water system**

API	Log *P*
Acetylsalicylic acid	1.2
Benzocaine	1.9
Methadone	3.9
Hydrocortisone	4.3

KEY POINTS

- The partition coefficient, *P*, measures the relative affinity of an API for aqueous and organic environments.
- The partition coefficient is constant for a particular API in a specific two-solvent system at fixed temperature.
- Hydrophobic APIs have positive log *P* values and hydrophilic APIs have negative log *P* values.

SELF CHECK 8.2

In a partitioning study of xamoterol, a cardiac stimulant, the concentration of the API in water and octanol phases was found to be 21 mM and 66 mM at 298 K. On this basis, what is the log *P* of xamoterol?

SELF CHECK 8.3

The octanol–water log *P* of caffeine is 0.0. On this basis, how would you classify caffeine?

8.3 Distribution coefficient

The partition coefficient (or partition ratio) describes the relative affinity of an API between aqueous and lipophilic phases at a particular temperature and pressure under ideal conditions. We have seen that it only applies to the partitioning of a single, definite form of an API between the two immiscible liquids. The partition coefficient remains constant for the given system and will be invariant with changes in other experimental conditions, such as the pH of the aqueous phase. The determination of *P* is straightforward when considering non-ionizable drug molecules, as only one form of the drug exists in dilute solution. However, the majority of APIs are acids or bases, and both the ionized and unionized species will exist in aqueous solution. For example, if we consider an API that is a weak acid (HA), it will partially dissociate in water to give the constituent ions and the undissociated form:

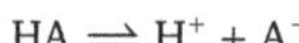

$$HA \rightleftharpoons H^+ + A^-$$

A change in pH will alter the equilibrium between the relative concentrations of the unionized and ionized forms, and the percentage ionization will change. In the above example, increasing the concentration of hydrogen ions (decreasing the pH), pushes the equilibrium to the left. This is in accord with **Le Chatelier's principle** and it will result in a greater proportion of the weak acid existing in the undissociated form (HA), decreasing the percentage ionization. Conversely, decreasing the hydrogen ion concentration (increasing the pH), pushes the equilibrium to the right. A greater proportion of the API is then in the ionized form.

For more information on percentage ionization, please refer to 'Degree of ionization of APIs' in Section 6.5.

For more information on Le Chatelier's principle, please refer to Section 5.6.

In general, ionized drug species do not partition significantly into the organic layer, so that only the unionized form of the API exists in the lipophilic phase. It is only the unionized form that is able to partition between both the aqueous and lipophilic phases. Experimentally, the total concentration of the API is measured in each of the aqueous and non-aqueous solvents. This includes the concentration of all of the species of the API in both liquids, including any ionized form. For this reason, it is convenient to define a **distribution coefficient**, *D*, sometimes referred to as a distribution ratio or apparent partition coefficient:

$$D = \frac{C_{HAo}}{C_{HAw} + C_{A_w^-}} \qquad (8.2)$$

where C_{HAo} is the concentration of the undissociated API in the lipophilic phase, C_{HAw} is the concentration of the undissociated API in the aqueous phase, and $C_{A_w^-}$ is the concentration of the dissociated API in the aqueous phase.

The IUPAC definition for the distribution ratio is:

> The ratio of the total analytical concentration of a solute in one phase (regardless of its chemical form) to its total analytical concentration in the other phase.

Unlike the partition coefficient, *D* does vary with pH and it is often also presented on a log scale (log *D*).

As pH is lowered, a greater proportion of our acidic drug (HA) will be in the unionized form that is able to partition into the non-aqueous phase. The distribution coefficient will increase as C_{HAo} increases at the expense of C_{HAw} and $C_{A_w^-}$. Conversely, as pH increases, the proportion of the unionized species in the aqueous phase will fall and the distribution coefficient will decrease also as C_{HAo} decreases. (These changes are summarized in Figure 8.2A).

Consider now a weakly basic API, B:

$$B + H^+ \rightleftharpoons BH^+$$

We can define a distribution coefficient in an analogous manner to equation 8.2:

$$D = \frac{C_{Bo}}{C_{Bw} + C_{BH_w^+}} \quad (8.3)$$

where C_{Bo} is the concentration of the unionized form of this basic API in the lipophilic phase, C_{Bw} is the concentration of the unionized API in the aqueous phase, and $C_{BH_w^+}$ is the concentration of the protonated form of the API in the aqueous phase.

As pH is lowered, the increase in hydrogen ion concentration will shift the basic equilibrium to the right. A greater proportion of the basic drug then will be in the ionized form, BH^+. As this is not able to partition into the non-aqueous phase, the distribution coefficient will decrease as $C_{BH_w^+}$ increases. Conversely, as pH increases, the basic equilibrium will shift to the left in an effort to generate more H^+ to counteract the change, in accord with Le Chatelier's principle. There will now be more of the unionized species, B, available to partition into the organic phase. The distribution coefficient will increase as C_{Bo} increases, at the expense both C_{Bw} and $C_{BH_w^+}$. These changes are summarized in Figure 8.2B. It can be seen that weakly acidic and basic drugs show opposite behaviour with regard to the variation of *D* with pH.

The pH of the aqueous phase can be controlled by the use of buffer solutions. As log *D* depends on pH, we might ask what pH should be chosen for measuring log *D*? The selection depends on the biological phenomenon of interest. If, for example, we wanted to study partitioning *in vitro* in order to simulate absorption from the acidic conditions of the stomach, then we would select a low pH. In this case, a buffered aqueous solution of pH 1–2 would be used to represent the physiological fluid within the stomach. The organic phase would then simulate the lining of the stomach, and octanol is generally used (see Section 8.6). An API found to have a high log *D* under these conditions might be expected to be readily absorbed by the stomach *in vivo*, although we will see later that other factors can be influential.

For more information on buffer solutions, please refer to Section 6.6.

Determination of the partition coefficient from the distribution coefficient

When quoting values for the distribution coefficient (*D*), the pH of the aqueous phase studied in the experiment must also be stated. The partition coefficient (*P*), which relates only to the unionized species, is invariant with pH (Figure 8.2). The log *P* of a drug molecule can be calculated from the log *D*. For acidic drugs with a known **acid dissociation constant, pK_a**, log *P* is given by:

$$\operatorname{Log} P = \operatorname{Log} D - \log\left(\frac{1}{1+10^{pH-pK_a}}\right) \quad (8.4)$$

For basic drugs, where the conjugate acid of the base (BH^+) has a known pK_a we may write:

FIGURE 8.2 Typical variation of *D* (—) with pH for (A) a weakly acidic API and (B) a weakly basic API. The partition coefficients (- - -) are shown for comparison

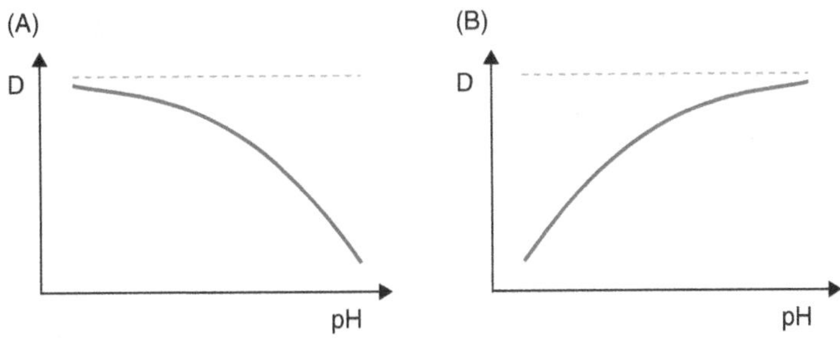

$$\text{Log}\,P = \text{Log}\,D - \log\left(\frac{1}{1+10^{\text{p}K_a-\text{pH}}}\right) \qquad (8.5)$$

If the final term in equations 8.4 and 8.5 is negligible, then log *P* is equivalent to log *D*. For weakly acidic APIs, this will occur when pH of measurement is significantly lower than the pK_a of the API. Thus, when pH is 3 units lower than pK_a, the final term in equation 8.4 is only 4.3×10^{-4}. Under these conditions, an acidic API will be almost entirely in the unionized form, so that the term $C_{\bar{A}_W}$ in equation 8.2 is almost zero. The measured value of *D* then is equivalent to *P*. For basic APIs, the pH of the aqueous phase can be buffered so that it is at least 3 units greater than the pK_a of the conjugate acid. Again, the drug will then be almost fully unionized and recorded value of *D* will be effectively equal to *P*.

If the pK_a of the API is not known, then the partition coefficient can be determined from the distribution coefficient using a graphical method. In this approach, distribution coefficients, *D*, are obtained for a series of controlled pHs, so that [H$^+$] is known. For a weakly acidic API, equation 8.4 rearranges to give:

$$1/D = K_a/P[\text{H}^+] + 1/P \qquad (8.6)$$

Thus, a plot of 1/*D* versus 1/[H$^+$] will yield a straight line graph with 1/*P* as the intercept and K_a/P as a gradient. *P* is then given by 1/intercept and the K_a of the acidic API is equal to gradient/intercept.

For weakly basic APIs, equation 8.5 rearranges to give:

$$1/D = [\text{H}^+]/K_aP + 1/P \qquad (8.7)$$

Thus, a plot of 1/*D* versus [H$^+$] will yield a straight line graph with 1/*P* as the intercept and $1/K_aP$ as a gradient. *P* is then given by 1/intercept and the K_a of the conjugate acid of the weakly basic API is then equal to intercept/gradient.

KEY POINTS

- The distribution coefficient, *D*, is the ratio of the total concentration of API in one phase to its total concentration in another phase. Total concentration includes all chemical forms of the API.
- The variation of *D* with pH for both acidic and basic APIs can be understood by the application of Le Chatelier's principle to ionization equilibria.
- Log *P* may be calculated from log *D* if the pK_a of the API is known.
- When pK_a is not known, both log *P* and pK_a can be determined by the graphical analysis of values for various pHs.

SELF CHECK 8.4

Consider a basic API. How is the distribution coefficient, *D*, expected to change as the pH of the aqueous medium is increased in a two phase oil-water system. Explain your answer.

SELF CHECK 8.5

In an investigation of the partitioning of salicylic acid between octanol and water, a student measured the distribution coefficient, *D*, at various pHs and at fixed temperature. A plot of 1/*D* versus 1/[H$^+$] was found to be linear and have a gradient of 1.0×10^{-5} M and an intercept of 1.0×10^{-2}. Determine the K_a and *P* for salicylic acid on the basis of these results.

8.4 Thermodynamics of partitioning

Partitioning can be understood in terms of the **chemical potential** of the solute. For a pure substance, the chemical potential is equivalent to **Gibbs free energy** per mole. The total free energy of a pure substance can then be calculated if the number of moles of substance and the chemical potential are known. For mixtures, the definition of chemical potential is more complex, but the total free energy of a mixture may still be calculated if the number of moles of each component and their respective chemical potentials are known.

For more information on Gibbs' free energy, please refer to Section 5.5.

The calculation of the chemical potential of each component in **mixtures** is complicated as it depends on the temperature, pressure and composition. From considerations of chemical potential and solute concentration, and the application of **Raoult's Law**, it can be shown how the chemical potential of water in an ideal aqueous solution, $\mu_{H2O(l)}$ is given by:

$$\mu_{H_2O(l)} = \mu^{\theta}_{H2O(l)} + RT\ln x_{H_2O}$$

where $\mu^{\theta}_{H_2O(l)}$ is the chemical potential of water in its standard, pure state, R is the **gas constant**, T is the **absolute temperature**, and x_{H_2O} is the **mole fraction** of water in solution.

For the derivation of this equation, please refer to Section 11.6.

It follows that the chemical potential of a solute in a liquid that we will identify as solvent 1, is given by:

$$\mu_{S(1)} = \mu^{\theta}_{S(1)} + RT\ln x_{S(1)}$$

where $x_{S(1)}$ is the mole fraction of the solute in solvent 1.

It then follows that in the second solvent the chemical potential of the solute is given by:

$$\mu_{S(2)} = \mu^{\theta}_{S(2)} + RT\ln x_{S(2)}$$

The solute will partition until its concentration in each phase remains constant. The condition for equilibrium is that $\Delta G=0$ i.e. there is no difference in the free energy of the solute in each phase and $\mu^{\theta}_{S(1)} = \mu^{\theta}_{S(2)}$. We may then write that:

$$\mu^{\theta}_{S(1)} + RT\ln x_{S(1)} = \mu^{\theta}_{S(2)} + RT\ln x_{S(2)}$$

This rearranges to give:

$$\frac{\mu^{\theta}_{S(1)} - \mu^{\theta}_{S(2)}}{RT} = \ln\left(\frac{x_{S(2)}}{x_{S(1)}}\right)$$

At constant temperature, all the terms of the left-hand side are constant. The right-hand side must also be constant and we can recognize that the ratio of the mole fraction of the solute in liquid 2 to liquid 1 is the partition coefficient of the solute:

$$\frac{\mu^{\theta}_{S(1)} - \mu^{\theta}_{S(2)}}{RT} = \ln P$$

When ideal solution behaviour cannot be assumed, as is usually the case with concentrated solutions, **activity** should be used in place of the mole fraction of solute.

For more information on the condition for equilibrium, please refer to Section 5.6.

For more information on Raoult's Law, please refer to 'Vapour pressure' in Section 4.2.

For more information on mole fraction, please refer to 'Units of concentration' in Section 3.4.

KEY POINTS

- The chemical potential of a solute in a solution depends on its concentration (mole fraction).
- Equilibrium is reached in a partitioning system when the chemical potential of the solute in one phase is equal to the chemical potential of the solvent in the second phase.
- The dependence of chemical potential on solute concentration can be used to understand why partition coefficients are expected to be constant at fixed temperature.

SELF CHECK 8.6

Consider an ideal two-phase liquid system in which a solute is present in both the aqueous and organic phases. If the chemical potential of the solute is greater in the aqueous phase than the organic phase, then how is this system expected to change over time, if at all?

8.5 Measuring the partition coefficient

The partition coefficient is commonly measured by the shake flask method, whereby the API is introduced into either the organic or the aqueous phase. These are then shaken together until equilibrium is reached. In some cases, the liquids have appreciable solubility in each other; for example, water and octanol. Because of this, the two liquids are typically pre-saturated with each other by shaking for 24 hours before starting the experiment. Once the API has been added and sufficient time has elapsed for the system to reach equilibrium, the concentration of the API in both phases is then assayed and the partition coefficient is calculated.

Although the shake flask method is a relatively simple experiment to perform in practical terms, it is difficult to measure the partition coefficients of very hydrophobic or very hydrophilic APIs. This is because compounds with log P values of less than –2 or greater than 4 will have a low solute concentration in one of the phases. The experiment is also time-consuming and requires a reasonable quantity of drug, which may be difficult to obtain in the early development stages of a **new chemical entity (NCE)**. As a result of these factors, other methods have been developed.

For more information on new chemical entity (NCE), please refer to Section 13.1.

Chromatographic techniques can provide more rapid measurements of P, particularly when the results of several APIs are required and only small amounts of each compound are available. Additionally, these techniques can extend the range over which log P values can be measured. Importantly also, several different computer programs have been developed that enable the calculation of log P, and one example is known as Clog P. The prediction of P is based on the calculation of the contributions from different structural groups that make up the drug molecule. The ability to calculate log P in this way is of particular use in the drug design process. It can be used to screen compounds designed to have activity at a target receptor but which have not yet been synthesized, so-called virtual screening. The calculation of log P can then be used to see if they are likely to have the appropriate physical properties for absorption. Calculated log P will be preferred when experimental partitioning data are unavailable and where there is a need to examine a large number of compounds.

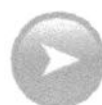

For more information on drug development and virtual screening, please refer to 'Modification of an existing molecule' in Section 13.1.

KEY POINTS

- The partition coefficient may be determined by the shake flask method or chromatographic techniques.
- Calculated log P values, Clog P, may be determined by computer and can be used to predict the hydrophobicities of compounds before they are synthesized.

SELF CHECK 8.7

The octanol–water log P value of a new chemical entity was determined using the shake flask method and was found to be 1.27. The Clog P value for the same compound was calculated to be 1.86. Which value should be used as a measure of the hydrophobicity of this compound?

8.6 Choice of the lipophilic phase

One of the key parameters for obtaining a partition coefficient is the selection of the organic, or lipophilic, phase. Any liquid that is immiscible with water may be used and the value of the partition coefficient for a particular API will depend on the nature of the organic phase. A wide number of different hydrophobic phases, including hydrocarbons, alcohols, ethers, and chlorinated hydrocarbons, have been used to investigate the partitioning behaviour of APIs. However, the selection of the hydrophobic phase ultimately depends on what the partition coefficient value is being used for. In the development of medicines, a phase that has relevance to biological activity and transport of drugs in the body is desirable. For this purpose, the aliphatic alcohol, octanol (Figure 8.3), is the most widely used and octanol–water partition coefficients have shown many excellent correlations with *in vivo* data.

FIGURE 8.3 Structure of octanol

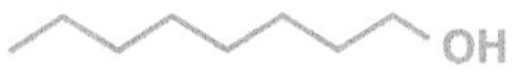

OH

Octanol is polar and partially miscible with water. This mutual solubility leads to more complex partitioning behaviour than occurs with less polar, anhydrous solvents, such as alkanes. Moreover, octanol exhibits hydrogen bonding acceptor and donor properties that are typical of biological macromolecules and constituents of cell membranes. Most molecules of interest, e.g. APIs and preservatives, have some degree of polarity. The partitioning of a polar solute into an inert, non-polar hydrocarbon solvent, e.g. hexane or heptane, is quite different to that for hydrogen-bonding solvents like octanol. For example, the octanol–water log *P* value of phenol is positive, indicating that this molecule prefers the lipophilic phase. In contrast, the hexane–water log *P* value of phenol is negative, indicating a preference for the aqueous phase.

Attempts have been made to fully understand the lipophilicity of solvents and these have looked at hydrogen bonding capabilities, solvent solubility parameters, interfacial tension, and dielectric constants. However, none of these approaches have been wholly successful or consistent. The factor that has been found to correlate best against solvent lipophilicity is the amount of water that the solvent contains at saturation. The relative inability of a solvent to carry water has been found to be a good measure of lipophilicity for a wide range of solutes.

The water content of the lipophilic phase modifies the solvent and it becomes more hydrophilic with increasing amounts of water. This would then be expected to increase the log *P* of a polar solute and reduce it for a lipophilic non-polar solute. In general, polar lipophilic solvents, like octanol, are preferred when attempting to correlate laboratory data with biological activity. Polarity may be quantified by measuring the amount of water that can be dissolved in a solvent. Thus, an organic solvent can be described as being less polar than octanol if it will dissolve less water than the equivalent amount of octanol.

Solvents that are less polar than octanol, e.g. heptane, are described as **hyperdiscriminating**, while those more polar than octanol, e.g. butanol and pentanol, are described as **hypodiscriminating**. These terms refer to the discriminating power of a lipophilic solvent used to study a series of structurally analogous solutes, e.g. 2-methylphenol, 3-methylphenol, and 4-methylphenol. In butanol-water, experimentally determined values of log *P* for similar solutes tend to be close together. In heptane-water, the differences in recorded log *P* are much greater and so this organic solvent may be described as being more discriminating. Octanol generally gives a range of log *P* values for different solutes that correlate well with data for drug absorption in the gastrointestinal tract (GIT).

Octanol remains the most widely used solvent for partitioning studies, but some have argued as to whether a single solvent can accurately model all cell and biological membranes. To fully model all the types of environment within the body, we would ideally want to determine log *P* in different classes of lipophilic solvent, such as:

- An inert solvent, e.g. cyclohexane.
- A hydrogen bond acceptor and donor, e.g. octanol.
- A hydrogen bond donor, e.g. chloroform.
- A hydrogen bond acceptor, e.g. propylene glycol dipelargonate.

For example, better correlations of blood–brain barrier (BBB) penetration can sometimes be achieved with consideration of both the octanol–water and cyclohexane–water partition coefficients, suggesting a solvent with reduced hydrogen bonding potential is a better model for this particular membrane. However, the use of a number of solvent models is hindered by:

- The experimental time required to generate data.
- A relative lack of published data of these systems.
- A limited capability to calculate log *P* values from molecular structures for solvents other than octanol.

For these reasons, octanol-water remains the main solvent system for log *P* measurement.

SELF CHECK 8.8

The partitioning of two structurally similar solutes was studied in octanol–water and it was found that their log *P* values were 0.32 units apart. If the experiment were repeated with a hypodiscriminating solvent in place of octanol, would the difference in log *P* be more than or less than 0.32?

KEY POINTS

- The water–octanol system is the most widely used when studying the partitioning of APIs and has shown many excellent correlations with *in vivo* data.
- Octanol exhibits hydrogen bonding acceptor and donor properties that are typical of cell membranes.
- Both the sign and magnitude of log *P* values depend on the nature of the lipophilic phase used with water.
- Solvent systems other than octanol–water may be useful when modelling specific phenomena, e.g. blood–brain barrier penetration, but are hindered by a lack of log *P* data.

8.7 Applications of partition coefficients

Partition coefficients have a wide application in the pharmaceutical sciences, from the analysis and purification of drug compounds to receptor binding, aqueous solubility, pharmacokinetics, formulation, and packaging. Here, however, we will focus on some of the applications most relevant to pharmaceutics, which includes drug delivery, formulation, and packaging.

Structure–activity relationships

A **quantitative structure–activity relationship (QSAR)** correlates a property of interest, e.g. drug potency or aqueous solubility, against selected physiochemical descriptors. These descriptors are numbers that quantify specific properties of a series of drug molecules. Thus, log *P* can be used as a physicochemical descriptor for hydrophobicity. The drug molecules correlated by a QSAR can be a relatively small homologous series of molecules, or a large collection of compounds with vastly different structural characteristics. QSAR models can also range from simple linear relationships, linking the property of interest to a single physiochemical descriptor, through to complex non-linear models using a number of different properties.

For more information on QSARs, please refer to Section 13.3.

Log *P* is one of the most commonly used physicochemical descriptors used in the construction of QSARs for pharmaceutical dosage forms. As mentioned in Section 8.5, log *P* values for molecules can now be calculated with computer software using molecular descriptors. These calculations are, in fact, a type of QSAR themselves and some QSARs have been developed that use these molecular descriptors rather than log *P*. Nonetheless, log *P* remains an important parameter, particularly for providing an understanding of the underpinning mechanism behind a particular biological process.

Transport across biological membranes

In order for an API to exert a pharmacological action it must first dissolve in the physiological fluids. This process, called **dissolution**, is a prerequisite step if the API is to ultimately reach the target receptor. The study of drug concentrations in the body with time, pharmacokinetics, is separated into four main phases:

- Absorption.
- Distribution.
- Metabolism.
- Excretion.

Drug hydrophobicity plays a role in each of these processes, sometimes referred to collectively as ADME.

Drug absorption often occurs by **passive diffusion** through a biological membrane, and this may be that of the GIT, the lung, or the skin (Figure 8.4). The absorption of an API that is dissolved in an aqueous physiological fluid is an example of partitioning. Previously, we have only used this term to describe a solute equilibriating between two immiscible liquids. The term partitioning applies equally well here because biological membranes have both a composition and behaviour comparable to a lipophilic solvent, albeit one that is more two-dimensional than three-dimensional in structure.

Once in the systemic circulation, the API will distribute to the tissues where it will act. These will include internal membranes, such as the blood–brain barrier, mammary glands, and individual cell membranes. Although the precise nature of these membranes varies, they typically present a hydrophobic barrier.

After absorption by one of the various membranes within the body, the API will then partition again from the lipophilic medium, back into an aqueous environment, be that a cell cytosol, interstitial fluid, or bloodstream. Thus, for effective delivery, APIs must have a balance of hydrophobic and hydrophilic properties to enable them to partition in to and out from the lipophilic environment of a membrane. If a molecule is too hydrophilic, then it will not partition sufficiently into the membrane. If an API is too hydrophobic, then it will tend to remain within the membrane.

As the partition coefficient provides a measure of a molecule's relative affinity for water and lipid phases, it is a useful indicator of whether a molecule is likely to passively diffuse across a membrane or not. One of Lipinski's rules of 5 for drug design states that APIs having a log P greater than 5 will be difficult to deliver. It is important to remember that this rule is a guideline and that many exceptions exist; nonetheless, the rules can be useful to gain an idea about the likely performance of a particular compound.

For more information on Lipinski's rules of 5, please refer to Section 13.2 in this volume and Chapter 12 'The molecular characteristics of good drugs' of the *Pharmaceutical Chemistry* book within this series.

Biological activity

Relationships between the narcotic activity of drug molecules and their oil–water partition coefficient were first reported around 1900. Since then, there has been a great interest in understanding the link between the biological activity of a molecule and its hydrophobicity. Such understanding can help underpin drug design, aiding the prediction of the biological activity of a particular molecule before it is synthesized. The relationship is not necessarily simple, as other factors, such as molecular size and shape, will have effects. Nonetheless, the ability of a molecule to interact with a receptor and cross cell membranes can

FIGURE 8.4 Passive diffusion across a biological membrane

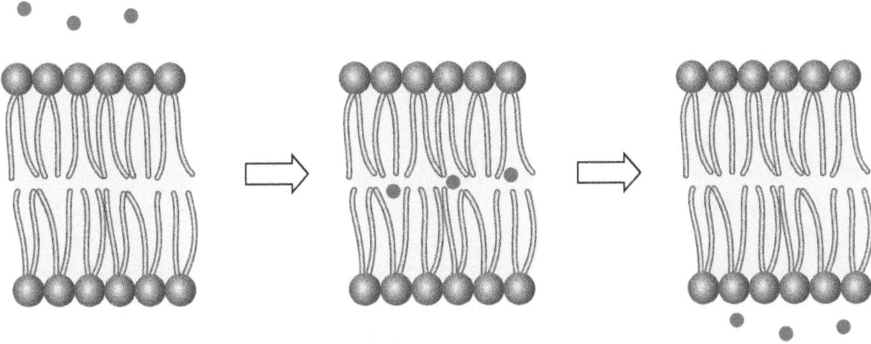

be linked to its hydrophobicity. Many of these relationships have been shown to be linear over a particular range of log *P* values, with an increase in the log *P* across a series of molecules often leading to increases biological activity. Such an effect may correlate with stronger binding of a drug at a particular receptor; for example, if hydrophobic interactions are important for binding. On expanding the number of molecules to include a wider log *P* range, a parabolic relationship is often noted where there is an optimum log *P* value. Above this value, increase in log *P* bring about a decline in biological activity.

Figure 8.5 shows the antifungal activity of a series of benzyldimethylalkylammonium chlorides plotted against the logarithm of the octanol–water partition coefficient. An optimal activity is observed at a log *P* of approximately 2, corresponding to a *P* value of around 100. In this study, activity is measured using log 1/*C*, where *C* is the concentration of API required to produce the desired pharmaceutical effect. It follows that highly active drugs will have low values for *C*, and correspondingly large values for log 1/*C*.

The decrease in antifungal activity with increasing log *P* above the optimal value is that predicted by the considerations of passive transport across biological membranes, above. Thus, highly hydrophobic agents will tend to remain in the cell membrane and will not pass through. However, other effects can also be involved. Figure 8.6A shows a signature parabolic activity relationship for a series of anticancer agents. Here, activity is measured using the concentration of API required to inhibit tumour growth by a factor one-half, or 50%. This value, known as the **half-maximal inhibitory concentration (IC_{50})**, will be lower for APIs that exert a stronger inhibitory effect. *In vivo*, the anticancer agents studied here can be inactive due to binding to other biological macromolecules. Alternatively, they can be unbound and active. When the data are re-plotted so that only the free, unbound API is considered (Figure 8.6B), a linear relationship is evident that shows that activity of the free API increases with increasing log *P*. We may conclude that the apparent decline in activity for derivatives with higher log *P* values (Figure 8.6A), is because these derivatives are more likely to exist in the bound, inactive form.

Drug absorption from the GIT

One of the most noted features of the GIT is the change in pH across its length. For example, the pH ranges from approximately 1.2 in the stomach to 6 in the duodenum and 7.4 in the colon. As the majority of APIs are acids or bases, this will affect the relative concentrations of the ionized and unionized forms in different regions of the GIT. A greater proportion of a weakly

FIGURE 8.5 Antifungal activity of a series of benzyldimethylalkylammonium chlorides against log *P*.
Source: From Hansch and Clayton (1973)

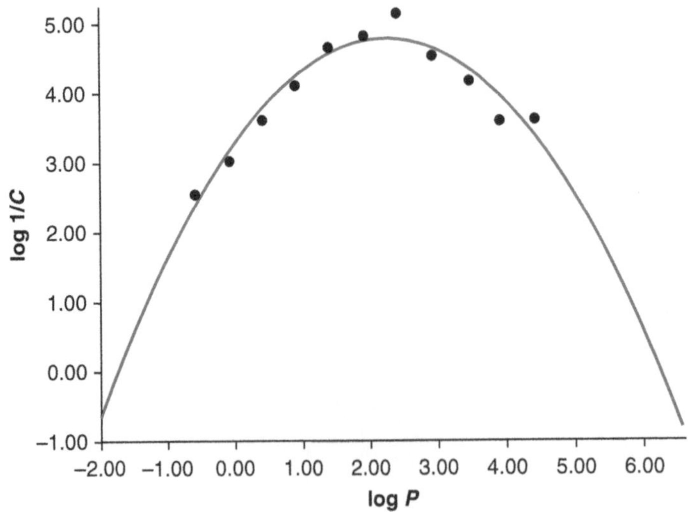

FIGURE 8.6 **Relationships between half-maximal inhibitory concentration and log *P* for the inhibition of tumour cells *in vitro* by gold phosphine derivatives, using (A) total API concentration and (B) concentration of free API only**
Source: Reused with permission from Springer Verlag from McKeage *et al.* (2000)

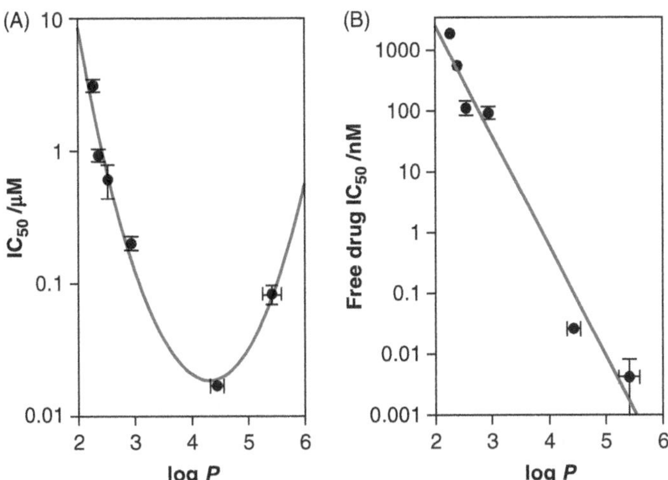

acidic API will be unionized in the acidic conditions of the stomach, with a larger degree of ionization in the more alkaline conditions of the small intestine. In contrast, basic APIs will have a greater proportion ionized in the stomach and unionized in the small intestine. As, in general, only unionized species will partition into the lipid of the cell membrane, this suggests that weakly acidic APIs will be preferentially absorbed in the stomach, whereas basic drugs will be better absorbed in the more alkaline regions of the GIT. This is known as the **pH-partition hypothesis** and it influences how some medicines should be taken (Case Study 8.1).

Whilst the pH-partition hypothesis is supported by some experimental evidence, it ignores several factors that limit its application, particularly for oral drug delivery. For example, the available surface area for absorption is much greater in the small intestine and

CASE STUDY 8.1

Ketoconazole is prescribed to prevent and alleviate fungal skin infections. It is often the first choice antifungal treatment for patients with deficiencies in their immune system; for example, due to chemotherapy. Ketoconazole is available in a variety of dosage forms, including those for topical application (shampoos, creams) and oral delivery (tablets). A patient prescribed ketoconazole tablets would be advised by the pharmacist to not take the medicine alongside an antacid or other indigestion remedy.

REFLECTION QUESTION

Why would the pharmacist advise against taking ketoconazole tablets with antacids or other indigestion remedies?

Answer

Ketoconazole is basic and, according to the pH-partition hypothesis, we would expect this drug to be preferentially absorbed in the alkaline regions of the GIT. However, the log P of ketoconazole is 3.7, indicating that this API is highly lipophilic and has low aqueous solubility in its unionized form. The API will only readily dissolve in the physiological fluids within the acidic conditions of the stomach and it is here where most of the drug is absorbed.

For absorption from the stomach to occur, it is essential that the stomach pH is maintained at the 'normal' level, around pH 1.2, so that the ionized form of the API is present in sufficient quantities to favour absorption. The presence of an antacid would raise the pH of the stomach, reducing the percentage ionization of ketoconazole. This, in turn, would result in reduced solubility and this would impair absorption.

many weakly acidic drugs, such as aspirin, are mainly absorbed there, rather than in the stomach.

The hypothesis also overlooks the importance of solubility. Before any absorption can occur, the API must first dissolve in the physiological fluids. These fluids are largely aqueous and so weak bases will generally dissolve under acidic conditions when they are predominantly ionized. In contrast, acidic compounds have better solubility in more alkaline conditions. For APIs with poor aqueous solubility, this may be the main factor restricting their absorption.

Drug absorption across skin

Similar to other biological membranes, the skin is known to present a hydrophobic barrier to the administration of drugs. The barrier resides in the very outermost layer of the skin with the deeper layers being more hydrophilic in nature. As before, a parabolic relationship between skin **permeability** and partition coefficient is often observed with an optimum log *P* of between 1 and 3. Any API applied topically to the skin would need sufficient hydrophobicity to partition into the hydrophobic layer, but also possess sufficient hydrophilic character so that it can migrate in sufficient concentration into the deeper, more hydrophilic, layers. Figure 8.7 demonstrates this parabolic relationship for a series of non-steroidal anti-inflammatory drugs (NSAIDs). Here, absorption of the drug into the skin is measured by the log of a permeability coefficient that describes the rate at which the API migrates through the skin per unit concentration. The higher the value of the permeability coefficient, the faster the API is able to diffuse through the skin.

There has been a lot of interest in trying to predict molecular structures that are likely to have good skin penetration properties. One of the commonest cited is the Potts and Guy equation, which relates the skin permeability of a particular compound to both its log *P* and the molecular weight. This equation indicates that skin permeability increases linearly with log *P*, whereas Figure 8.7 suggests a parabolic relationship. As discussed previously, with regard to correlations involving biological activity, the range of log *P* values that are considered is critical. Thus, if the skin permeability of NSAIDs with log *P* values in the range 0–3 are considered, then skin permeability does indeed appear to increase with log *P*. It is only when the log *P* range of the APIs studied is expanded that the parabolic relationship become evident. The Potts and Guy equation is still very useful in drug development when there is a need to quickly establish if a new chemical entity is a likely candidate for crossing the skin barrier, or for identifying which one of a series of new chemical entities is most likely to become a candidate drug.

FIGURE 8.7 Relationship between skin permeability and log *P* for a series of NSAIDs and phenol
Source: From Singh and Roberts (1994)

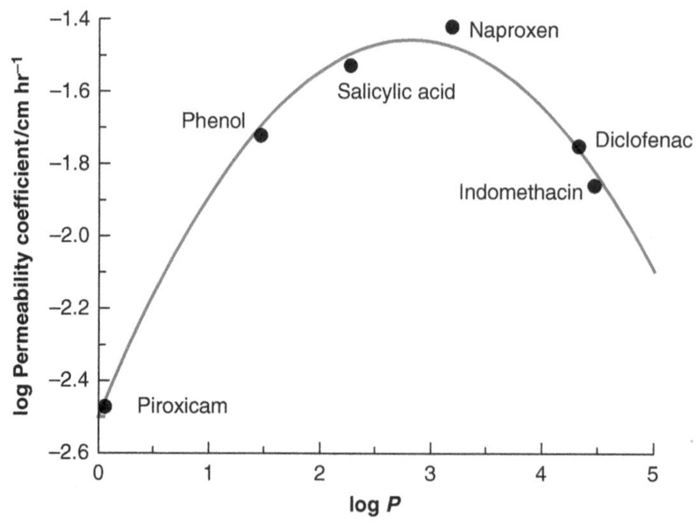

The pH-partition hypothesis is often applied to the delivery of drugs across skin, with APIs being formulated such that they are predominately in their unionized form to ensure that they partition sufficiently into the skin. This is one of the reasons why APIs for transdermal use are often formulated in the free acid or base form, rather than as a salt, which is often preferable for other routes of administration. For example, fentanyl, an opioid analgesic, is formulated as the free base form in transdermal patches, whereas the citrate salt is preferred for the nasal spray and buccal tablets. Again, similar exceptions to the pH-partition hypothesis to that discussed for the GIT have been observed from studies of absorption by skin. Poor absorption can result if the pH of the medication is selected to ensure that the API is mostly unionized, as this can be accompanied by poor aqueous solubility. Improved absorption from aqueous formulations can sometimes be achieved by modifying the pH to that where a greater proportion of the drug is ionized, improving solubility.

The blood–brain barrier (BBB)

Within the peripheral circulation, blood vessels have relatively open clefts that allow the interchange of a wide range of molecules with the surrounding tissues. In contrast, the cells in the blood vessels of the brain (the cerebrovascular system) are particularly tightly connected and they restrict absorption. This region is referred to as the blood–brain barrier (BBB) and it has an important role in regulating brain function. Only relatively small lipophilic molecules are able to passively diffuse across the BBB, some more polar molecules relying on **active transport**. A reasonably good correlation has been achieved between cerebrovascular permeability and the log *P* of a range of molecules. In Figure 8.8 there is a linear relationship, with APIs having a higher log *P* demonstrating improved permeability across the BBB. The points that seem to not follow this linear trend, shown in black, are known to have active transport mechanisms, which remove them from the cerebrospinal fluid. This impairs their ability to permeate the cells in the cerebrovascular system.

Drugs in breast milk

A large proportion of mothers wish to breastfeed their children, as it is associated with enhanced health outcomes and improved bonding between the mother and her child. There is limited clinical data, however, on the extent to which any drugs taken by the mother may enter the breast milk. Of course, breastfeeding mothers would not wish to expose an infant to unnecessary medication through their milk. However, they

FIGURE 8.8 Cerebrovascular permeability for a series of compounds, ○=not involved in active transport, ●=involved in active transport.

Source: Reproduced with permission of Blackwell Publishing Asia from Saunders *et al.* (1999)

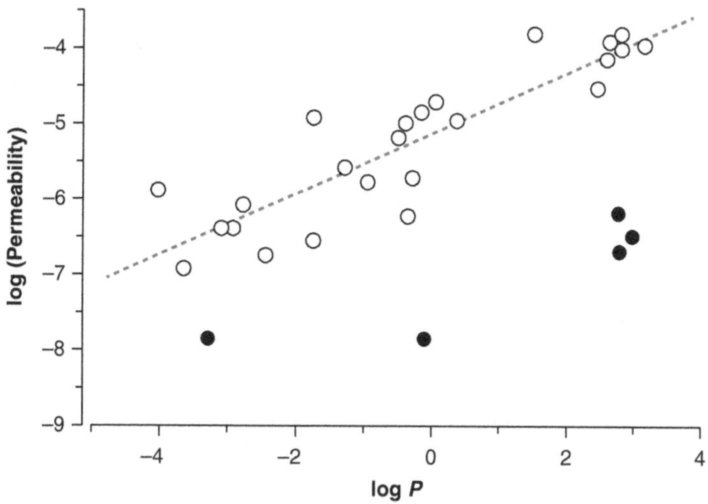

may prefer to continue breast feeding if data was available allowing them to make a decision based on the risks associated with infant exposure to a particular drug (which may be negligible). Understanding the distribution of drugs in milk is complex as the API can reside in either the aqueous portion of the liquid, fat droplets, or be bound by the milk proteins present in the aqueous phase.

As a result of the lack of clinical data, a QSAR has been developed to predict the likely expression of a drug in milk. The QSAR suggests that this is, in part, dependent on the log *P* of the API. Subsequent clinical data for drugs such as buprenorphine, citalopram, and venlafaxine, have shown good agreement with that predicted by the QSAR. This suggests that the model can be useful for estimating the exposure of a drug to an infant when there is limited clinical data on its safety for this purpose.

Emulsions and preservatives

Many pharmaceutical products that contain water are subject to degradation through hydrolysis and microbial growth. In order to ensure an adequate shelf life, the addition of chemical preservation agents is common. These can prevent the growth of microorganisms and are used in **emulsions**, such as creams for topical application. Emulsions consist of two immiscible phases, one of which is dispersed in the other, either as oil droplets dispersed in water or as water droplets dispersed in oil.

For more information on hydrolysis, please refer to 'Hydrolysis' in Section 12.1.

For more information on emulsions, please refer to 'Emulsions' in Section 10.2.

Consideration of the partition coefficient of any emulsion preservative is important, as the preservative would be expected to partition between both the oil and aqueous phases. In order to be effective, an adequate concentration in the appropriate phase is required. In particular, the concentration of the preservative in the aqueous phase is important as it is here, and at the oil–water interface, that the majority of microorganisms reside. If the preservative is too lipophilic, it may partition into the oil phase to such an extent that an insufficient concentration is present in the aqueous phase to prevent microbial spoilage.

A number of different oil phases may be used in pharmaceutical emulsions and a particular preservative would be expected to have different partition coefficients in the different oil phases. Table 8.2, for example, shows the partition coefficients for a number of preservatives in liquid paraffin and arachis oil. The values for arachis oil are considerably higher than that of the paraffin. This indicates that considerably more preservative is required in arachis oil emulsions to have a sufficient concentration in the aqueous phase. Another factor that should not be overlooked is the relative volumes of both phases, as this will also affect how much preservative is needed.

As a thermodynamic function, the partition coefficient should always be measured at a defined temperature. Changes in temperature would be expected to alter the value obtained. For drug absorption and distribution in the body, the temperature is relatively constant. In contrast, pharmaceutical products may be subject to more dramatic fluctuations in temperature prior to their administration. Changes in the storage temperature of an emulsion could have significant effects on the partitioning behaviour, potentially changing the concentration of a preservative in the aqueous phase sufficiently, such that it becomes ineffective. Table 8.3 compares the effect on log *P* on a number of preservatives at two temperature extremes that a product might feasibly be subjected to, 5 and 45 °C. It can be seen that the effect is very dependent on the particular system, depending not only on the preservative, but also the oil phase. In some cases, an

TABLE 8.2 **Partition coefficient at 25 °C of some preservatives in liquid paraffin and arachis oil**

	Partition coefficient	
Preservative	Liquid paraffin/water	Arachis oil/water
Phenol	0.067	5.6
Chlorocresol	1.53	116.7
Thymol	–	447
Phenylmercuric acetate	0.23	–

From Bean *et al.* (1965).

TABLE 8.3 Change in partition coefficient on increasing the temperature from 5 to 45 °C for some preservatives in liquid paraffin and arachis oil

Preservative	Oil phase	Percentage increase in *P*
Phenol	Liquid paraffin	+260 %
Chlorocresol	Liquid paraffin	+170 %
Chlorocresol	Arachis oil	+103%
Phenylmecuric acetate	Liquid paraffin	-50 %

From Bean *et al.* (1965).

increase in temperature increases the partition coefficient and other cases it decreases it.

It is clear, therefore, that the addition of chemical preservation agents to emulsions requires careful consideration to ensure a suitable shelf life is achievable.

Absorption into packaging

Another example to which knowledge of partition coefficients is useful is the phenomenon of a drug absorbing into the packaging of a formulation. This can occur prior to the administration of **intravenous (IV)** infusions if the API partitions out of the infusion fluid into the polymeric bag containing it, lowering the dose given to the patient. This is a particular concern for APIs with a narrow **therapeutic window**, where the difference between a toxic and ineffective dose is small and may have serious consequences.

APIs that have been found to have problems with infusion bags include glyceryl trinitrate, diazepam, isosorbide dinitrate, and warfarin. Particular issues have been discovered with polyvinylchloride (PVC) bags with, for example, 70% of diazepam being lost after 24 hours. This is not unexpected as the octanol–water partition coefficient for diazepam indicates a preference for non-aqueous environments.

Drug losses have also been observed to correlate with the pH-partition hypothesis. Thus, a greater proportion of warfarin is lost when the pH of the infusion fluid is 4.9, in comparison to a pH of 5.6. At higher pH, a greater proportion of the API is ionized and is therefore less likely to partition out of the water phase. To address this issue, other plastics have been investigated as materials for infusion bags, including polypropylene. Efforts have also been made to coat PVC infusion bags to try to minimize drug losses.

Drug adsorption to other parts of the infusion apparatus is also possible. For example, **catheters** may be made from a variety of polymers, or be coated with a particular polymer to give desirable properties. Figure 8.9 shows the loss of chlormethiazole to three different catheter types against time. The catheters were:

- An uncoated catheter manufactured from polyurethane.
- A catheter manufactured from polyurethane and coated with polyvinylpyrollidone. This water-soluble polymer can ease insertion of the catheter into the body and reduce bacterial adhesion.
- An uncoated catheter manufactured from Topecon™, a type of polyurethane.

The contact time of an API with a catheter will vary depending on the infusion rate, but can be between a few minutes and several hours. Over extended periods, the losses due to catheter type can be significant but can be mitigated by the material used to manufacture the catheter.

FIGURE 8.9 The loss of chlormethiazole edisylate from solution to uncoated (——), coated (- - -), and Topecon™ (–·–·) catheters at 37 °C
Source: Reproduced with permission from Pergamon from Smith *et al.* (1996)

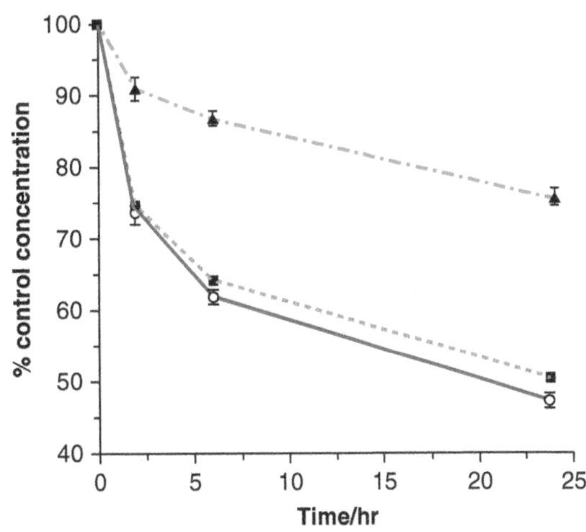

FIGURE 8.10 **Uptake of 5 APIs from a 0.4 nM solution by an uncoated Pellethane™ catheter at 37 °C**
Source: Reproduced with permission from Pergamon from Smith *et al.* (1996)

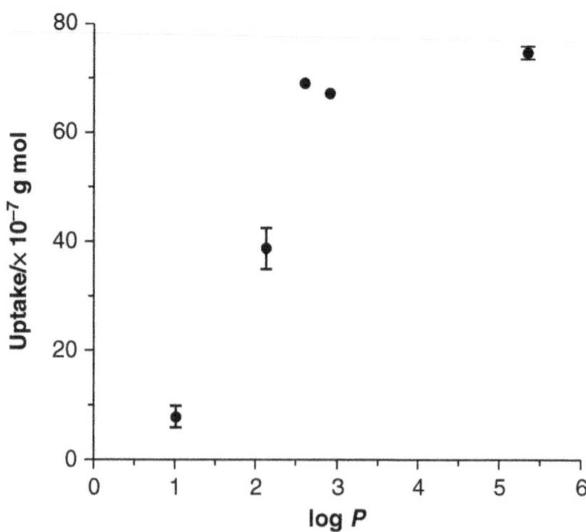

Drug loss to catheter can be related to the octanol–water partition behaviour of the API. One study has investigated the absorption of various APIs into a catheter made of Pellethane™, a medical grade polyurethane. A considerable increase in the loss has been observed for APIs with log *P* values ranging from 1 to 3 (Figure 8.10). Further increases in log *P* had a less pronounced effect. It is clear that knowledge of the partition coefficient of a compound can be used to provide an indication of the likelihood of losses to a particular packaging, and can help ensure appropriate doses of medications are administered to patients.

KEY POINTS

- Partition coefficients can used to understand pharmaceutically relevant phenomena, including drug delivery, formulation, and packaging.
- The passive diffusion of an API dissolved in aqueous physiological fluid to a lipophilic cell membrane is an example of partitioning.
- APIs must have a balance of hydrophobic and hydrophilic properties to enable them to partition in to and out from the lipophilic environment of a membrane. This is often apparent by a parabolic relationship between drug activity and log *P*, the peak activity being recorded for the optimum log *P* value.
- The pH-partition hypothesis predicts that the absorption of acidic and basic drugs will be favoured when the local pH is such that the API is largely in an unionized form.
- The pH-partition hypothesis does not take into account the size of the surface area over which the drug may absorb, or that APIs are more likely to dissolve in physiological fluids when they are ionized.
- The partitioning of preservatives must also be considered when designing dosage forms and this is a particular consideration for emulsions.
- Pharmaceutical containers should be designed to minimize the possibility of the API partitioning from the dosage form into the packaging.

SELF CHECK 8.9

One of Lipinski's rules of 5 of drug design states that APIs having a log *P* greater than 5 will be difficult to deliver. Why should this be so?

SELF CHECK 8.10

Explain why the analgesic fentanyl is formulated in the free base form within transdermal patches, but as the citrate salt within a nasal spray.

CHAPTER SUMMARY

- An API added to a two-phase system of immiscible liquids will partition into each phase.
- The two liquids can normally be classified as aqueous and organic, the solute concentrating in the phase for which it has the greatest affinity.
- The partition coefficient, *P*, is the ratio of the concentration of a particular form of a solute in organic and aqueous media.

- The distribution coefficient, *D*, is the ratio of the sum of concentrations of all forms of a solute in organic and aqueous media.
- The partition coefficient is independent of pH. For weakly acidic drugs, the distribution coefficient decreases as pH increases. For weakly basic drugs, the distribution coefficient increases as pH increases.
- When an API has partitioned between two phases and reached equilibrium, the chemical potential of the solute within each phase is the same.
- The shake flask method is the most common technique for the determination of the partition coefficient.
- The aliphatic alcohol, octanol, is the most widely used lipophilic phase when determining log *P* for APIs. Octanol–water partition coefficients have been found to correlate well with *in vivo* data.
- A quantitative structure–activity relationship (QSAR) correlates a property of interest against physiochemical descriptors.
- The absorption of an API that is dissolved in physiological fluid can occur through partitioning in to and out from a lipophilic biological membrane.
- A structurally similar series of APIs often exhibit an optimum log *P* value that affords the maximum biological activity.
- The pH-partition hypothesis states that weakly acidic APIs will be preferentially absorbed in acidic regions of the body, while weakly basic APIs will be preferentially absorbed in alkaline regions of the body.
- The pH-partition hypothesis does not take into account other factors. The aqueous solubility of the API, for example, can sometimes be a dominant factor in determining absorption *in vivo*.
- The partitioning of preservatives is an important consideration in biphasic formulations such as emulsions.
- APIs in aqueous solution may partition into lipophilic containers. This is a consideration for the storage of solution for IV infusion.

FURTHER READING

Florence, A.T. and Attwood, D. *Physicochemical Principles of Pharmacy*, (4th edn). London: Pharmaceutical Press, (2006).

Considers partitioning and the pH-partition hypothesis in a chapter devoted to oral delivery that includes a discussion of the mechanisms of absorption.

Monynihan, H. and Crean, A. *The Physicochemical Basis of Pharmaceuticals*. Oxford: Oxford University Press, (2009).

Emphasizes the importance of phase transitions, including dissolution and partitioning, in understanding drug delivery.

Begg, E.J., Atkinson, H.C., and Duffull, S.B. Prospective evaluation of a model for the prediction of milk–plasma drug concentrations from physicochemical characteristics. *British Journal of Clinical Pharmacology* (1992). 33(5): 501–5.

El Tayar, N., Tsai, R.S., Testa, B., Carrupt, P.A., and Leo, A. Partitioning of solutes in different solvent systems the contribution of hydrogen-bonding capacity and polarity. *Journal of Pharmaceutical Sciences* (1991). 80(6): 590–8.

Guy, R.H. and Potts, R.O. Structure-permeability relationships in percutaneous penetration. *Journal of Pharmaceutical Sciences* (1992). 81(6): 603–4.

Lipinski, C.A., Lombardo, F., Dominy, B.W., and Feeney, P.J. Experimental and computational approaches to estimate solubility and permeability in drug discovery and development settings. *Advanced Drug Delivery Reviews* (2001). 46(1–3): 3–26.

Rice, N.M., Irving, H., and Leonard, M.A. Nomenclature for liquid–liquid distribution (solvent-extraction) (IUPAC Recommendations 1993). *Pure and Applied Chemistry* (1993). 65(11): 2373–96.

REFERENCES

Bean, H., Heman-Ackah, M., and Thomas, J. The activity of antibacterials in two-phase systems. *Journal of the Society of Cosmetic Chemists* (1965). 16: 15–30.

Hansch, C. and Clayton, J.M. Lipophilic character and biological-activity of drugs. 2. Parabolic case. *Journal of Pharmaceutical Sciences* (1973). 62(1): 1–21.

McKeage *et al.* Role of lipophilicity in determining cellular uptake and antitumour activity of gold phosphine complexes. *Cancer Chemotherapy and Pharmacology* (2000). 46(5): 343–50.

Saunders, N.R., Habgood, M.D., and Dziegielewska, K.M. Barrier mechanisms in the brain, I. Adult brain. *Clinical and Experimental Pharmacology and Physiology* (1999). 26(1): 11–19.

Singh, P. and Roberts, M.S. Skin permeability and local tissue concentrations of nonsteroidal anti-inflammatory drugs after topical application. *Journal of Pharmacology and Experimental Therapeutics* (1994). 268 (1): 144–51.

Smith, J.C., Davies, M.C., Melia, C.D., Denyer, S.P., and Derrick, M.R. 1996. Uptake of drugs by catheters: the influence of the drug molecule on sorption by polyurethane catheters. *Biomaterials* (1996). 17: 1469–72.

9

Surface phenomena

IMRAN SALEEM AND ALI AL-KHATTAWI

This chapter will discuss the behaviour of molecules at interfaces. These are regions where there is a boundary between two adjacent **phases**. The interface between a solid and a gas, or a liquid and a gas, is commonly referred to as the surface (see Figure 9.1). It is important to understand the behaviour of molecules in these interfacial regions as it is different to that in the bulk of each phase. For example, imagine a beaker that contains a layer of oil above a layer of water. In this system, the water molecules beneath the oil/water boundary will behave differently to those molecules at the interface.

All physical entities, such as humans, cells, and pharmaceutical preparations, possess a boundary with their surroundings. The phenomena occurring at the boundaries can be utilized in the development of drug delivery systems. This includes the solubilization and dispersion of APIs in liquid media, understanding the stability of **suspensions** or **emulsions**, and controlling the adsorption of drugs on to different substrates, such as packaging containers.

Learning objectives

Having read this chapter you are expected to be able to:

- Understand the principles of surface phenomena and their importance in pharmaceutics.
- Know the different techniques used to measure surface tension and interfacial tension.
- Understand the role of surfactants in the formulation of different dosage forms and the development of drug delivery applications.

FIGURE 9.1 Types of interface and surface boundaries within example dosage forms

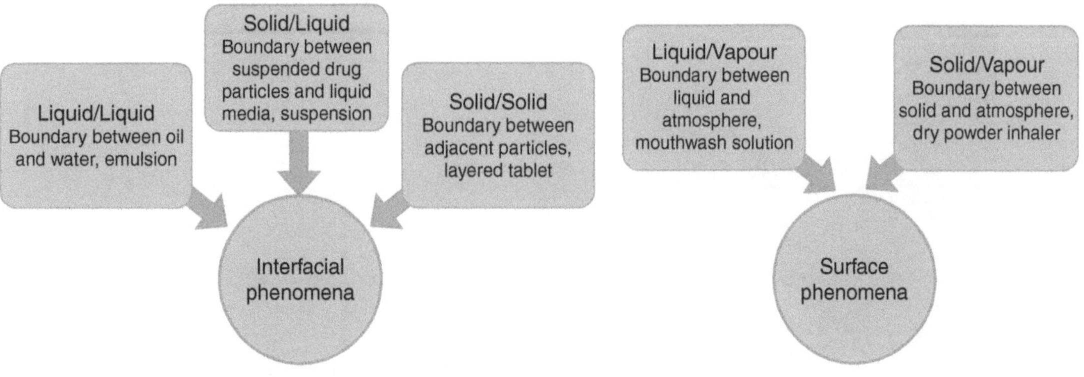

9.1 Surface and interfacial tension

We are familiar with insects, such as pond skaters (see Figure 9.2A), that are able to walk on water. It is the **surface tension** of the water that allows them to perform this function without sinking. In fact, surface tension plays an integral role in our daily lives, from washing and cleaning processes to the use of lubricants in car engines and cosmetics.

The symbol for surface tension is γ. As surface tension always arises at an interfacial region, it is common to use subscripts to identify the two adjacent phases. Thus, we might use γ_{LV} to indicate the surface tension of a liquid (L) at its interface with a vapour (V). The surface tension of water, for example, is normally measured in air and we might use γ_{LV} to represent its value. Often, however, subscripts are only used when the phases being considered are potentially ambiguous.

Liquid–gas surface tension

In the liquid state, molecules that reside in the bulk of a pure liquid are surrounded by molecules of the same kind. Thus, they experience equal attractive **cohesive forces** from all directions, resulting in no net force (see Figure 9.2B). In contrast, molecules at the surface, or liquid–gas interface, are not equally surrounded by other liquid molecules. Hence, they can only form attractive cohesive forces with molecules below or adjacent to them (see Figure 9.2B). Molecules at the liquid surface experience a force pulling them into the bulk liquid. Cohesive forces that would normally attract molecules above in the bulk liquid instead reinforce the attraction to neighbouring molecules at the interface. Consequently, surface molecules move closer together (Figure 9.2B), resulting in a contraction of the surface. The interfacial region becomes denser and is resistant to stretching or breaking. It is more difficult to move an object through the surface than the bulk liquid. It is for this reason that objects that are denser than the liquid can remain on the surface.

The **surface tension** (γ) is the force that develops across the surface at the liquid–gas interface (γ_{LV}) to prevent the surface molecules from entering the bulk liquid. It can be measured as the contracting force per unit length around the perimeter of the liquid surface. Surface tension has the units of newtons per metre ($N\,m^{-1}$) expressed in **SI units**. You may also encounter surface tension expressed in units of dyne (dyn) per centimetre, where $1\,dyn\,cm^{-1}$ is equivalent to $1\,mN\,m^{-1}$ (1 millinewton per metre).

By looking at Figure 9.3, it is possible to show why surface tension is expressed as a force per unit length. The diagram shows an n-shaped wire frame with a

FIGURE 9.2 (A) Image of a pond skater on water. © AZ/istock. (B) The intermolecular attractive forces between molecules within a liquid and on the surface of a liquid

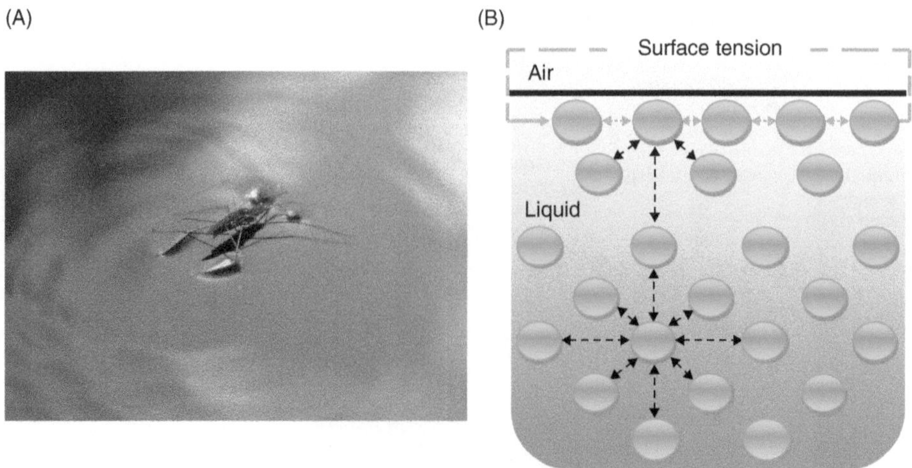

FIGURE 9.3 The pull exerted on the slider as a result of surface tension

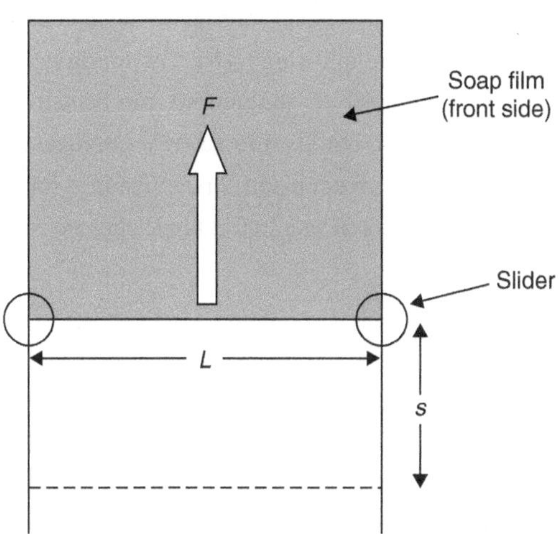

slider wire that may move freely back and forth. The frame contains a thin film of liquid formed by soap and water. The force (F) generated by the surface tension will pull the slider so that the surface area of the film is reduced to a minimum. The slider represents an interface between soap film (top) and air (bottom) and has a length of $2L$ due to the soap film having two liquid–air interfaces, at the front and back. Surface tension (γ_{LV}) depends on the length of this interfacial perimeter and the magnitude of the contracting force, equation 9.1:

$$\gamma_{LV} = \frac{F}{2L} \qquad (9.1)$$

For example, the surface tension of water at 20 °C is 72.8 mN m⁻¹. This represents a contracting force of 0.0728 newtons per metre of the surface perimeter.

Surface free energy

Each molecule in the bulk of a pure liquid is surrounded by the same kind of molecules and experiences equal attractive cohesive forces. At the liquid–gas surface boundary, however, molecules are not equally surrounded. Interactions with neighbouring molecules are limited and are weaker as a consequence. There will be, for example, reduced van der Waals (VDW) attractive forces between molecules at the surface compared to molecules in the bulk of liquid. This results in surface molecules having a higher **Gibbs free energy**, known as the surface free energy. All surfaces have a positive free energy of formation ($\Delta G > 0$). In other words, work must be done to create a new surface e.g. breaking a solid tablet in two.

For more information on van der Waals (VDW) interactions, please refer to 'Intermolecular forces' in Section 2.1 in this volume and Chapter 2 'Organic structure and bonding' of the *Pharmaceutical Chemistry* book within this series.

For more information on Gibbs free energy and work, please refer to Section 5.5.

Similarly, for liquids, work must be done to move a molecule from the inner bulk liquid to the boundary layer and increase the surface area. Consequently, energy and surface area are minimized by allowing the maximum number of surface molecules to enter the bulk of the liquid. It is for this reason that liquid droplets are spherical in shape, as a sphere has the smallest surface area per unit volume. In order to increase the surface area of the liquid, work must be done against the surface tension.

Suppose the slider in Figure 9.3 is moved to a new position depicted by the dashed line. The work, w, required to pull the slider a distance, s, against a constant force, F, is given by the equation:

$$w = Fs$$

From equation 9.1, it follows that:

$$w = \gamma_{LV}.2L.s$$

Increase in surface area, ΔA, is equal to $2L.s$:

$$w = \gamma_{LV}\Delta A$$

By rearrangement, we obtain equation 9.2:

$$\gamma = \frac{w}{\Delta A} \qquad (9.2)$$

If $\Delta A = 1\ m^2$ then w represents the surface free energy (in joules per metre squared) and this equation then shows that it has the same value as the surface tension (in newtons per metre).

KEY POINT

Molecules that exist at the liquid–gas boundary are not equally surrounded by like molecules as in bulk liquid, thus interactions with neighbouring molecules are weaker than molecules in the bulk liquid. Consequently, molecules at the boundary layer have a higher free energy compared to molecules in the bulk liquid.

KEY POINT

The higher free energy of molecules in the boundary layer is called the surface free energy. Molecules at the surface of a liquid will move into the bulk liquid until this Gibbs free energy is minimized. This in turn causes a contraction of surface, generating surface tension. The surface free energy (in joules per metre squared) has the same value as the surface tension (in newtons per metre).

SELF CHECK 9.1

Define the term surface free energy.

Liquid–liquid interfacial tension

Molecules at a liquid–liquid interface can experience attractive forces from molecules in the adjacent phase. If the attractive forces are stronger than their own, then the two phases will be **miscible** and mix together, like alcohol and water. We know from experience that some liquid pairs are **immiscible** and do not mix together, e.g. oil and water. At the boundary between the phases there will be an interfacial tension similar to surface tension, and this resists the mixing of the two liquids. By vigorous shaking, we can transform a pair of immiscible liquids into a single homogeneous phase, known as an emulsion. An emulsion is formed when tiny droplets of one liquid are dispersed in the other liquid.

For more information on emulsions please refer to 'Emulsions' in Section 10.2.

Emulsions tend to be unstable and they revert to their separate phases over time. This is the reason why medicinal emulsions, such as Oilatum®, are shaken before use. Stability can be achieved by mixing the two phases using **amphiphilic** molecules, which have an affinity for both phases due to their **hydrophobic** and **hydrophilic** components. This type of molecule is termed a surface active agent (or **surfactant**; see Section 9.5) and reduces the interfacial tension by placing itself at the interface allowing the two phases to mix.

SELF CHECK 9.2

Define the term surface tension as applied to a liquid–gas system.

SELF CHECK 9.3

Define the term interfacial tension between two liquids.

9.2 Contact angle

The **contact angle** is the angle between a liquid (L)/vapour (V) interface and a substrate (S) surface. It can be observed when a liquid drop is placed on a solid surface (Figure 9.4), the vapour phase being the surrounding air. This angle is important in understanding the behaviour of liquid pharmaceutical preparations upon contact with solid surfaces. Contact angle measurement is usually carried out in an ideal system that employs an homogenous, horizontal, and smooth solid surface.

FIGURE 9.4 Contact angle of a liquid drop on horizontal solid surface

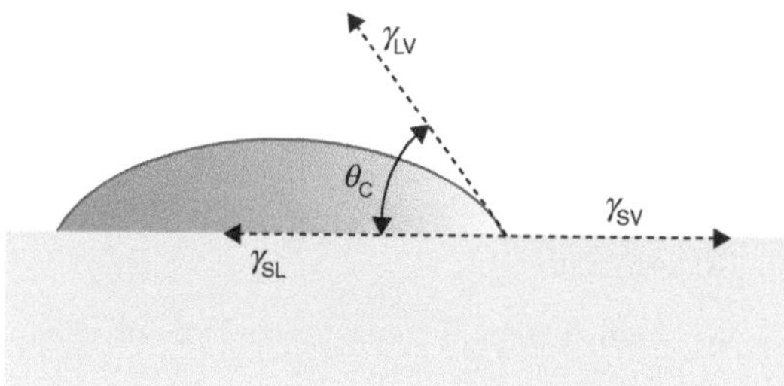

For a drop of liquid lying on an ideal substrate (Figure 9.4), the forces represented by γ_{SV}, γ_{SL}, and γ_{LV} are at equilibrium, according to Young's equation:

$$\gamma_{SV} = \gamma_{SL} + \gamma_{LV}\cos\theta \tag{9.3}$$

Remember that the force resulting from the surface tension acts around the entire interfacial perimeter, not just the cross section shown in Figure 9.4.

The work of adhesion (w_{AD}) is the energy per unit area required to separate two materials at their interface, creating two new surfaces. Separating a liquid drop from a solid surface removes the substrate–liquid (SL) interface, but creates both a liquid–air (LV) and substrate–air interface (SV). The work of adhesion between the substrate and the liquid can then be calculated using the Dupre equation:

$$w_{AD} = \gamma_{SV} + \gamma_{LV} - \gamma_{SL} \tag{9.4}$$

Combined with Young's equation, by substituting γ_{SV} from equation 9.3 into equation 9.4, we obtain the Young–Dupre equation:

$$w_{AD} = \gamma_{LV}(1+\cos\theta) \tag{9.5}$$

The **wettability** of a pharmaceutical solid material can be estimated based on the contact angle it forms with liquids such as water. **Hydrophobic** materials tend to form contact angles of more than 90° with water and are not readily wetted. **Hydrophilic** substrates form contact angles of less than 90° with water. If the contact angle value is close to zero, then the material is described as being highly wetted. For example, lactose powder is a commonly used excipient and forms a contact angle of only 30° with water. This confirms that lactose has good wettability and this is attributable to its hydrophilic structure. In contrast, the excipient magnesium stearate has a hydrophobic nature and the powder is difficult to wet, the contact angle with water being 121°.

For more information on hydrophilic and hydrophobic materials, please refer to Section 8.1.

There are various methods for determining the contact angle of powdered solids with water. Some of these techniques require that the powder is compressed into flat and smooth plates. Consequently, this may not reflect the real contact angle of the material because the compacted material could have different properties to the original powder.

Granulation is a common processing step in pharmaceutical tablet production where fine particles are converted into **granules**. It involves mixing of powder and a granulating agent, such as water, liquid glucose, or alcohol. Granulating agents must be able to adequately wet the solid particles and they can be selected by measuring the contact angle with the powder bed. A good granulating agent will give a contact angle close to zero and this may be determined using the Washburn capillary rise method. This technique does not require the compaction of powder during assessment. Instead, the measurement of wettability takes place directly using a capillary tube inserted into a wetted powder bed.

For more information on granulation, please refer to 'Compressed and layered tablets' in Section 2.5.

When **suspensions** are formulated, wetting of the powders can be complicated due to powder particles being hydrophobic. They may form large clumps or remain floating at the surface. A high interfacial tension and large contact angle value between the powder and the liquid would cause low adhesion of the hydrophobic powder. This problem can be overcome if the interfacial tension and the contact angle are decreased by using appropriate suspending agents.

For more information on suspending agents, please refer to 'Suspensions and nanosuspensions as dosage forms' in Section 10.7.

KEY POINT

Contact angle is useful in determining the wettability of solid materials and in identifying their hydrophobic or hydrophilic nature. Most hydrophobic materials form contact angles of more than 90° with water while most hydrophilic materials form contact angles of less than 90° with water.

SELF CHECK 9.4

Determine which material (a, b, or c) could be used as a wetting agent in a hydrophobic drug formulation?

(a) A material that forms contact angle of 90° with water.

(b) A material that forms contact angle of more than 90° with water.

(c) A material that forms contact angle of less than 90° with water.

9.3 Spreading of liquids

There are three possible observations when oil, a liquid (L), is placed on the surface of water, a substrate (S):

- The oil may spread as a film over the water surface (see Figure 9.5A).
- A liquid globule may form if the oil cannot spread over the water surface (see Figure 9.5B).
- A combination of the above, where a **monolayer** film may form with areas of globules on the surface. Here, the monolayer film saturates the water surface (see Figure 9.5C).

KEY POINT

A monolayer is a film that has a thickness of one molecule.

In order to spread and form a film, the forces of adhesion between oil and water molecules must be greater than the **cohesive forces** between the oil molecules. The **adhesive force** is related to the work of adhesion, w_{AD}. This is the energy required to separate a substrate (S) and liquid (L) of a unit interfacial area to form substrate–vapour and liquid–vapour interfaces (see Figure 9.6A). We can use the Dupre equation (9.4) to calculate w_{AD}.

The cohesive force between the oil molecules is related to the work, or energy, required to pull apart a volume of the spreading liquid (L) with a unit cross-sectional area to create two new liquid–air interfaces (LV) (see Figure 9.6B). Thus the work of cohesion (w_{CO}) is represented by equation 9.6:

$$w_{CO} = \gamma_{LV} + \gamma_{LV} = 2\gamma_{LV} \qquad (9.6)$$

FIGURE 9.5 Indicates two immiscible liquids representing (A) spreading of oil over water, (B) formation of globules when no spreading occurs, (C) saturation leading to monolayer film with areas of globules

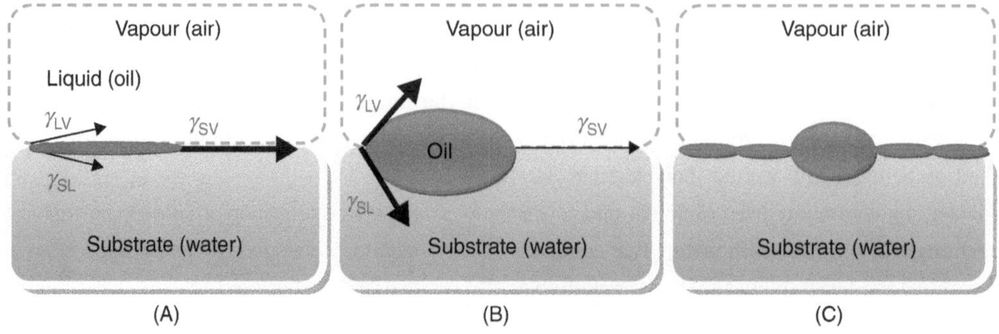

FIGURE 9.6 Represents the formation of new liquid–air interfaces with: (A) work of adhesion to separate two immiscible liquids; (B) work of cohesion to create two new surfaces

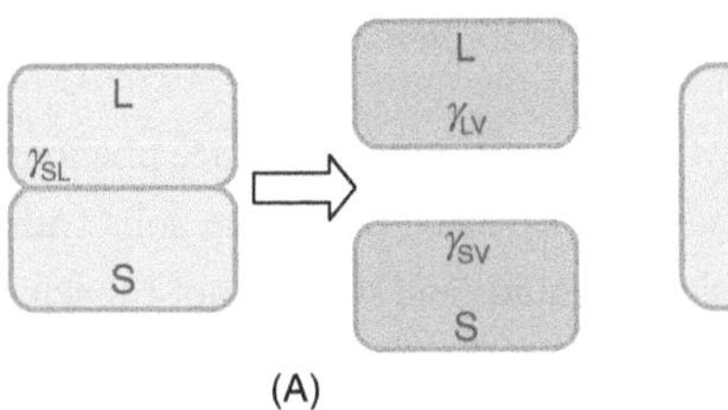

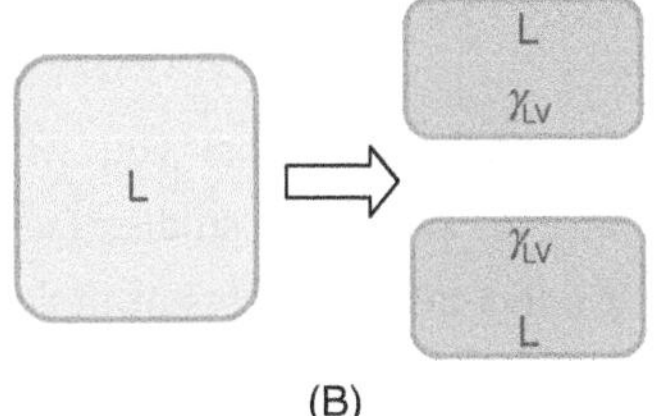

For the spreading of oil to occur over water, the forces of adhesion must be greater than the forces of cohesion. This requires that the work of adhesion must be greater than the work of cohesion. The spreading coefficient, S, is the difference between these two quantities:

$$S = w_{AD} - w_{CO} \tag{9.7}$$

By substitution of equations 9.4 and 9.6 we obtain:

$$S = \gamma_{SV} - \gamma_{LV} - \gamma_{SL} \tag{9.8}$$

If the spreading coefficient is greater than zero then spontaneous spreading will occur.

Looking at Figure 9.5A, spreading occurs ($S>0$) when the surface tension of the substrate (i.e. water, γ_{SV}) is greater than the sum of surface tension of the spreading liquid (i.e. oil, γ_{LV}) and the interfacial tension between substrate and spreading liquid (γ_{SL}). However, if $\gamma_{LV}+\gamma_{SL}$ is greater than γ_{SV}, then the oil forms a globule and does not spread across the surface of the water ($S<0$) (see Figure 9.5B).

In two-layer oil/water systems, some of the oil will dissolve in the water, and some of the water will dissolve in the oil. The spreading liquid (oil) and substrate liquid (water) will become saturated with each other over time, reducing the surface and interfacial tension. This can cause the spreading coefficient to become negative ($S<0$). Consequently, initial spreading may occur on a liquid surface, but as saturation is reached the spreading stops, leaving a monolayer film with globules in certain areas (see Figure 9.5C).

Spreading is an important concept that applies to lotions, creams, and cosmetics that are applied to the skin. To exert their effect they must spread as a thin film over the sebum, a thin oily liquid that covers the skin, which is produced by the sebaceous glands.

KEY POINT

Spreading occurs when the surface tension of the substrate (γ_{SV}, e.g. water) is greater than the sum of surface tension of the spreading liquid (γ_{LV}, e.g. oil) and the interfacial tension between substrate and spreading liquid (γ_{SL}). If ($\gamma_{LV}+\gamma_{SL}$) is greater than γ_{SV} then the oil forms a globule and does not spread across the surface of the water.

KEY POINT

At the saturation point of two liquids with some mutual solubility, the surface and interfacial tension are lowered when compared to the pure liquids. This can cause the spreading coefficient to become negative ($S<0$). Consequently, initial spreading may occur on the liquid surface, but as saturation is reached the spreading stops, leaving a monolayer film with globules in certain areas.

SELF CHECK 9.5

What conditions are required for a liquid that is immiscible in water, such as oleic acid, to spread over the surface of water?

SELF CHECK 9.6

Calculate the spreading coefficient of benzene over water, if the surface tension of water and benzene are 72.8 dyn cm^{-1} and 28.9 dyn cm^{-1}. The interfacial tension between the liquids is 35.0 dyn cm^{-1}. Does spreading occur?

SELF CHECK 9.7

Benzene and water have some mutual solubility and this lowers the surface tension of both water and benzene to 62.2 dyn cm^{-1} and 28.8 dyn cm^{-1}. The interfacial tension between the liquids is 35.0 dyn cm^{-1}. What is the value of the spreading coefficient and will spreading occur?

9.4 Adsorption

Adsorption is an important concept that you will come across throughout your pharmacy studies (see Integration Box 9.1). It refers to the process of molecules (adsorbate) binding to the surface (adsorbent) of solids and liquids. It is different to absorption, in which a molecule penetrates into the bulk of the absorbing medium, such as water being absorbed by a sponge. The process of adsorption is termed a surface phenomenon and occurs at the interface. Hence, adsorption can be understood by the application of the principles of surface tension and surface energy of the adsorbent (Section 9.1). As molecules at the surface of the adsorbent are not surrounded equally by like molecules, they attract molecules from the adsorbate, forming bonds. The type of bonds formed determines the type of adsorption:

- **Physisorption** is a reversible process utilizing weak van der Waals forces and can lead to **multilayer** adsorption.
- **Chemisorption** involves strong covalent or ionic bonds formed by the exchange of electrons between the adsorbate and adsorbent. Chemisorption only allows for **monolayer** adsorption to occur.

INTEGRATION BOX 9.1

Adsorption in pharmaceutical preparations

Containers used to package solutions have the potential to adsorb the API, reducing its concentration in solution and decreasing the dose delivered. Preservatives may also be adsorbed on to the surface of containers, leaving the preparation susceptible to microbial attack. Adsorption onto packaging is a particular problem for volatile medicines. For example, glyceryl trinitrate is a drug used to treat angina. It vaporizes at room temperature when formulated as sublingual tablets. The vapour of the drug can be adsorbed by the container, again leading to a loss of potency.

Adsorption is a surface phenomenon and it can occur between a liquid and solid. Adsorption of gases onto liquids and solids is not considered in this chapter.

For more information on adsorption of gases, please refer to 'Adsorption of gases' in Section 4.2.

Liquid–solid systems

The adsorption of a solute from a solution on to a solid surface is described by mathematical relationships such as the Langmuir and Freundlich **isotherms** (see Figure 9.7). Experimental data that follows the predictions of the Langmuir isotherm indicates the formation of a monolayer (type I behaviour). This is indicative of chemisorption on the solid surface, although the Langmuir isotherm can also be used to model physical adsorption on to solids with a fine pore structure. Freundlich isotherms indicate multilayer physical adsorption resulting from weak van der Waals forces.

KEY POINT

In adsorption, molecules of an adsorbate bind to the surface of an adsorbent. Monolayer and multilayer adsorption may occur.

FIGURE 9.7 Typical Langmuir and Freundlich adsorption isotherms

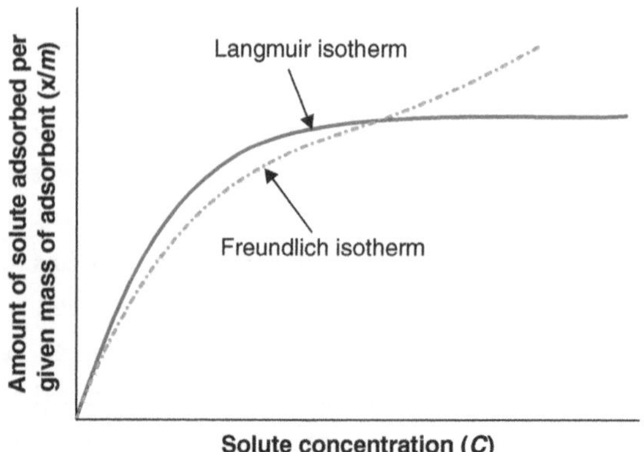

The Langmuir isotherm for solid–liquid systems is represented by equation 9.9:

$$\frac{X}{m} = \frac{abC}{1+abC} \Rightarrow \frac{X}{m} = \frac{abC}{1+bC} \tag{9.9}$$

where X is the mass of solute adsorbed, m is the mass of solid, C is the solute concentration, a is a constant relating to the amount of solute that has to be adsorbed to form a monolayer, and b is a constant relating to the enthalpy of adsorption.

This is generally rearranged into a linear equation as represented by equation 9.10:

$$C/(X/m) = \frac{1}{ab} + \frac{C}{a} \tag{9.10}$$

Plotting a graph of $C/(X/m)$ against concentration (C) will produce a straight line and the constants a and b can be determined from the intercept, $1/ab$, and slope, $1/a$.

The Freundlich isotherm for solid–liquid systems is shown in equation 9.11:

$$\frac{X}{m} = KC^{1/n} \tag{9.11}$$

where K and n are empirical constants for each adsorbent–adsorbate pair at a given temperature.

Once again, the equation can be rearranged to produce a linear equation 9.12:

$$\log\frac{X}{m} = \log K + \frac{1}{n}\log C \tag{9.12}$$

Plotting log (X/m) against log C should produce a straight line with log K representing the intercept and $1/n$ the slope.

Multilayer adsorption may not always be modelled by the Freundlich isotherm. Thus, sigmoidal isotherms (Type II behaviour) are better modelled using the Brunauer-Emmett-Teller (BET) equation. There are several factors that affect the adsorption of solute from solution and they include the following:

- Solubility: There is an inverse relationship between the solubility of a solute in solution with its adsorption onto a solid surface. The solubility of an acid or base is affected by the pH of the solution, which affects its degree of ionization. In aqueous solution, unionized drugs have low solubility and thus a higher degree of surface adsorption.
- Temperature: Adsorption is exothermic and, in accordance with **Le Chatelier's principle**, lowering the temperature will enhance the surface adsorption.

For more information on type II isotherms, please refer to 'Adsorption' in Section 4.2.

- Surface area: The extent of adsorption of the adsorbate is directly proportional to the surface area of the adsorbent. Hence, for maximum adsorption to occur we want the adsorbent of a given mass to have maximum surface area. The surface area of the adsorbent could be increased by reducing the particle size or making particles porous.

These principles can be used in the design of **dosage forms**. An example of this is in the use of activated charcoal as an antidote to poisoning. The adsorption of toxic substances to the carbon surface is improved by increasing the surface area per gram of charcoal. The term 'activated' relates to the process by which carbon is processed to produce a highly porous material. Around 15 grams of activated carbon has a surface area equivalent to a football pitch.

KEY POINT

The correlation of experimental data with the Langmuir isotherm indicates the formation of a monolayer on the solid surface and this is indicative of chemisorption. Systems that follow the Freundlich isotherm generally involve multilayer physical adsorption through weak van der Waals forces.

SELF CHECK 9.8

State the difference between adsorption and absorption.

SELF CHECK 9.9

State the difference between **physisorption** and chemisorption.

9.5 Surfactants

Surface active agents are more commonly known as **surfactants** and are molecules or ions that have affinity for both **polar and non-polar solvents**. These substances are generally stable at the interface between two immiscible solvents, having both **hydrophilic** ('water-loving') and **hydrophobic** ('water-hating') or **lipophilic** ('lipid-loving') characteristics (see Figure 9.8). The hydrophobic portion, or 'tail', of a surfactant molecule is usually composed of a hydrocarbon chain. The nature of the hydrophilic 'head' can be used to classify the agent:

- Non-ionic surfactants (no charge). Common examples fall in to three main categories and their uses are dependent on the hydrophile–lipophile balance (see later in this section):
  (a) Sorbitan esters (Spans) have low solubility in water, e.g. Span 20.
  (b) Polysorbates (Tweens) have good solubility in water, e.g. Tween 80.
  (c) Poloxamers (Pluronics) consist of both hydrophobic and hydrophilic chains. The ratio of the chain lengths dictates the physical state of pluronics (solid, liquid, or paste). This class of surfactants tend to be used as emulsifiers or wetting agents during preparation of microparticles or nanoparticles.
- Cationic surfactants (positively charged). Quaternary ammonium cationic surfactants are used in a wide range of pharmaceutical preparations due to their bactericidal activity against Gram–ve and some Gram+ve organisms. For this reason, they are often used in wound cleaning preparations and as preservatives in pharmaceutical formulations, most notably in eye preparations. A common example is benzalkonium chloride.

For more information on quaternary ammonium cationic surfactants, please refer to Chapter 5 'Alcohols, phenols, ethers, organic halogen compounds, and amines' of the *Pharmaceutical Chemistry* book within this series.

- Anionic surfactants (negatively charged). Sodium lauryl sulphate (SLS) is an example of an anionic surfactant and it is also known as sodium dodecyl sulphate (SDS). It is commonly used in preoperative skin cleaner preparations, due to its antibacterial (bacteriostatic) activity against Gram+ve bacteria, and it is also found in medicated shampoos. SLS is used in some encapsulation techniques and can improve the uniformity of gelatin capsules during manufacture.

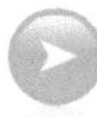

For more information about sodium lauryl sulphate, please refer to Chapter 8 'Inorganic chemistry in pharmacy' of the *Pharmaceutical Chemistry* book within this series.

- Zwitterionic surfactants (**zwitterions** are both positively and negatively charged).

For more information on zwitterions, please refer to 'Zwitterions' in Section 6.5.

At gas–liquid interfaces, surfactants will arrange themselves at the surface of a polar liquid to minimize the exposure of the hydrophobic parts of the surfactant to the liquid. Similarly, surfactants will orientate themselves at the interface between two immiscible liquids such that the hydrophobic tail is associated with the non-polar (typically organic) phase, and hydrophilic head is associated with the polar (typically aqueous) phase. The associated reduction in interfacial tension may lead to the formation of an emulsion and is important for the action of soap (Box 9.1).

For more information on emulsions, please refer to 'Emulsions' in Section 10.2.

FIGURE 9.8 The components of a single surfactant molecule

Hydrophilic head

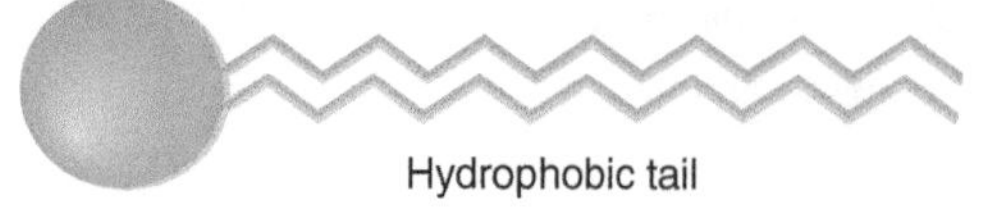

Hydrophobic tail

BOX 9.1

The action of soap

Modern soap is a combination of germicidal materials (which kill the bacteria and germs) and surfactants. The surfactants reduce the surface tension of the solution, which help it to spread efficiently into the minute crevices and spaces of the object being disinfected. This increases the concentration of the germicidal materials on the cell walls of bacteria.

The chemical structure of a surfactant determines its surface activity. In simple terms, an increase in the length of the hydrocarbon tail leads to an increase in surface activity, i.e. a greater reduction of surface tension is recorded. Traube's rule states that for a homologous series of surface active agents in water, the concentration of surfactant required to yield a particular surface tension is inversely proportional to 3^n, where n is the number of CH_2 groups in the hydrocarbon chain. Thus, the potency of a surfactant is increased by a factor of three for each additional methylene group in the tail.

Surfactants are found naturally in the alveoli of human lungs. Phospholipoprotein complexes form a lining over a liquid layer present in the alveoli and function to reduce the interfacial tension between the liquid–air interface, protecting the alveoli from collapse during expiration.

Hydrophile–lipophile balance (HLB) classification

Surfactants have various applications in the pharmaceutical industry as solubilizing, emulsifying, wetting, and spreading agents, depending on the balance between their hydrophilic and hydrophobic regions. The hydrophile–lipophile balance (HLB) classification is an arbitrary scale that records the relative hydrophilic–hydrophobic character of surfactants. From the scale shown in Figure 9.9 you can clearly see that an increase in HLB value is related to the material being more hydrophilic and *vice versa*.

Table 9.1 lists some important examples of surfactants used in pharmaceutical formulations. Span 20 is used as a wetting agent because of its low HLB value.

FIGURE 9.9 Classification of surfactants according to HLB scale

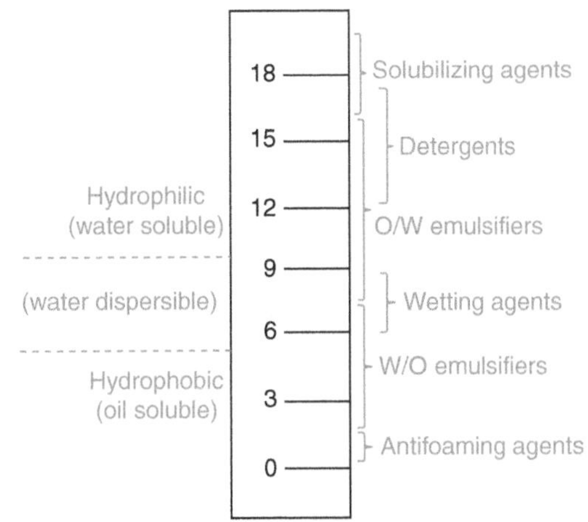

TABLE 9.1 Selected surfactant molecules and their HLB values

Compound	HLB
Sodium oleate	18.0
Polysorbate 20 (Tween 20)	16.7
Polyethylene glycol 400 monolaurate	13.1
Sorbitan monolaurate (Span 20)	8.6
Sorbitan monooleate (Span 80)	4.3
Oleic acid	1.0

In contrast, a material such as Tween 20 has a high HLB value and is used as a detergent.

Micelles

The behaviour of surfactants in a liquid is dependent on their concentration. As this rises, the number of surfactant molecules at the interfacial region gradually increases until it becomes saturated. After this point, any more added surfactant molecules will aggregate to form spherical structures called **micelles** (see Integration Box 9.2). In aqueous solution, micelles form to shield hydrophobic tails from the surrounding water molecules (Figure 9.10). The minimum concentration at which micelles start to form is referred to as the **critical micelle concentration (CMC)** and it is evident in a plot of solution surface tension versus surfactant concentration (Figure 9.11). Below the CMC,

FIGURE 9.10 **Micelles formation upon increasing surfactant concentration in solution**

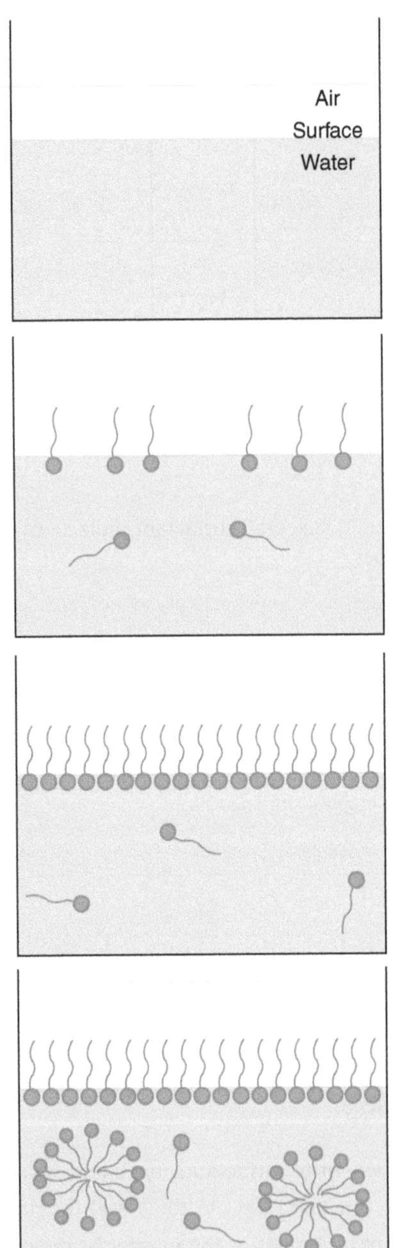

FIGURE 9.11 **Plot of solution surface tension versus surfactant concentration**

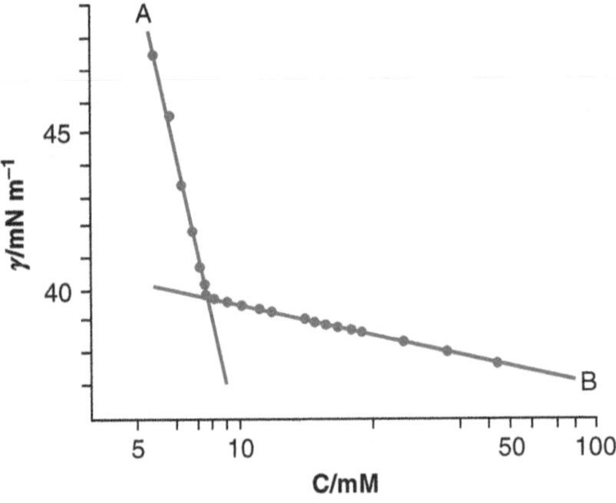

surface tension decreases as the surfactant concentration increases. Above the CMC, the surface tension shows little further change.

The CMC can also be observed in other solvents, aside from water. In a non-polar organic medium, reverse micelles can form where the hydrophilic heads of the surfactant molecules position themselves into the core of the micelle, with the hydrophobic tails on the outside.

INTEGRATION BOX 9.2

Micelles and their applications in drug delivery

Pharmaceutical scientists have tried attaching different molecules and chemical groups to the surface of micelles to deliver drugs to their targets in the human body. Targeting molecules, such as folate residues, have been attached to the surface of drug-loaded micelles. These micelles can deliver anticancer drugs to cancerous cells, which over-express receptors to folate residues. The increased specificity of targeting may enhance the outcome of treatment, as well as reducing the toxicity to normal tissues.

Liposomes

Liposomes are surfactant-based vesicles formed mostly from phospholipids, which have a phosphate hydrophilic head group and a hydrophobic tail. They have been investigated as drug delivery vehicles since the 1960s. In comparison to micelles, liposomes have one or multiple lipid bilayers, whereas micelles have a monolayer. Look at Figure 9.12, which shows the structure of a liposome.

Liposomes have gained considerable interest in drug-delivery research and pharmaceutics, as they have a similar bilayer structure to that of cell walls. Accordingly, they could be used to transfer drug molecules into cellular targets and would have enhanced

FIGURE 9.12 Liposome

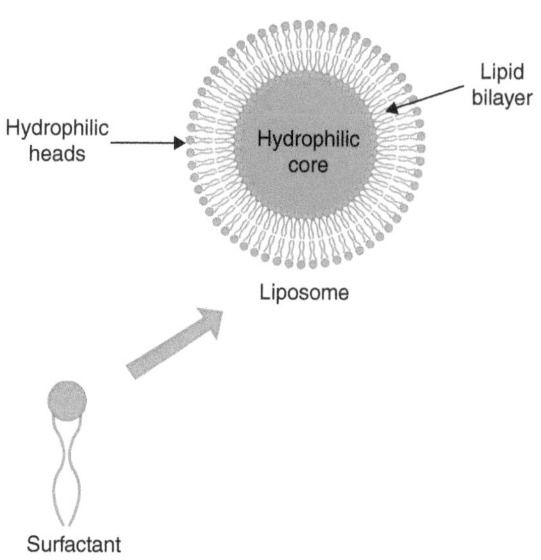

TABLE 9.2 Examples of liposomal formulations available in the market

Trade Name	Drug	Indication
Myocet	Doxorubicin	Breast cancer
AmBisome	Amphotericin B	Antifungal Infections
Epaxal	Inactivated hepatitis A virus	Hepatitis A vaccine

From Perrie and Rades (2010).

permeability into cells. The uses of liposomes as anticancer agents, and as carriers of DNA molecules and genes within vaccines, have been investigated.

Liposomes are a flexible delivery system. Thus, hydrophilic drugs can be entrapped in the hydrophilic core, while hydrophobic drugs can be embedded in the hydrophobic bilayer. Most of the liposome formulations available in the market are administered via the **intravenous** route (IV), while few of them are available in other forms. Examples of liposomal formulations are given in Table 9.2.

KEY POINT

Surfactants can be utilized in drug delivery as they form systems such as micelles and liposomes. Surfactant-based delivery systems can be used for different objectives, such as improving the solubility of hydrophobic drugs, masking the taste of bitter-tasting drugs, or delivering biomolecules and proteins, which are easily degraded in gastrointestinal tract (GIT) if unprotected.

9.6 Surface charge and zeta potential

Adsorption at the surface is a key process in determining the behaviour and stability of dispersed particles, including colloidal systems such as nanosuspensions. If dispersed particles possess a negatively charged surface in solution, positive ions will adsorb strongly on to the negative surface to form a dense layer called the Stern layer. Once this adsorption is complete, free ions (cations and anions) create a diffuse layer around the Stern layer called the Gouy–Chapman layer. These two layers contribute to the electrical double layer and this is represented in Figure 9.13.

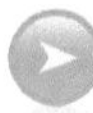
For more information on colloidal systems, please refer to 'Colloidal dispersions' in Section 10.1.

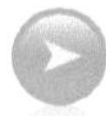
For more information on nanosuspensions, please refer to 'Suspensions and nanosuspensions as dosage forms' in Section 10.7.

When two charged colloidal particles approach each other in an aqueous medium, an electrostatic repulsion force is generated as a result of the particles' electrical double layers. Whether particles are able to form stable associations will depend on the balance of these repulsive electrostatic forces and the attractive van der Waals forces between particles. This can be quantitatively understood by using DLVO theory.

For more information on DLVO theory, please refer to Section 10.8.

FIGURE 9.13 The electrical double layer surrounding a negatively charged colloidal particle

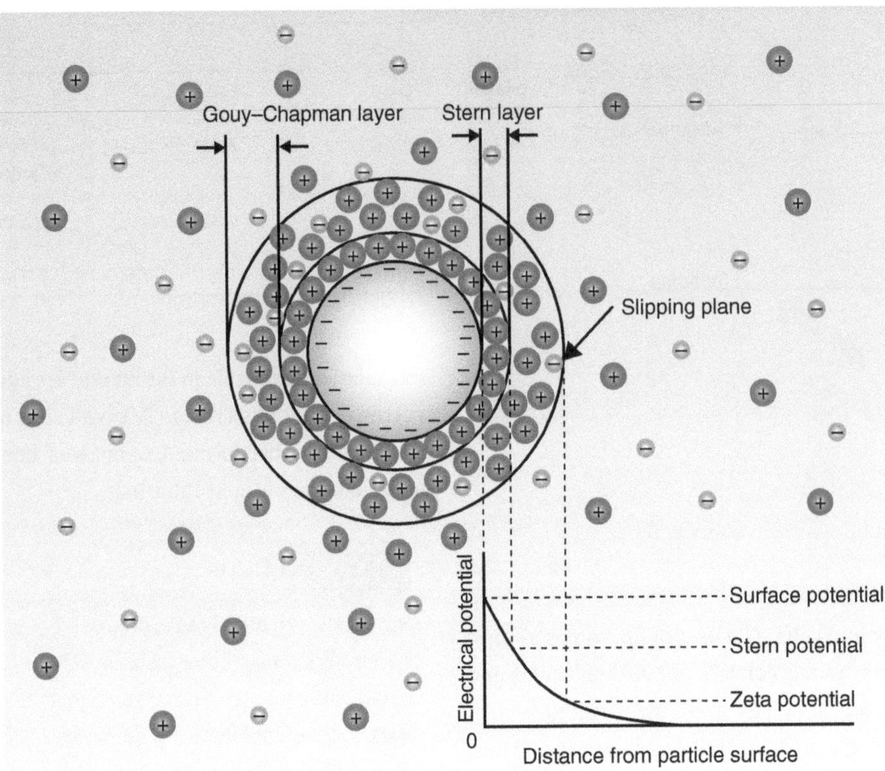

Attractive van der Waals forces are always present between particles. Therefore, to prepare a stable colloidal dispersion it is necessary to introduce repulsive interactions between particles that oppose attractive forces. The most common way to do this is to enhance the electrical potential of the double layer by adding ionic surfactants or polymers that adsorb onto the surface. It is also possible to achieve particle stabilization by coating particles with long, non-ionic polymer chains. Particles will then have reduced tendency to associate due to a steric repulsive force (Box 9.2). A combination of the two mechanisms is also possible, so-called electrosteric stabilization.

The electrical potential within the electrical double layer has the maximum value on the particle surface, or Stern layer (Figure 9.13). This potential drops with increasing distance from the surface and reaches zero at the boundary of the electrical double layer. When a colloidal particle moves in the dispersion medium, a layer of the surrounding liquid remains attached to the particle. The outer surface of this layer is called the slipping plane and it represents the outer boundary of the Gouy–Chapman layer.

The value of the electric potential at the slipping plane is called the **zeta potential** (ζ). It is a very

BOX 9.2

Origin of the steric repulsion force

The steric repulsion force is predominantly entropic in origin. As two polymer-coated domains come close together, the long chains adsorbed on one particle will interpenetrate into those adsorbed onto the neighbouring particle. Interpenetration results in the polymer chains losing entropy and this is not a favourable process, being manifest as a repulsive force. In a similar fashion, wriggling the fingers on your hands represents a high entropy state. However, clasping your hands together by interlocking your fingers restricts their freedom and represents a lower entropy state.

important parameter in the theory of interaction of colloidal particles as it is related to the strength of the electrostatic repulsion force between particles. Zeta potential has applications in the research and development of new drugs and dosage forms. In general, formulations that have high zeta potentials are more stable as their particles tend to aggregate less because of the high electrostatic repulsion forces between them. In practice, zeta potential can be measured indirectly using suitable analysers to determine the stability of the prepared formulations. Colloidal formulations with zeta potentials less than 5 millivolts (mV) will rapidly flocculate and are unstable, while those with zeta potentials greater than 30 mV are generally considered to be stable.

For more information on flocculation, please refer to 'Flocculation' in Section 10.5.

KEY POINT

Measuring the zeta potential of liquid pharmaceutical formulations can be helpful in determining the stability of these systems. It is important that the pharmaceutical formulations have adequate stability to withstand storage conditions.

SELF CHECK 9.10

What happens to the electrical potential around a particle in a liquid medium with increasing the distance away from the particle?

9.7 Gibbs adsorption isotherm

In 1878, Gibbs derived an equation to calculate the amount of surfactant adsorbed on the surface of a liquid, or at the interface between two immiscible liquids. The equation can be used to predict how surface tension varies with the concentration of surfactant and the Gibbs' adsorption isotherm is shown (equation 9.13):

$$\frac{d\gamma}{d(\ln C)} = -RT\,\Gamma \qquad (9.13)$$

where $d\gamma/d\ln C$ is the rate of change of surface tension of the solution with the natural log of surfactant concentration in the bulk of the liquid, Γ is the surface concentration of the surfactant per unit area of the surface (mol m^2), R is the **gas constant** (which has a value of 8.314 J K^{-1} mol^{-1}), and T is the **absolute temperature** in kelvin (K).

The negative sign in equation 9.13 indicates that surface tension is anticipated to decrease with an increase in surfactant concentration, in accordance with experimental observation, Figure 9.11. We may define Γ_{Max} as the maximum surfactant concentration at the surface, or saturation point.

Gibbs derived his equation theoretically. However, scientists have quantitatively validated the equation practically using a microtome. This instrument is capable of cutting a thin layer on the surface of a liquid to enable the determination of surfactant concentration. The results obtained are very close to the values calculated from Gibbs' equation which was proposed years before the microtome was introduced.

KEY POINT

Surface tension decreases when surfactants are added to a liquid phase.

KEY POINT

Surfactants normally arrange themselves at the surface or interface, however, if their concentration is increased, the surface or interface becomes saturated leading to formation of micelles.

SELF CHECK 9.11

As surfactant concentration is increased, what is reached first, Γ_{Max} or the CMC?

9.8 Measurement of surface and interfacial tension

There are several approaches that can be used to determine surface or interfacial tension. Here we will describe four of the most commonly used methods. These are:

- Drop weight or drop volume.
- Capillary rise.
- Wilhelmy plate.
- Du Noüy ring.

In addition, there are other methods such as bubble pressure, pendant drop, and sessile drop. There is no single optimum method, but certain considerations need to be taken into account such as:

- Whether surface or interfacial tension is to be measured.
- The accuracy required.
- The size of the sample to be analysed.
- Whether the effect of time on surface tension is to be investigated.

Another important consideration is temperature. The surface tension of most liquids is inversely proportional to temperature, i.e. as temperature increases the surface tension decreases (see Figure 9.14). This gives more effective wetting (Section 9.2) and is one reason, for example, why hot water is used for cleaning rather than cold water. The literature values for surface/interfacial tension of pure liquids always quote the temperature of the reference liquid, e.g. the surface tension of water is 72.8 mN m^{-1} at 20 °C, while it is 71.9 m Nm^{-1} at 25 °C. In fact, water has one of the highest surface tensions and is only exceeded by mercury, which has a surface tension of 486.5 m Nm^{-1} at 20 °C and 485.5 m Nm^{-1} at 25 °C.

FIGURE 9.14 The effect of temperature on the surface tension of water

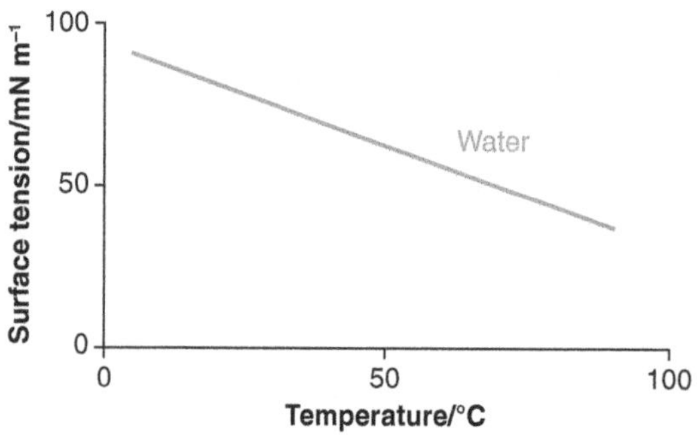

Drop weight or drop volume method

The surface or interfacial tension can be determined from the volume or weight of a liquid droplet falling from an aperture of known radius. Figure 9.15 A shows a typical experimental set-up. It is important that the drop should be formed slowly and that the tip of the dropper is completely wetted by the liquid under analysis to eliminate the drop climbing up the outside of the tip. Equation 9.14 is used to calculate the surface or interfacial tension:

$$\gamma = \frac{\phi mg}{2\pi r} = \frac{\phi V \rho g}{2\pi r} \tag{9.14}$$

where γ is the surface or interfacial tension (N m^{-1}), r is the radius of the tip (m), m is the mass of the drop (kg), V is the volume of the drop (m^3), g is the gravitational constant (9.81 ms^{-2}), ρ is the density of the liquid (kg m^{-3}), and ϕ is a correction factor.

The correction factor is required as not all the drop will leave the tip. It is dependent on the apparatus and is determined by using the experimental set-up with liquids of known density and surface tension.

Capillary rise method

If a uniform circular glass tube is placed in water, the liquid will rise a certain distance up the inside of the tube. The liquid molecules experience strong

FIGURE 9.15 (A) Measuring surface tension using drop weight or drop volume method. (B) Measuring surface tension using capillary rise method; h represents the height to which liquids rise inside a glass tube due to capillary action. (C) An example of a liquid that forms a convex meniscus in a capillary tube

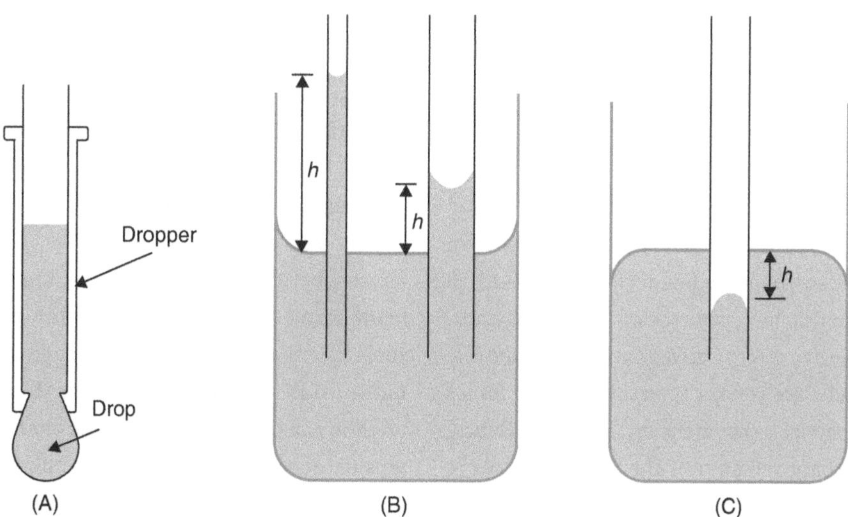

cohesive forces between each other and **adhesive forces** with unlike molecules. In the example shown in Figure 9.15B, the adhesive forces between the molecules of liquid and the walls of the tube are stronger than the cohesive forces between the molecules of water. This leads to the liquid wetting the inside surface of the tube, spreading over it and contributing to capillary action.

Capillary action is the result of adhesion and surface tension. Adhesion of liquid to the walls of a uniform circular tube will cause an upward force on the liquid at the edges and result in a concave **meniscus**. The surface tension acts to hold the surface intact, so instead of only the edges moving upward, the whole liquid surface is dragged upward. Capillary action will always occur when the adhesion to the walls is stronger than the cohesive forces between the liquid molecules.

The height to which capillary action will raise a liquid in a uniform circular tube depends upon both the mass and the surface tension of the liquid. Since capillary rise method is weight limited, the liquid will rise higher in a tube with a smaller diameter (see Figure 9.15B). This can be predicted by equation 9.15, which is derived in Box 9.3:

$$h = \frac{2\gamma}{r\rho g} \text{ or } \gamma = \frac{rh\rho g}{2} \tag{9.15}$$

BOX 9.3

Derivation of capillary rise method equation

The upwards force moving the liquid up in the capillary tube is given by the equation:

$$\text{Upwards force} = 2\pi r\gamma \cos\theta$$

where r is the radius of the capillary, γ is the surface tension and θ is the contact angle between the surface of the liquid and capillary wall (Section 9.2).

The downwards force caused by gravity is given by the equation:

$$\text{Downwards force} = \pi r^2 h\rho g$$

Where h is the height of liquid in the capillary and g is the gravitational constant.

At equilibrium, the upwards force and the downwards force are equal. At this point, the level of liquid in the capillary tube will neither rise nor fall and we may write:

$$2\pi r\gamma \cos\theta = \pi r^2 h\rho g$$

For most liquids at equilibrium, θ equals zero and $\cos\theta$ equals 1 so that this term can be ignored.

By simplification:

$$2\gamma = rh\rho g$$

$$h = \frac{2\gamma}{r\rho g} \text{ or } \gamma = \frac{rh\rho g}{2}$$

where :

- h=height (m)
- γ=surface tension ($N m^{-1}$)
- ρ=density of the liquid ($kg m^{-3}$)
- r=radius of the tube (m)
- g=gravitational constant ($9.81 m s^{-2}$)

A convex meniscus will form when the height of liquid inside a uniform circular capillary tube is lower than the level of the surrounding liquid (see Figure 9.15C). The liquid metal, mercury, shows this behaviour. Here, the adhesive forces between the liquid and the walls of the tube are weaker than the cohesive forces between the particles that make up the liquid. Hence, the liquid does not spread over the inside surfaces of the tube.

Wilhelmy plate method

The Wilhelmy plate method can be used to measure both surface and interfacial tension. The apparatus consists of a thin plate, such as a glass microscope slide or a platinum plate, suspended from a balance (see Figure 9.16A). The plate is placed vertically so that it touches the surface of the liquid. The surface of the plate is wetted and a liquid meniscus forms around its perimeter. The force required to pull the plate from the surface is proportional to the surface tension of the liquid, the length and thickness of the plate used (equation 9.16).

$$F = 2(L+T)\gamma \text{ or } \gamma = \frac{F}{2(L+T)} \quad (9.16)$$

where F is the force required to pull the plate from the surface (N), γ is the surface tension of the liquid ($N m^{-1}$), L is the length of plate used (m), and T is the thickness of plate used (m).

It is also possible to determine the interfacial tension between two immiscible liquids, the plate being immersed so as to touch the interface. The surface of the plate is normally rough so that the liquid spreads readily over the plate. In addition, this method can be used to determine changes in surface tension over time, by measuring the force required to keep the plate at a constant depth. This is useful for assessing the stability of emulsions which tend to separate to their original phases over time through **coalescence**.

Du Noüy ring method

This method is used to measure both surface and interfacial tension. It employs a platinum–iridium ring connected to a microbalance (see Figure 9.16B). Similar to the Wilhelmy method, the ring is brought into contact with the liquid surface or interface. The force required to detach the ring is proportional to the

FIGURE 9.16 Measuring surface tension using (A) the Wilhelmy plate method (B) the Du Noüy ring method

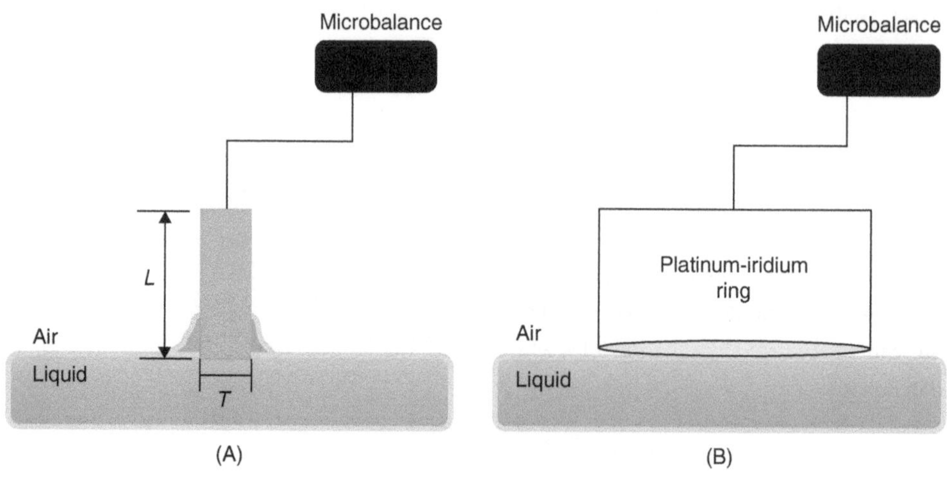

surface or interfacial tension, as represented using the equation 9.17:

$$\gamma = \frac{F\beta}{2(R1 + R2)} \tag{9.17}$$

where F is the force required to detach the ring (N), γ is the surface or interfacial tension ($N\,m^{-1}$), $R1$ is the inner radius of the ring (m), $R2$ is the outer radius of the ring (m), and β is a correction factor.

A correction factor is required as the equation does not take into account the volume of liquid lifted by the wire ring or the cross-sectional shape of the wire. Standard solutions with known surface tension are chosen to determine the correction factor, and values can be found in the International Critical Tables.

The du Noüy ring method has the following disadvantages:

- The platinum–iridium ring is prone to shape changes even from gentle impact, which can affect the measurements being performed.
- It is difficult to obtain accurate surface tension measurements for liquids with high viscosity.
- The apparatus is not suited to determining changes in surface tension over time.

SELF CHECK 9.12

Using the capillary rise method, calculate the surface tension of methanol which rose to a height of 3.42 cm at 20 °C in a capillary tube with an inside diameter of 0.2 mm? The density of methanol at 20 °C is 0.7914 g cm^{-3}.

SELF CHECK 9.13

Briefly state how capillary action causes a liquid to rise up a uniform circular tube.

SELF CHECK 9.14

Why does mercury form a convex meniscus in a glass capillary?

SELF CHECK 9.15

How is the correction factor determined in the du Noüy ring method?

CHAPTER SUMMARY

- When two phases are adjacent, a boundary exists between them. The boundary formed between two phases of solid–solid, solid–liquid, or liquid–liquid is generally termed the interface, while the boundary between solid–air or liquid–air is termed surface.
- The molecules existing at the boundary layer are not surrounded by like molecules from all sides, and hence have different properties to molecules within the bulk material.
- These different properties relate to cohesive forces between molecules at the boundary layer. This prevents surface molecules from moving into the bulk material and is termed surface or interfacial tension.
- Molecules at the boundary layer have a higher Gibbs free energy compared to molecules in the bulk liquid and this is called the surface free energy.
- The surface free energy (in joules per metre squared) is so defined that it has the same value as the surface tension (in newtons per metre).
- The contact angle is the angle between a liquid (L)–vapour (V) interface and a substrate (S) surface.
- Spreading occurs when the surface tension of the substrate (e.g. water) is greater than the sum of surface tension of the spreading liquid (e.g. oil) and the interfacial tension between substrate and spreading liquid.

- Adsorption refers to the process of molecules (adsorbate) binding to the surface (adsorbent) of solids and liquids.
- Physisorption is a reversible process utilizing weak van der Waals forces and can lead to multilayer adsorption
- Chemisorption involves strong covalent or ionic bonds formed and only monolayer adsorption can occur.
- Surfactant molecules can have different pharmaceutical applications depending on their HLB values.
- Micelles and liposomes are useful as drug delivery vehicles due to their surfactant-based nature composed of both hydrophilic and hydrophobic parts.
- An electrical double layer is formed when a solid particle in immersed in a liquid and it represents the arrangement of positive and negative charges around the particle surface. The electrical potential formed is called zeta potential which can be employed to predict the stability of a pharmaceutical suspension.
- A number of techniques may be used to measure surface and interfacial tension.

FURTHER READING

Adamson, A.W. *Physical Chemistry of Surfaces*, (6th edn). New York: John Wiley & Sons, Inc. (1997).

This book provides a thorough account of the basics in liquid–gas and liquid–solid interface physical chemistry, with details of measuring surface tension by various methods.

Erbil, H. *Surface Chemistry of Solid and Liquid Interfaces*. Chichester: John Wiley & Sons, Ltd, (2006).

This book provides a concise introduction to the subject area associated with solid and liquid interfaces.

Malmsten, M. *Surfactants and Polymers in Drug Delivery*. New York: Marcel Dekker, (2002).

This book features the physicochemical aspects of surfactants and polymers which are important in drug delivery such as micellar systems, block copolymers, liposomes, and microemulsions.

Rosen, M.J. and Kunjappu, J.T. *Surfactants and Interfacial Phenomena*, (4th edn). Hoboken: John Wiley & Sons, Inc. (2012).

This book contains detailed information of the different types of surfactants based on their charge and chemical structure; it also explains concepts such as electrical double layer and Gibbs' adsorption equation.

REFERENCE

Perrie, Y. and Rades, T. *Carriers for Drug Targeting*, in *Pharmaceutics—Drug Delivery and Targeting*, London: Pharmaceutical Press, (2010).

10

Disperse systems

JAYNE LAWRENCE

Dosage forms that consist of two or more gases are always single-phase systems. Other types of mixtures involving solids, liquids, and gases can also be homogenous. Thus, solid sodium carbonate will dissolve in liquid water to yield a colourless solution that may be used as an antacid. Magnesium hydroxide is also a solid and, like sodium carbonate, is used in the treatment of indigestion. However, when magnesium hydroxide is added to water, a suspension is obtained because the solid has limited aqueous solubility. The resulting mixture is a white liquid and is sold over the counter as 'milk of magnesia' (Figure 10.1A). Two-phase systems consisting of a liquid phase and suspended solid particles are an example of a disperse system.

An understanding of disperse systems can help us to control their physical properties so that they are appropriate to specific formulations. For example, the solid particles in milk of magnesia tend to settle to the bottom of the container under the influence of gravity and this is not ideal. Some suspensions show little tendency to settle, however, an example being blood, which is revealed to consist of more than one phase only after centrifugation (Figure 10.1B). A dispersion of sodium carbonate in water would never separate in this way as it is a true solution. We will see that we can understand the behaviour of suspensions in terms of the characteristics of the dispersed phase. Dispersions are not just limited to solid in liquid suspensions, however, and we will we encounter solid, semi-solid, liquid, and gaseous vehicles that can deliver active pharmaceutical ingredients (APIs).

FIGURE 10.1 (A) Milk of magnesia, an example of a disperse system formed by a solid dispersed phase and a liquid continuous phase (B) Blood before and after centrifugation
Source: (A) copyright Alice Mumford.

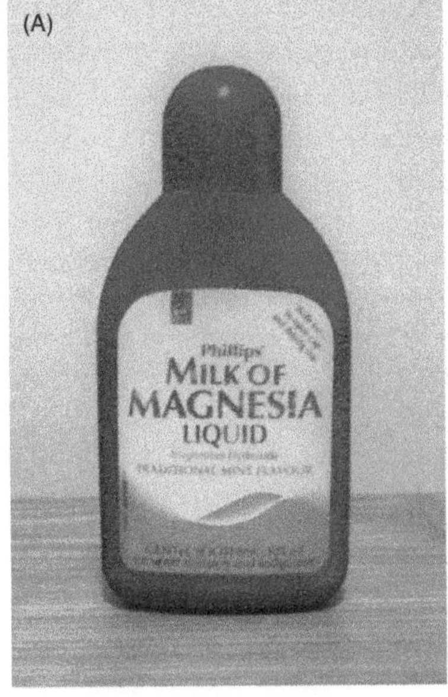

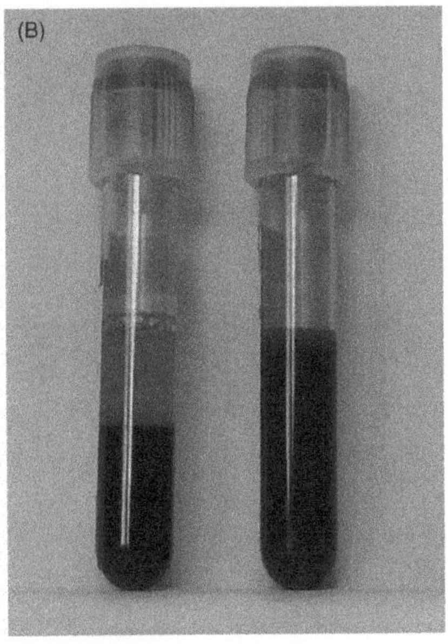

Learning objectives

Having read this chapter you are expected to be able to:

- Describe a disperse system and be able to differentiate between a colloidal and coarse dispersion.
- Name the types of disperse system that may be formed from combinations of solid, liquid, and gas.
- Appreciate the role of stabilizing agents in the preparation of dispersions.
- Outline the top-down and bottom-up approaches used in the preparation of dispersions.
- State some of the principal properties of dispersions and how they are dependant on the composition of the system.
- Understand why some types of dispersion are unstable and identify general approaches that may be used to stabilize dispersions.
- Know how the various types of dispersions are used in pharmacy for the purposes of drug delivery.

10.1 Classifications of disperse systems

A number of dosage forms are disperse systems and they can be classified according to the size of the **domains** in the dispersed (or internal) phase. There are three types (Figure 10.2):

- Coarse dispersions.
- Colloidal dispersions.
- Molecular dispersions.

In each of these classifications, the continuous phase may be variously referred to as the external phase, dispersion medium, or vehicle. Coarse or colloidal dispersions may also be classified as **monodisperse** or **polydisperse**, depending on the distribution of particles sizes in the dispersed phase (Figure 10.2).

Dispersions can also be classified according to their physical stability and this may be thermodynamic or kinetic in origin:

- A thermodynamically stable dispersion has a negative **Gibbs** free energy of formation. As the free energy of the dispersion is lower than the separate phases, it has no tendency to breakdown.
- A kinetically stable dispersion is one that is not thermodynamically stable. However, the rate of breakdown is small and the system will persist in a largely unchanged form for long periods (perhaps months).
- An unstable dispersion is one that has neither thermodynamic nor kinetic stability.

It is worth emphasizing that we will use these descriptions to refer to physical stability. Pharmaceutical dispersions are formulated to have a high chemical stability and their chemical composition generally remains constant during their lifetime.

Coarse dispersions

Coarse dispersions have dispersed phase domains with sizes greater than 1000 nm (or 1 μm). They are physically unstable when the continuous phase is a liquid or gas, and dispersed solid or liquid domains

FIGURE 10.2 The three classes of dispersions arranged according to the size of the domains that make up the dispersed phase. The colloidal system shown is polydisperse, while the coarse system is monodisperse

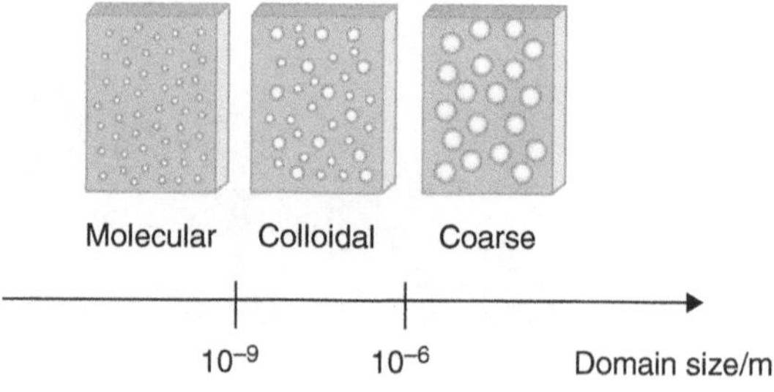

will have a tendency to settle under the influence of gravity. The appearance of fluid dispersions therefore changes over time and the two phases present can normally be separated by standard laboratory filter paper.

Colloidal dispersions

Colloidal dispersions (or **colloids**) have dispersed phase domains with sizes between 1 and 1000 nm and these cannot be trapped using standard laboratory filter paper. Colloids are generally more physically stable than coarse dispersions. Colloids have kinetic stability and we shall see that they can be thermodynamically stable in some instances. **Micelles** represent a special type of colloidal particle and are referred to as association colloids. This reflects the fact that these particles are formed when **surfactant** molecules cluster together.

For more information on micelles, please refer to 'Micelles' in Section 9.5.

Colloids can also be referred to as submicron systems, given that the domain size is less than 1 μm. The term nanoparticle is used when the size of a colloid is less than 100 nm. Significantly, many nanoparticles behave very differently from their corresponding bulk material and they can have very different physical and biological properties (see Box 10.1). During your general reading, you may encounter a lack of consistency over the term nanoparticle. In some areas of pharmaceutical science, the terms nanoparticle and colloid are used interchangeably, even though the latter includes the particles in the size range 100–1000 nm.

BOX 10.1

Nanoparticles and bulk materials

The differing properties of nanoparticles, compared to the bulk material, are not just of interest in pharmaceutics. For example, copper nanoparticles are very hard, in contrast to bulk copper, which is malleable and ductile. Carbon nanotubes of a few nanometres diameter are mechanically strong, flexible, conduct electricity, and are 100 times stronger than steel but are only 1/6th of the weight. It should be noted, however, that not all substances with particles sizes less than 100 nm exhibit such distinctive changes in their behaviour.

Molecular dispersions

Molecular dispersions have dispersed phases with domain sizes less than 1 nm in size and they are thermodynamically stable systems. They are sometimes called true solutions to distinguish them from colloidal systems. Sodium carbonate dissolved in water is an example of a true solution and this class of dispersion is widely used to deliver drugs orally or by intravenous injections. Solutions of gases are more commonly referred to as gas mixtures and include Entonox.

For more information on solutions, please refer to 'Solutions' in Section 3.4.

For more information on Entonox, please refer to 'Medical gases' in Section 4.4.

KEY POINTS

- Disperse systems may be classified as coarse, colloidal, or molecular dispersions according to the size of the domains within the dispersed phase.
- In a monodisperse system, particles are of uniform size. In a polydisperse system, particles size varies.
- Colloids are generally stable, whereas coarse dispersions are not stable and will separate over time.

SELF CHECK 10.1

A dispersion is found to contain fine solid particles suspended in water. The particles sizes range from 10 nm to 100 nm. What is the best description of this system?

(a) Monodisperse and coarse.

(b) Monodisperse and colloidal.

(c) Polydisperse and coarse.

(d) Polydisperse and colloidal.

SELF CHECK 10.2

A student mixed flour and water to form a cloudy liquid. Over a few minutes, the flour settled to the bottom of the mixture. After shaking and pouring the mixture into a filter funnel, the flour was trapped by the filter paper. On the basis of these observations, is this a molecular, colloidal, or coarse dispersion?

10.2 Types of disperse system

Dispersions are formed from dispersed and continuous phases, each being formed from solid, liquid, or gas. As there are three classifications of dispersion, and nine different ways to pair solids, liquids, and gases, we might suppose that there are 27 different descriptions for disperse systems. The actual number is less than this as some combinations are not observed in nature and some commonly used terms may be applied to more than one class of dispersion (Table 10.1).

You will have encountered most, if not all, of these types of dispersions in your day-to-day life. Thus, fog is an aerosol of water in air and fizzy drinks are solutions of carbon dioxide gas in water. Milk is an emulsion formed by an oily butterfat phase dispersed in water, while butter is an example of a gel or solid emulsion. Most seating and bedding relies on solid foams to provide comfort and support, perhaps using a porous polyurethane polymer as the continuous phase. In addition to these generalized examples, you will have also encountered medicines that are dispersions and we will come across some of these later in this chapter.

Gas solutions and aerosols

Mixtures of gases are always molecular dispersions as gases are always mutually soluble. **Aerosols** are suspensions of either liquid droplets or fine solid particles dispersed in a gaseous continuous phase, and the terms 'liquid aerosol' and 'solid aerosol' may be used, respectively.

For more information on mixtures of gases and aerosols, please refer to Section 4.5.

Foams

A foam consists of bubbles of gas dispersed throughout a liquid or solid continuous phase. A **foaming agent**, typically a surfactant, is required for stable foam formation and this lowers the **surface tension** between the gas and the continuous phase. Although foaming agents tend to be **surfactants**, not all surfactants can stabilize foams. In the absence of a suitable foaming agent, water will not foam upon shaking in air as its high surface tension will rip any bubbles apart as soon as they form. A surfactant which stabilizes a foam containing an aqueous continuous phase adopts a particular orientation at the gas–water interface. The **hydrophilic** head group remains in the continuous phase, while the hydrophobic chains protrude into the dispersed, gaseous phase. In this way, the **hydrophobic** tails of the surfactant molecules are shielded from the water.

TABLE 10.1 Types of disperse system

Continuous phase	Dispersed phase	Coarse dispersion	Colloidal dispersion	Molecular dispersion
Gas	Gas	Not observed	Not observed	Gas solution
	Liquid	Liquid aerosol	Liquid aerosol	Not observed
	Solid	Solid aerosol	Solid aerosol	Not observed
Liquid	Gas	Foam	Foam	Solution
	Liquid	Emulsion	Microemulsion, nanoemulsion	Solution
	Solid	Suspension	Sol, nanosuspension	Solution
Solid	Gas	Solid foam	Solid foam	Solid solution
	Liquid	Gel, solid emulsion	Gel, solid emulsion	Solid solution
	Solid	Solid suspension	Solid sol	Solid solution

For more information on surfactants, please refer to Section 9.5.

The fraction of the total foam volume that is composed of the bubbles of gas (or phase volume) is typically high at between 0.5 and 0.9. Foam systems are generally very polydisperse and bubbles can range in size from small to extremely large, i.e. mm in size. At the lower end of the volume fraction range (~0.5), the bubbles are more or less spherical in shape. At higher volume fractions (~0.9), the bubbles are irregularly sized polyhedrons (Figure 10.3). This arrangement allows the high volume of trapped gas to minimize the surface area between the gas and the continuous phase.

Emulsions

When **miscible** liquids are combined, a single-phase solution or molecular dispersion is formed. The term emulsion describes dispersions with continuous and dispersed phases that are **immiscible** liquids, such as oil and water. An emulsion in which the oil is dispersed as droplets in an aqueous continuous phase is described as normal or oil-in-water (o/w). When the continuous phase is oil and the water is dispersed as droplets, then the system is called a reverse or water-in-oil (w/o) emulsion. In addition to these types of emulsions, it is possible to prepare multiple emulsions, i.e. emulsions of water-in-oil-in-water (w/o/w) and oil-in-water-in-oil (o/w/o).

Emulsions are not thermodynamically stable systems and an **emulsifier** can be added to confer some stability. This might be a surfactant, perhaps with additional surfactants (co-surfactants) to optimize the properties of the system. Surfactants orientate at the water–oil interface, such that the hydrophilic head groups remain in the water, while the hydrophobic chains form a monolayer around the oil droplets in an o/w emulsion (Figure 10.4).

Microemulsions and nanoemulsions

Colloidal disperse systems formed from two immiscible liquids are referred to as microemulsions or nanoemulsions (see Box 10.2). In contrast to what these SI prefixes suggest, the size of the dispersed phase domains in a microemulsion are smaller (~2–100 nm) than those present in a nanoemulsion (~20–200 nm). It should be noted, however, that the size ranges quoted for each type of emulsion vary within the literature and there are historical reasons for these discrepancies.

There is no distinct change in physical properties so as to differentiate a nanoemulsion from an

FIGURE 10.4 Formation of an o/w emulsion

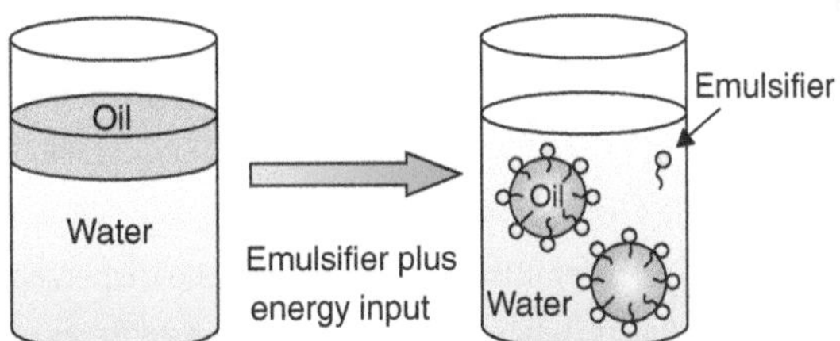

FIGURE 10.3 (A) Low-phase and (B) high-phase volume foams
Source: (A) © Portishead1/iStockphoto. (B) © Kuricheva/iStockphoto

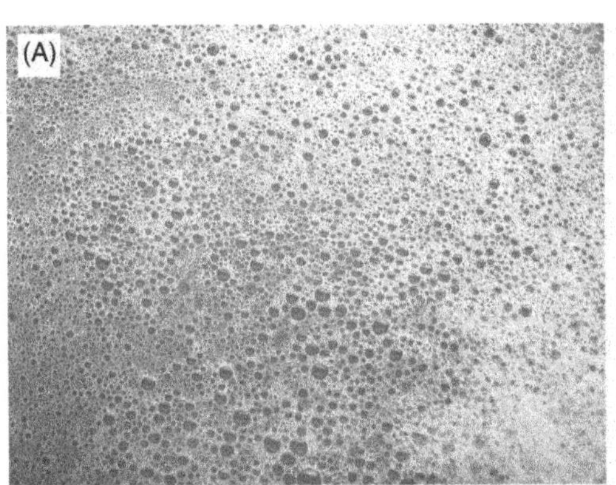

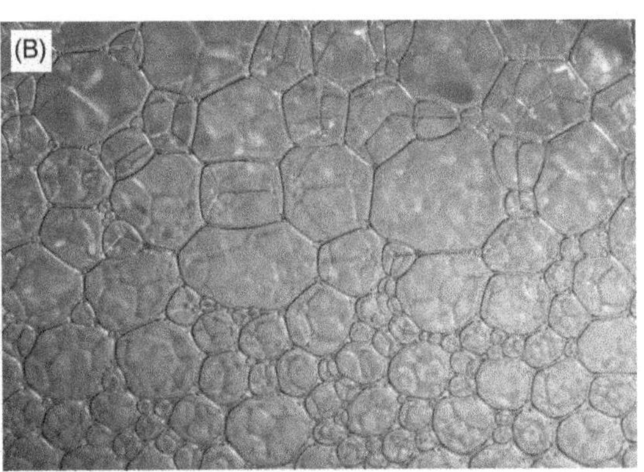

BOX 10.2

Origin of the term microemulsion

When microemulsions were first named by Schulman and colleagues in 1959, they did not know the size of the regions of dispersed phase. It was understood that the size of dispersed phase domains were smaller than those present in the emulsion (~0.1–10 μm) from which the microemulsions were originally prepared. Hence, the prefix micro- was used. More recently, emulsions have been prepared with droplets in the size range 50–500 nm. Although this size range extends beyond that of the typical range for microemulsions, the prefix nano- or mini- is used to denote the small size of the dispersed phase.

emulsion. The distinction due to the size of droplets in the dispersed phase is arbitrary, with values of 100, 200, and 500 nm being variously suggested. Although both microemulsions and nanoemulsions are surfactant/co-surfactant stabilized oil/water dispersions, microemulsions are thermodynamically stable systems, while nanoemulsions are not thermodynamically stable. This will be explored further in Section 10.6.

For more information on SI prefixes, please refer to Section 1.5.

In a w/o microemulsion, the shape of the dispersed water droplets is dependent on the relative volumes of the dispersed and continuous phases. When the volume of the dispersed phase is low, spherical structures predominate (Figure 10.5A). As the volume of the oil phase increases, the droplet shape changes to ellipsoidal and elongated, cylinder-like shapes (Figure 10.5B). As the volumes of the two phases become comparable, planar-like or sponge-like structures are observed. These two types of microemulsion structures are termed bicontinuous because of the 'channels' of oil and water running throughout the system (Figure 10.5C). They represent a transitional stage between a w/o and an o/w microemulsion, the latter being formed as more oil is added (Figure 10.5D). The spherical, ellipsoidal, and cylinder-like structures in microemulsions can be observed in both normal and reverse systems.

Due to the small size of the droplets, the total surface area of the dispersed phase domains in a microemulsion is very large when compared to an emulsion. This requires a correspondingly high surfactant to dispersed phase ratio for microemulsion formation. Consequently, while it is possible to prepare microemulsions, nanoemulsions, and emulsions from exactly the same ingredients, different ratios of the various components are required. This may be summarized on a three-component phase diagram for a typical reverse emulsion (Figure 10.6). This diagram highlights the portion of the phase diagram where the fraction of oil exceeds the fraction of water in the dispersion and w/o systems are favoured. The arrow on the diagram represents emulsions where the mole fraction of oil is 0.7. As we progress in the direction of the arrow, the mole fraction of surfactant increases from 0 to 0.3, while the mole fraction of water decreases from 0.3 to 0. It is noteworthy that as the fraction of surfactant increases, the preferred form of the system changes from emulsion to nanoemulsion to microemulsion.

FIGURE 10.5 The effect of increasing the proportion on oil in a water-in-oil emulsion showing: (A) spherical structures, (B) cylinder-like shapes, (C) the bicontinuous structure, and (D) an oil-in-water emulsion

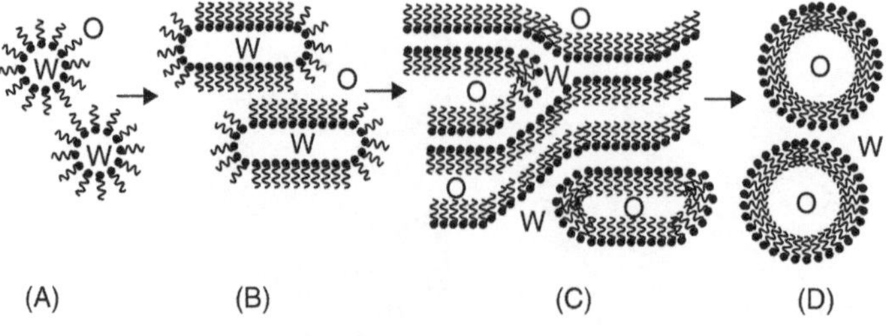

FIGURE 10.6 A three-component phase diagram for a typical o/w system showing three regions: (A) emulsion, (B) nanoemulsion, and (C) microemulsion. The arrow on the diagram represents emulsions where the mole fraction of oil is 0.7

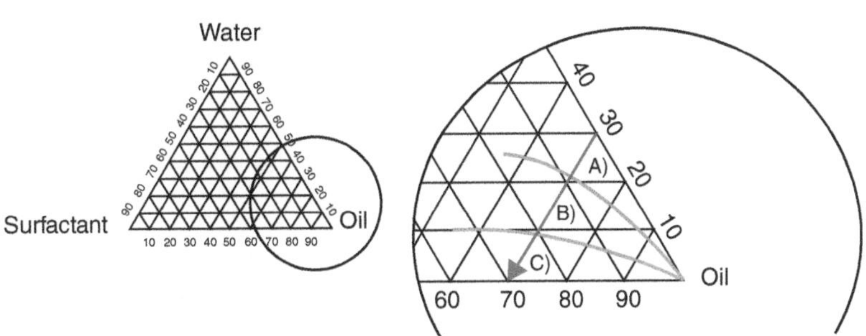

For more information on three-component phase diagrams, please refer to Section 7.7.

Suspensions and nanosuspensions

A **suspension** is a dispersion of solid particles in a liquid solvent in which the solid particles have little or no solubility. Colloidal suspensions are known as sols, although the term nanosuspension is generally preferred within pharmaceutics.

For more information on suspensions, please refer to 'Suspensions and emulsions' in Section 3.4.

The solid particles of a suspension can be stabilized by a coating of **suspending agent**, typically a surfactant or polymer, that minimizes **agglomeration**. Its main function is to completely wet the solid domains. Coating the particles provides a physical barrier to the agglomeration of the suspended particles. The choice of agent is dependent on the nature of the dispersed phase and whether it is to be suspended in an aqueous/non-aqueous polar phase, or an oil phase.

For more information on wetting, please refer to Section 9.2.

Gels

A gel is a semi-solid, 'jelly-like' material that does not flow when inverted and can have properties ranging from soft and weak to hard and tough. Gels have a solid continuous phase, or gelling agent, composed of a 3-D network of interconnected nanostructures with a dispersed liquid phase. The amount of continuous phase in a gel can be very low and gels tend to be mostly liquid by weight and typically exhibit the density of a liquid. The formation of a 3-D network after combining a gelling agent and liquid may be an irreversible or reversible process.

When a gel contains a network of small, discrete particles, it is described as a two-phase system. In contrast, where there are no apparent boundaries between the dispersed particles and the liquid, then it is known as a single-phase dispersion. Gels containing organic macromolecules uniformly distributed throughout a liquid, for example, are often single-phase gels.

SELF CHECK 10.3

Coarse dispersions with gaseous dispersed and continuous phases are not observed in nature. Why not?

SELF CHECK 10.4

Using the three-component phase diagram in Figure 10.6, determine whether the mixtures with the following % (w/w) concentrations will be an emulsion, nanoemulsion, or microemulsion:

(a) 70% oil, 5% surfactant, and 25% water.

(b) 70% oil, 25% surfactant, and 5% water.

(c) 80% oil, 10% surfactant, and 10% water.

KEY POINTS

- The name used to describe a disperse system depends on the physical state of the dispersed and continuous phases, and whether the dispersion is coarse, colloidal, or molecular.
- Aerosols are suspensions of either liquid droplets or fine solid particles dispersed in a gaseous continuous phase.
- A foam consists of bubbles of gas dispersed throughout a liquid or solid continuous phase.
- Emulsions, nanoemulsions, and microemulsions have continuous and dispersed phases that are immiscible liquids.
- Unlike nanoemulsions, microemulsions are thermodynamically stable and they generally have smaller dispersed domains.
- Suspensions and nanosupsensions are dispersions of insoluble solid particles in a liquid solvent.
- Gels have a solid continuous phase composed of a 3-D network of interconnected structures with a dispersed liquid phase.

10.3 Preparation of dispersions

There are two general approaches for the preparation of a dispersion, namely the top-down and the bottom-up techniques (Figure 10.7).

Top-down methods

The top-down technique involves either the size reduction of large particles down to the required size, or alternately the dispersion of one phase using techniques such as **milling**. These processes are scalable and are capable of producing large amounts of dispersion. However, due to their mechanical nature, these techniques have some disadvantages:

- They are usually very time-consuming and require significant energy.
- Processing can introduce contamination from the milling media or the homogenization chamber.
- The ratio of **amorphous** to **crystalline** forms of an API may be increased, leading to a reduction in stability.

Despite this, such methods are typically used to prepare solid-in-gas aerosols, emulsions, and nanoemulsions. In the case of emulsions, mechanical agitation may be through the use of high speed mixers, homogenizers, or ultrasound generators.

FIGURE 10.7 Preparation of nanoparticles using the top-down and down up approaches

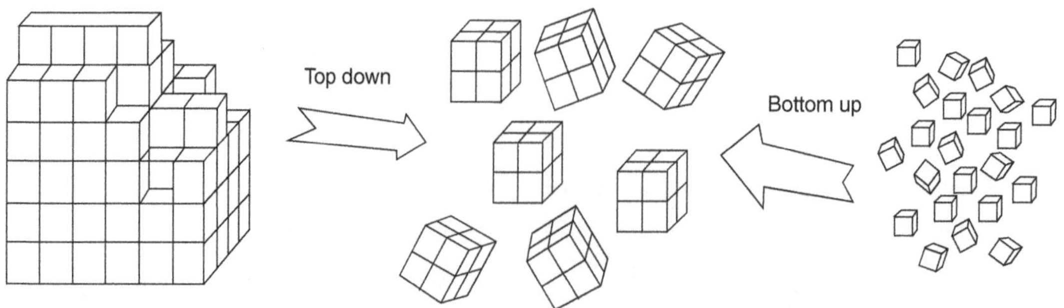

For more information on milling, crystals, and amorphous forms, please refer to Chapter 2.

Suspensions, nanosuspensions, and foams may also be produced by top-down methods. Suspensions are generally prepared by mixing the solid particles with a solution of the surfactant and/or polymer. Nanosuspensions are more complex to prepare and generally involve mixing a solid with a surfactant/polymer solution under conditions in which the solid particles are broken up. This may be, for example, by wet milling in the presence of ceramic beads or high-pressure homogenization in order to reduce particle size to within the nanoscale range. Liquid foams are formed when a liquefied gas expands as it is being forced through a liquid containing an **amphiphilic** foaming agent, typically a surfactant.

Bottom-up methods

These methods are used to prepare dispersions by the condensation, precipitation, or self-assembly (e.g. micelles) of materials dissolved in a true solution into larger particles. The bottom-up technique has advantages over top-down technique:

- It tends to produce particles with fewer defects and of a more homogenous composition.
- It gives better control over particle properties, e.g. size, morphology, and where appropriate, crystallinity.
- The mechanical energy required is generally minimal.

A colloid may be formed from a molecular dispersion by controlled precipitation (or crystallization), evaporation, or altering the concentration of the dispersed phase.

KEY POINTS

- In the top-down technique, a dispersion is prepared by reducing large particles down to the required size.
- The top-down technique requires a significant amount of energy and can impair the quality of the final product.
- In bottom-up methods, the dispersion is prepared by the condensation, precipitation, or self-assembly of materials dissolved in solution.
- The bottom-up technique can produce more uniform dispersions than the top-down technique and can give more control over the properties of the final product.

10.4 Properties of dispersions

The behaviour of dispersions is different from the behaviour of the bulk forms of dispersed and continuous phases. This can be understood in terms of their properties, including:

- Surface area.
- Appearance.
- Viscosity.

Although the pure forms of each phase have constant physical properties under fixed conditions, the properties of a disperse system will be dependent on the composition of the dispersion, the shapes and sizes of the dispersed domains (and their respective distributions).

Surface area

An important consequence of decreasing the size of the domains in the dispersed phase is the corresponding increase in surface area. Figure 10.8 shows how the percentage of atoms at the surface decreases as particle size increases. Indeed, in very small particles with diameters less than 5 nm, the majority of the atoms

FIGURE 10.8 Relationship between nanoparticle size and percentage of the particles atoms at the surface

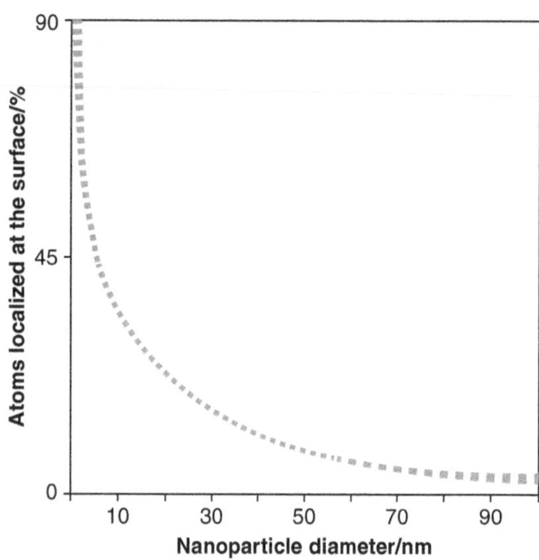

in a particle are located on the surface. Consequently, surface effects are more important in colloids than in coarse dispersions.

Surface area and particle radius

The surface area ($A_{surface}$) and volume (V) of a spherical particle are related to its radius, r:

$$A_{surface} = 4\pi r^2$$

$$V = (4/3)\pi r^3$$

If a monodisperse system consists of spherical particles of 1 mm radius, then the surface area and volume of each particle will be 1.3×10^{-5} m^2 and 4.2×10^{-9} m^3, respectively. Imagine that one of these particles is then split into smaller spherical particles that each have a radius that is 10-times smaller, 0.1 mm. It follows that the volume of each of these smaller spheres will be 1000 (10^3) times smaller. Thus, a single spherical particle of radius 1 mm could be split into 1000 particles of radius 0.1 mm. Each new particle would have a surface area of 1.3×10^{-7} m^2, and the total surface area of all the particles will therefore be 1000 times this value, 1.3×10^{-4} m^2. Thus, a 10-fold decrease in radius yields a 10-fold increase in surface area. This trend continues as particles become smaller. Thus, a 100-fold decrease in radius results in a 100-fold increase in surface area. This has important implications for dispersions as their behaviour, including their stability, is determined by the surface area of the dispersed phase.

Appearance

A property of colloidal and coarse dispersions that distinguishes them from true solutions is their ability to scatter light (Figure 10.9). In other words, if a light beam passes through these disperse systems, then some or most of the light is deflected by the dispersed phase. The amount of scattering is dependent upon three factors:

- The sizes and shapes of the dispersed domains.
- The dispersed phase concentration (i.e. the number of domains per mL).
- The difference in the refractive indexes of the dispersed and continuous phases.

The scattering of light by disperse systems is known as the Tyndall effect. In contrast, when a light beam passes through a true solution (e.g. sodium carbonate in water) there is so little scattering of light that it cannot be detected.

FIGURE 10.9 Light will pass through a molecular dispersion (left) but will be scattered by larger particles in a coarse dispersion (right)

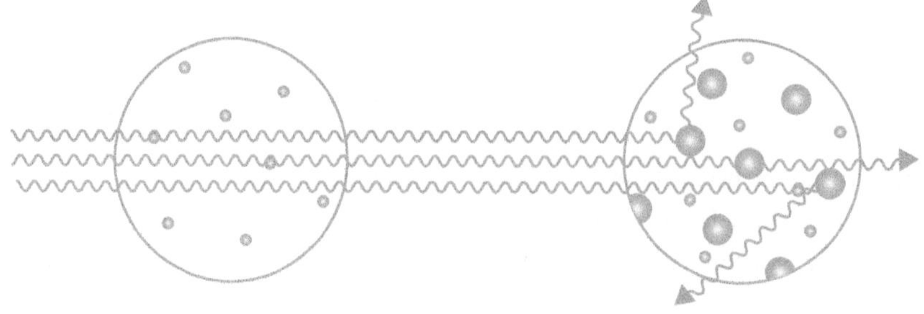

The particles in a coarse dispersion are sometimes large enough to be seen by the naked eye and certainly by an optical microscope. Colloids variously appear transparent through to translucent, cloudy, and ultimately milky white, depending on the factors above. Dispersions of nanoparticles (<100 nm) are often clear in appearance as they do not scatter light to a significant extent.

The particles in a colloidal dispersion are normally too small to be seen in an optical microscope. Instead a specialized device, such an electron microscope, is needed to see these very small particles. If there is no difference in refractive index between the dispersed and the continuous phases, then it is not possible to detect the dispersed particles as they will not scatter light, an effect known as **contrast matching**.

Water is the most commonly used liquid continuous phase in dosage forms and it has a low refractive index (~1.33). Contrast matching rarely occurs in pharmaceutically relevant dispersions as most dispersed phases have refractive indexes greater than 1.4.

Viscosity

Viscosity is a measure of the resistance of a fluid to flow: The higher the resistance to the flow of a fluid, the greater its viscosity. The viscosity of a dispersion depends largely upon the sizes and shapes of the dispersed domains, the number of domains per unit volume, and the viscosity of the continuous phase. For a particular dispersed and continuous phase at fixed temperature, a positive linear trend is often observed between the volume fraction of the dispersed phase and the recorded viscosity. In addition, those dispersions with non-spherical domains tend to be more viscous than those with spherical domains.

For pharmaceutical dispersions with a liquid continuous phase, viscosity-increasing excipients may be added to slow the rate at which the dispersed and continuous phases separate. A balance must be reached where separation is slowed without inhibiting the ability to re-disperse the formulation by shaking before use. Ideally, liquid suspensions should display pseudoplastic flow properties, where the fluid behaves in a **non-Newtonian** fashion, i.e. viscosity decreases with increasing shear rate. This yields a vehicle with greater viscosity during storage (low shear rate), and this will disfavour separation. Upon dispensation (high shear rate) the viscosity of the formulation decreases so that pouring can occur more readily.

For more information on pseudoplastic flow and viscosity, please refer to 'Non-Newtonian fluids' in Section 3.3.

KEY POINTS

- The surface area, appearance, and viscosity of dispersions can be very different from that of the bulk forms of dispersed and continuous phases.
- For a dispersion with spherical domains, each 10-fold reduction in the radius of the domains leads to a 10-fold increase in their total surface area.
- The scattering of light by coarse and colloidal disperse systems is known as the Tyndall effect.
- The viscosity of a dispersion depends upon the sizes and shapes of the dispersed domains, the number of domains per unit volume, and the viscosity of the continuous phase.

SELF CHECK 10.5

Calculate the surface area (in m^2) and volume (in m^3) of a spherical particle in a colloidal suspension that has a radius of 10 nm.

10.5 Types of physical instability

The particles forming the dispersed phase of an aerosol, suspension, or emulsion exhibit random, continuous movement known as Brownian motion. This arises due to collisions between the dispersed domains and the constantly moving molecules of the continuous phase. It is Brownian motion which causes the bubbles, droplets or particles of the dispersed phase to come into contact. This is often the first stage of the collapse of thermodynamically unstable dispersions and the various types of physical instability will now be considered.

Flocculation

This is a process in which two or more droplets or particles cluster together without losing their individual identity, rather like individual grapes joining together to make a bunch (Figure 10.10). The term agglomeration may also be used, although **flocculation** is sometimes preferred when the process is prompted by the addition of an agent. Flocculation is the main mechanism for the collapse of dispersions that have dispersed phase volume fraction of < 0.05 and domain sizes less than 1 mm. The process is generally reversible and droplets and particles that have flocculated can generally be re-dispersed upon shaking. However, flocculation is often the precursor to coalescence/aggregation.

Coalescence/aggregation

This occurs when two or more dispersed domains collide with each other, resulting in the formation of one larger domain (Figure 10.11). The original identity of each domain is lost, rather like when globules of oil in a shaken mixture of oil and water join together to reform a distinct oil layer. **Aggregation** dominates when the volume fraction of the dispersed phase is high. The term **coalescence** tends to be reserved for emulsions and involves the irreversible breaking of the interfacial film between droplets.

FIGURE 10.10 Flocculation of particles in a dispersion

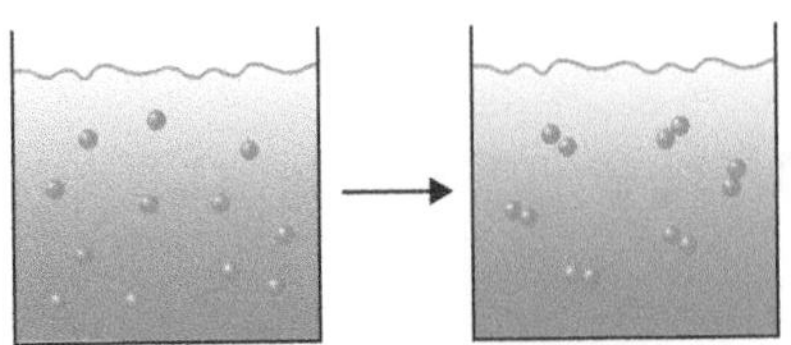

FIGURE 10.11 Coalescence of particles in a dispersion

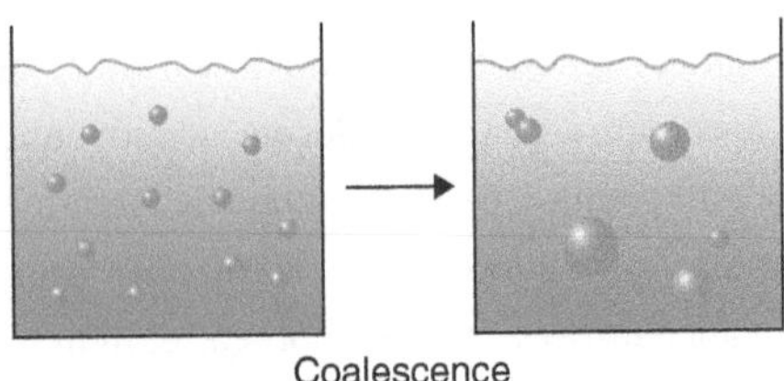

Ostwald ripening

This type of physical instability occurs in dispersions containing **polydisperse** domains of droplets or particles (Figure 10.12). Collisions between two domains can lead to one bigger domain and one smaller domain. Small domains become smaller and eventually dissolve in the continuous medium. **Ostwald ripening** requires that the dispersed phase has a measurable solubility in the continuous phase.

Sedimentation

In a coarse dispersion, such as a suspension, the dense particles may very rapidly settle under the influence of gravity to leave a clear dispersion medium. This process is called **sedimentation** and the rate at which it occurs is described by Stokes' Law, which takes into account:

- The size of the dispersed domains.
- The viscosity of the dispersion medium.
- The difference in density of the dispersed and continuous phases.

According to Stokes' Law, large particles dispersed in a medium of low viscosity will sediment very quickly, while small particles in a highly viscous medium will settle very slowly.

Creaming

Creaming occurs when the dispersed phase floats and concentrates at the top of dispersion (Figure 10.13). This will happen when the dispersed domains are less dense than the surrounding continuous phase. Downward creaming (sedimentation) will occur if the density of the dispersed phase is greater than that of

FIGURE 10.12 Ostwald ripening of particles in a dispersion

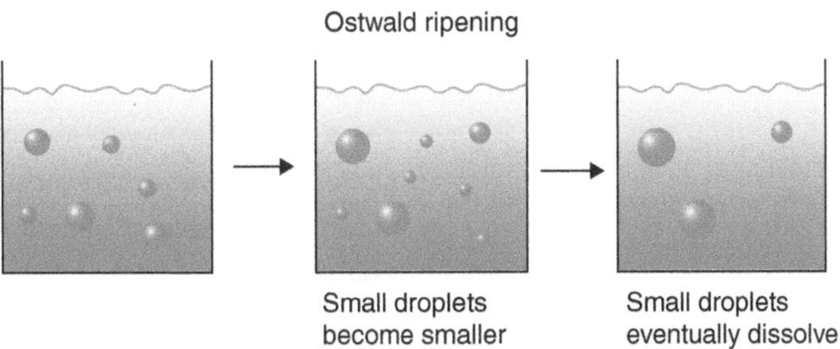

the dispersion medium. For creaming and sedimentation, the greater the difference in densities, the more rapidly the particles will separate and the lower the kinetic stability of the dispersion.

The rate of creaming can be lowered by:

- Reducing the droplet/particle size.
- Lowering the density difference between the two phases.
- Increasing the viscosity of the medium.

The creaming rate is dependent on the volume fraction of the dispersed phase and is usually slow in concentrated dispersions.

FIGURE 10.13 Creaming of particles in a dispersion

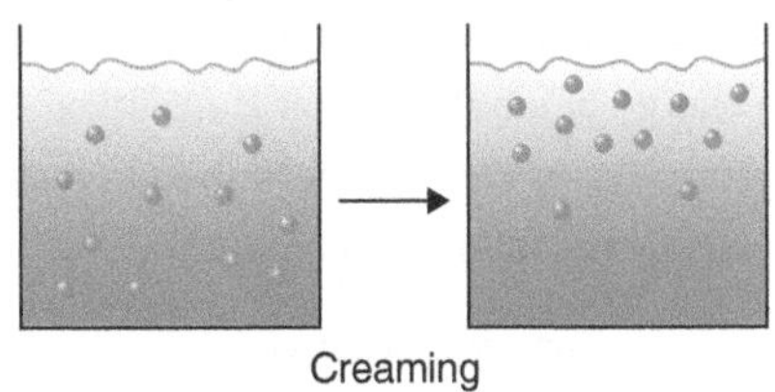

KEY POINTS

- Flocculation (or agglomeration) is where dispersed particles cluster together without losing their individual identity.
- In coalescence or aggregation, dispersed particles join together and lose their individual identity.
- In Ostwald ripening, a collision between two domains leads to one bigger domain and one smaller domain.
- Sedimentation occurs when dense particles rapidly settle under the influence of gravity. If the dispersed phase is less dense than the continuous phase then it will rise and creaming will occur.

SELF CHECK 10.6

What is the difference between flocculation and coalescence?

10.6 Physical stability of different types of dispersions

Molecular dispersions of solids, liquids, and gases are always stable due to the large **entropy** gain associated with **dissolution**. Although coarse and colloidal dispersions with a solid continuous phase may not necessarily be thermodynamically stable, bubbles, droplets, and particles are trapped in a solid lattice. This immobilizes the dispersed phase and gives a very high kinetic stability. For fluid dispersions, i.e.

those with a gas or liquid continuous phase, stability is determined by the classification of the dispersion and the presence of stabilizing agents. In general, colloids tend to have higher kinetic stabilities than coarse dispersions.

For more information on entropy, please refer to Section 5.4.

Stability of foams

Foams are not thermodynamically stable, even in the presence of a foaming agent. Gas bubbles aggregate over time and the foam ultimately collapses, although this process is slowed by a foaming agent and the dispersion will have some kinetic stability. Instability results from the large interface between the bubbles and dispersion media. Bubble growth is spontaneous, as it reduces the extent of the surface area between the bubbles and continuous medium, lowering the **Gibbs free energy** of the system. As a consequence of their instability, foams are sometimes considered to be 'transition states'. Experimentally, it is observed that the rate at which a foaming agent lowers surface tension is an important factor in determining whether a foam is formed, and not the overall reduction in surface tension that the agent causes.

Stability of emulsions and nanoemulsions

Emulsions and nanoemulsions are always thermodynamically unstable, these liquid-in-liquid dispersions having a higher Gibbs free energy than the two separated phases. It follows that for these systems, the free energy of emulsification is positive requiring that work must be done for an emulsion to be formed, e.g. through a high-speed mixer. Once formed, there are a number of different processes that can be involved in the collapse of an o/w emulsion, including flocculation, coalescence, and Ostwald ripening. These processes will ultimately result in a planar interface between the oil phase and the aqueous phases and the system reverts to separate liquid layers.

The rate of collapse of nanoemulsions can be very low and take months, such that they are often considered to be kinetically stable. The very small size of the dispersed phase inhibits droplet flocculation and coalescence, so that the rate of Ostwald ripening alone governs the destabilizing process. As the oil phase typically has a very low solubility in the aqueous phase, this process occurs very slowly. A whole variety of factors can affect the physical stability of an emulsion, including:

- **pH**.
- Dissolved salts.
- Phase–volume ratio.
- Temperature.
- Properties of the interfacial film.
- Solubility of the emulsifier.
- Emulsifier concentration.

The presence of an emulsifier can only ever increase the kinetic stability of emulsions and nanoemulsions.

Stability of microemulsions

Microemulsions are defined by the fact that they are thermodynamically stable dispersions. This can be understood by considering the free energy change, ΔG, accompanying the formation of an emulsion from two layers of immiscible liquids, such as oil and water. Any emulsion will be thermodynamically stable if the free energy of emulsification is negative. At fixed temperature, T, this can be determined to reasonable accuracy using the following equation:

$$\Delta G = \gamma_{\mathrm{LL}}\Delta A - T\Delta S \qquad (10.1)$$

where γ_{LL} is the interfacial surface tension between the oil and liquid phases, ΔA is the change in the interfacial surface area, and ΔS is the entropy of emulsification (see Box 10.3).

In a chemical process, ΔS measures the reaction entropy change, which results from changes in the composition of the system from reactant to product. During emulsification, there is no change in the composition of the system as no chemical reaction occurs. ΔS therefore measures the configuration entropy change that results from the physical change from an ordered two-layer liquid system, to a relatively chaotic dispersion. Accordingly, the

BOX 10.3

The origin of $\Delta G = \gamma_{LL}\Delta A - T\Delta S$

The free energy change, ΔG, for homogeneous chemical and physical processes at temperature, T, can be determined using:

$$\Delta G = \Delta H - T\Delta S$$

where ΔH is the enthalpy change and ΔS is the entropy change.

By definition, Gibbs free energy is the maximum non-expansion work that a process can do. Thus, when ΔG is negative, the system can do work on the surroundings in a spontaneous process. When ΔG is positive, the surroundings must do work on the system and constant pressure for change to occur and the process is then described as non-spontaneous.

Maximum non-expansion work means the maximum work that the system can do after subtracting any work that the system must do due to changes in volume of the system. When a reaction produces a gas, for example, work needs to be done to push back the atmosphere and this cannot, therefore, be classified as 'free' or available energy.

For heterogeneous systems, we must also take into account changes in free energy due to contributions from the work, w, required to change the size of interfacial areas. We may write:

$$\Delta G = \Delta H - T\Delta S + w$$

For reactions that occur in homogeneous solution, w is negligible and can be ignored. During emulsification, the interfacial area between the two phases changes markedly and w is significant.

Enthalpies of emulsification, ΔH, are generally endothermic due to the disruption of the hydrogen bond network in bulk water that results from the creation of the dispersion. ΔH is generally small, however, as no covalent bonds are broken during the process. If we assume that ΔH is zero, rearrangement of the equation above gives:

$$\Delta G = w - T\Delta S$$

Work is related to surface free energy and can be calculated using:

$$w = \gamma_{LL}\Delta A$$

where γ_{LL} is the interfacial surface tension between the oil and liquid phases and ΔA is the change in the interfacial surface area.

This area will, in turn, be related to the number, size, and shape of oil droplets produced during emulsification.

By substitution of the expression for w, we obtain:

$$\Delta G = \gamma_{LL}\Delta A - T\Delta S$$

entropy of emulsification in equation 10.1 is always positive.

Whether or not an emulsion is thermodynamically stable will depend on the relative magnitudes of $\gamma_{LL}\Delta A$ and $T\Delta S$ in equation 10.1. In a microemulsion, the interfacial tension between the oil and water phases, γ_{LL}, is small due to the presence of surfactant. The entropy of emulsification is comparatively large due to the formation of numerous fine droplets. In this case, $T\Delta S$ is then greater than $\gamma_{LL}\Delta A$ and, consequently, ΔG is negative. Microemulsions therefore have a lower free energy than the two separated phases and are stable (Figure 10.14A). They can be formed spontaneously by the simple mixing of the constituent phases, although the application of heat and/or agitation may often speed up microemulsion formation. The increase in entropy during nanoemulsion formation is not sufficient to compensate for the work done as a result of increases in interfacial area. Consequently, nanoemulsions are thermodynamically unstable with respect to the separate phases (Figure 10.14B).

Stability of suspensions and nanosuspensions

Both suspensions and nanosuspensions are not thermodynamically stable systems and the dispersed domains will generally flocculate and settle over time. Ostwald ripening is quite common in these systems, as the dispersed phase normally has a little solubility in the continuous phase. The presence of a suspending agent can slow these processes and increase the kinetic stability of suspensions and nanosupensions.

FIGURE 10.14 Schematic diagram of the free energy of (A) nanoemulsion and (B) microemulsion systems compared to their constituent, separate phases

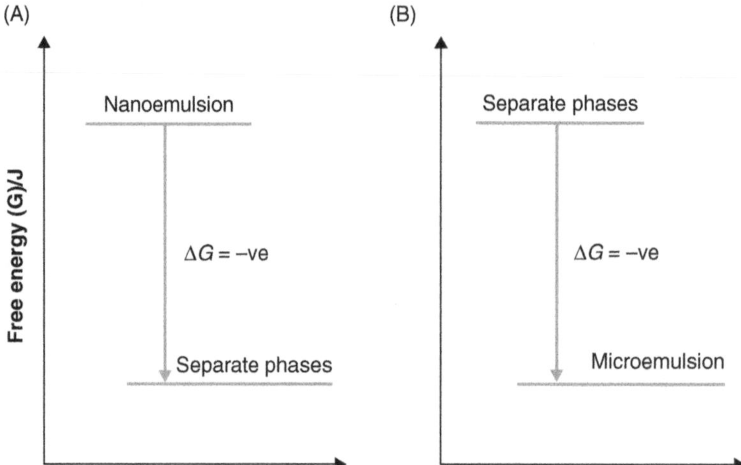

KEY POINTS

- Foams are not thermodynamically stable. Bubble growth reduces the surface area between the two phases, lowering free energy.
- Emulsions and nanoemulsions are always thermodynamically unstable. Their kinetic stability can be enhanced by the use of emulsifiers.
- Microemulsions are thermodynamically stable due to the large increase in entropy accompanying the formation of very small droplets.
- Both suspensions and nanosuspensions are not thermodynamically stable, but kinetic stability can be enhanced by the use of suspending agents.

SELF CHECK 10.7

The label on a bottle of milk of magnesia states that it should be shaken before use. Why is this necessary in thermodynamic terms?

10.7 Disperse systems used to deliver APIs

This section describes the various disperse systems used in drug delivery, concentrating on those classified as colloidal and coarse dispersions. Dosage forms may have solid, liquid, or gaseous continuous phases, water being the most commonly used liquid vehicle. Table 10.2 gives examples of some of the more commonly used disperse systems in drug delivery and the means by which they deliver the API.

In these dispersions, the API may be one of the components of one of the phases, although we will also encounter systems where the dispersed phase is composed almost entirely of the API. It is not uncommon to find the API in both phases. When the API is present in the dispersed phase of a coarse or colloidal suspension, for example, a small amount of the API will also dissolve in the continuous phase. Thus, magnesium hydroxide in a milk of magnesia suspension has limited, but some, solubility in water. Similarly, if an API is located in the continuous phase of dispersion, some of the API may also dissolve in the dispersed phase of the system.

TABLE 10.2 **Commonly used disperse systems in drug delivery and the means by which they deliver APIs**

Continuous phase	Dispersed phase	Dispersion	Routes of Administration
Gas	Gas	Gas solutions	Lung (pulmonary) delivery
	Liquid	Aerosols	Lung, nasal, sub-lingual, and throat delivery
	Solid	Aerosols	Lung, nasal, sub-lingual, and throat delivery
Liquid	Gas	Foams	Skin, rectal, vaginal, and nasal delivery, burn dressings
	Liquid	Emulsions	Skin, eye, ear, nose, vagina, rectal, oral, and intravenous delivery
	Solid	Suspensions	Oral, ear, eye, nose, skin, intramuscular, subcutaneous, rectal, and intravenous delivery
Solid	Gas	Solid foams	Skin delivery, burn dressings
	Liquid	Gels	Skin, eye, mouth (oral mucosa) and vaginal delivery
	Solid	Solid solutions	Oral delivery

Gas solutions and aerosols

Mixtures of gases are always molecular dispersions. It is not unusual for a gaseous API to be combined with other gases or volatile materials in pharmaceutical applications. A pharmaceutical aerosol is a suspension of either liquid droplets or fine solid particles of the API dispersed in a gaseous, continuous phase.

For more information on gas solutions and aerosols as dosage forms, please refer to Section 4.4.

Foams as dosage forms

Solid foams, which are also known as dry foams, xerogels, or sponges, are formed when a liquid continuous phase solidifies. They can be used as dressings for wounds and, in this application, disinfection agents, antibiotics, or steroids may also be present.

Liquid foams are more commonly used as dosage forms and they typically employ a gaseous hydrocarbon as the dispersed phase. This gas is also known as the propellant and examples include propane, butane and isobutene. Other gases such as hydrofluoroalkanes, nitrogen, oxygen, helium, argon, and carbon dioxide may also be used. If a cooling effect is required at the site of application of the foam then a slower evaporating gas can be added. This is known as secondary propellant and examples include pentane, isopentane and isobutene.

The continuous phase of pharmaceutical foams is generally water, although **hydroethanolic** solvents, oils, emulsions, and non-aqueous polar solvents such as propylene glycol and glycerol are also used. The API is generally contained in the continuous phase, either in solution or suspended.

Examples of **amphiphilic** molecules that are used as foaming agents include anionic surfactants such as sodium stearate, sodium oleate, sodium dodecyl sulphate, and dioctyl sulfosuccinate. Generally the concentration of surfactant required for foam formation is low at less than 1% (w/v). Although surfactants are commonly used as foaming agents, occasionally proteins, such as collagen, may be used.

Regardless of the combination of materials used, it is essential that liquid foams remain stable for the intended duration of use. When a foam is used for rectal and vaginal administration, for example, this issue can be addressed by producing the gas *in situ* using formulations that effervesce upon on contact with mucosal secretions.

Liquid foams are aesthetically pleasing formulations and are becoming increasingly popular as drug-delivery vehicles. In addition, they are very easily spread, which is of considerable benefit when treating large areas of hairy and/or inflamed skin. The need to apply pressure or maintain prolonged contact with the surface being treated is reduced when a foam is applied. Currently, however, there is little evidence of any improvement in the delivery of an API from a foam, as compared to other topical dosage forms. As with aerosols, the relatively high cost associated with foam production limits the wide spread pharmaceutical use of this delivery vehicle. As a consequence, alternative technologies, such as pump sprays, are being developed to allow foam production in the absence of propellants.

Emulsions as dosage forms

Although water is typically the continuous phase in pharmaceutical emulsions, a wide variety of other media can also be used, including:

- Hydroethanolic solvents.
- Water/polar co-solvent mixtures.
- Oils, such as triglycerides.

A similar range of solvents to those used as the continuous phase can be used as the disperse phase. Any API incorporated into an emulsion is generally dissolved or dispersed in the dispersed phase and/or the interfacial region. The amount of dispersed phase present is normally about 10–20% (w/v). Emulsions are more commonly used in external applications, and are only used in oral liquids when the emulsion is in the oil in water form.

Generally, hydrophilic surfactants, such as dodecyl sulphate, are required to produce o/w emulsions, while lipophilic surfactants such as dioctyl sulfosuccinate and dimethyldodecylammonium bromide are needed for production of w/o or reverse emulsions (Figure 10.15A).

In the case of microemulsions, the stabilizing agent is typically a low molecular weight surfactant. Sometimes this is in combination with a short chain co-surfactant, such as butanol, although microemulsions can be prepared using a single surfactant, such as dioctyl sulfosuccinate or Brij 96 (Figure 10.15B). Compared to microemulsions, nanoemulsions and emulsions can be prepared using a wider variety of surface active molecules including:

- Low molecular weight surfactants.
- Polymeric surfactants.
- Proteins and polysaccharides.
- Solids, such as aluminium hydroxide and bentonite.

As with microemulsions, when a surfactant is used, a co-surfactant is often also required. In the case of emulsions and nanoemulsions, the co-surfactant is typically a long chain alcohol or a sterol, such as cholesterol.

APIs have been delivered via emulsions for many years and such dispersions are relatively cheap to prepare. They can be used for a wide variety of purposes, including local application to the skin, eye, ear, nose, vagina, or rectum. For example, o/w emulsions are used for the oral delivery of oils such as castor or cod liver oil. Soybean oil-in-water emulsions, stabilized by phospholipids, have been used for the intravenous delivery of emulsified fat. This example of parenteral nutrition is used with patients who cannot absorb or

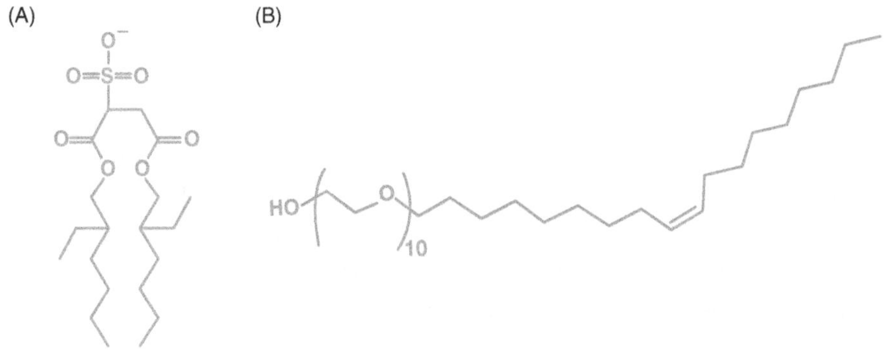

FIGURE 10.15 Example emulsifiers: (A) dioctyl sulfosuccinate, a short dichain, anionic surfactant; and (B) Brij 96, a non-ionic surfactant

metabolize fat through oral administration. Such lipid formulations have a two-year shelf life and an excellent stability and safety record, being readily sterilized by heat sterilization. They have recently been used as a vehicle for drugs; including, for example, the poorly soluble intravenous anaesthetic propofol.

For more information on parenteral delivery, please refer to 'Parenteral delivery' in Section 1.2.

The viscosity of an emulsion can vary from thin and runny low viscosity systems to very thick and viscous emulsions called creams, which are classed as semi-solids. Creams contain an excess of surfactant/co-surfactant, which results in planar-like phases in the bulk liquid (Figure 10.5C), giving the emulsion its high viscosity. Non-greasy creams are o/w emulsions that hydrate the skin and leave a thin layer of oil on the surface, limiting further loss of water. Greasy creams are w/o emulsions, the nature of the continuous phase meaning that a thick layer of oil is deposited on the skin after application. Un-medicated non-greasy and greasy creams are used to treat a variety of skin conditions, particularly xeroderma (dry skin).

Suspensions and nanosuspensions as dosage forms

With the exception of molecular dispersions, a suspension is considered to be the most bioavailable form of an API. In particular, nanosuspensions have been used to increase the bioavailability of poorly water-soluble drugs after oral administration. Although suspensions are not thermodynamically stable systems, pharmaceutical dispersions of this type are generally formulated so that they can be readily re-dispersed through gentle shaking, e.g. milk of magnesia. The aesthetics of a suspension are also important from a consumer point of view, and homogeneity is also important in this respect.

Typically, the dispersed phase of a pharmaceutical suspension is the API, either in the form of the free drug or its salt. The form selected will depend on the suspending solvent used, although, whichever form is chosen, crystalline APIs are preferred to ensure stability when suspended. Although it is possible to adsorb APIs on to insoluble carrier particles, this is less common in dosage form design.

The dispersion medium is typically a solvent in which the dispersed phase is insoluble or poorly soluble. Indeed, the poorer the solubility of the dispersed phase in the solvent of choice, the better the stability of the resulting suspension. A wide range of suspending agents can be used to stabilize pharmaceutical suspensions including:

- Phospholipids.
- Non-ionic surfactants, such as the polysorbates and poloxamers.
- Polymers such as the polysaccharides and polyvinylpyrrolidone.

The amount of suspending agent required depends upon the amount of API administered but it is low, being typically around 1% (w/v) for a nanosuspension. As coarse suspensions have a larger particle size, they have a smaller surface area per unit mass of solid. Consequently, they require less stabilizer to completely wet the dispersed particles. In addition to the amount added, the physicochemical properties of the stabilizing agent will have a pronounced effect on the physical stability and the *in vivo* behaviour of all types of suspension.

Being liquids, colloidal suspensions for pharmaceutical use have similar advantages to molecular dispersions or true solutions. Both suspensions and nanosuspensions can be used to deliver poorly soluble APIs by a range of routes of administration including:

- Orally.
- Topically to the skin, ear, eye, nose, and rectum.
- Parenterally, including intramuscular, subcutaneous, and intravenous injection.

When pharmaceutical suspensions are intended for intramuscular administration, the solvent is typically an oil, such as ethyl oleate. This ensures that the injection remains at the site of administration and does not spread through the muscle. It can also provide a sustained release of drug from the formulation.

Ointments are a class of semi-solid dosage forms that includes formulations where the API is suspended as solid particles (or dissolved) in a highly viscous organic liquid, called the base. A variety of bases are available, including pharmaceutical grade soft paraffin wax, and the choice of base is ultimately informed by the intended use of the medicine. In general, the term ointment is generally reserved for oil-based topical formulations and this includes greasy creams.

The greasy nature of ointments makes them suited to the water-insoluble APIs and they are used in both ocular and otic delivery, and for direct application to the skin. Pastes and ointments are, in essence, the same thing with the only real difference being the concentration of API present. Pastes usually contain greater than 50% (w/w) of API, whereas, in comparison, the concentration present in ointments is much lower.

Gels as dosage forms

Pharmaceutical gels are semi-solid dosage forms where the continuous phase, or gelling agent, is typically a suspension made up of either:

- small inorganic lipophobic particles, e.g. insoluble clay particles formed from aluminium magnesium silicate, aluminium silicate, and magnesium or aluminium hydroxide; or,
- large organic macromolecules, e.g. naturally occurring polysaccharides and synthetic polymers.

Any API incorporated into a gel is generally located in the liquid dispersed phase. Although gels for pharmaceutical use commonly use an aqueous solvent, alcohols and oils may also be used. For example, mineral oil can be combined with a polyethylene resin to form an oily (oleaginous) ointment base.

There are a variety of different types of gel:

- Hydrogels, containing a network of hydrophilic polymer chains and water. They are sometimes called an aquagel.
- Organogels, composed of an organic liquid entrapped in a 3-D cross-linked network.
- Xerogels, being a solid formed from a gel by drying. They usually retain high porosity and enormous surface area along with an extremely small pore size.

Gels, and in particular hydrogels, can be used to administer an API topically or into body cavities. Gels for application to the nasal passages and eye are often sustained release formulations. It is possible to prepare environmentally sensitive hydrogels, also known as 'smart' or 'intelligent' gels. These semi-solids have the ability to detect changes of pH, temperature, or the concentration of metabolite, and release their load as result of such a change.

KEY POINTS

- Pharmaceutical dispersions may have solid, liquid or gaseous continuous phases, water being the most commonly used liquid vehicle.
- It is not uncommon for the API to be present in both phases.
- Solid foams can be used as dressings for wounds. Liquid foams are more common and they have advantages over semi-solids in topical applications to sensitive areas.
- Emulsions can be used for a wide variety of purposes including topical applications and parenteral nutrition.
- Both suspensions and nanosuspensions can be used to deliver poorly soluble APIs enterally, topically and parenterally.
- Gels can be used to administer an API topically or into body cavities.

SELF CHECK 10.8

An aerosol for topical application to skin burns contains benzocaine and pentane. What is the purpose of these two ingredients?

SELF CHECK 10.9

Why might a foam be preferred to a cream when treating a large area of inflamed skin on the legs of an adult male?

10.8 DLVO theory

Intermolecular forces exist between the dispersed phase and the continuous phase, as well as between the domains that make up the dispersed phase. Whether or not dispersed particles flocculate will depend on the balance of attractive and repulsive forces between the dispersed particles. If the repulsive forces are stronger than the attractive forces then the particles will show no tendency to aggregate and the dispersion will be stable.

Attractive van der Waals (VDW) interactions act between the dispersed domains and these forces promote the aggregation of particles. VDW forces are short-range and are the result of the interaction of two dipoles that may be permanent or induced/temporary. Fluctuations in electron density give rise to temporary dipoles in a particle and this can induce dipoles in particles nearby. The temporary dipole and the induced dipoles are then attracted to each other. Repulsive electrostatic charges at the surface must also be considered and the origin of these can be understood using the model of an electrical double layer.

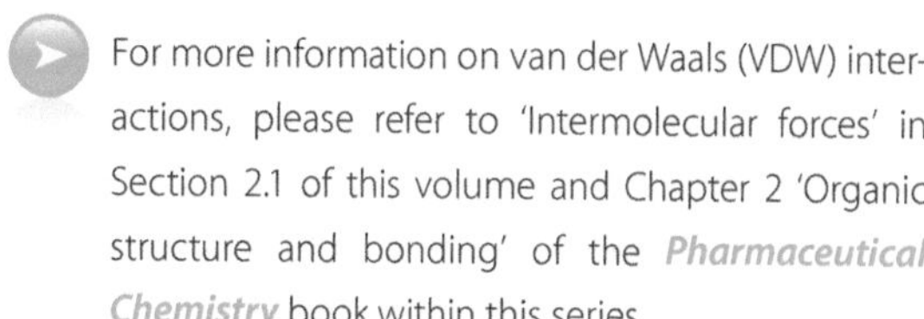

For more information on van der Waals (VDW) interactions, please refer to 'Intermolecular forces' in Section 2.1 of this volume and Chapter 2 'Organic structure and bonding' of the ***Pharmaceutical Chemistry*** book within this series.

For more information on the electrical double layer, please refer to Section 9.6.

In the 1940s, Deryagin, Landau, Vewey, and Overbeek (DLVO) developed a theory of the stability of colloids that took into account the balance between the attractive and repulsive forces present in a dispersion. The DLVO theory assumes that the dispersion is dilute and that only two forces act on the dispersed particles, these being attractive VDW forces and repulsive electrostatic forces. It is assumed that the electric charge and other properties are uniformly distributed over the solid surface and that the distribution of charged domains is determined by electrostatic forces, Brownian motion and entropy considerations. The DLVO theory provides a good explanation of the interaction between two particles as they approach each other.

According to DLVO theory, colloidal stability is influenced by two contributions:

- The energy of the attractive interaction due to van der Waals forces (V_A).
- The energy of the repulsive electrostatic interaction (V_R).

The energy of the particles (V_T) can then be expressed in terms of the these contributions:

$$V_T = V_A + V_R \tag{10.2}$$

For spherical particles, the VDW attractive energy is inversely related to the distance (d) between the particles, while the electrostatic repulsive energy decays exponentially with distance. It is possible to plot a diagram showing how the interaction potential varies with distance as shown in Figure 10.16. Three features on the resulting energy-distance curve are important in explaining colloid stability, namely:

- The secondary minimum.
- The primary maximum.
- The primary minimum.

At large distances of separation, the particles experience a minimal attraction which is greatest at the secondary minimum. At this point, the forces of attraction are weak and do not generally lead to a permanent coalescence/aggregation of the droplets/particles. At this interparticle distance, for example, flocculation may occur but the system can be re-dispersed upon shaking.

As particles come even closer together they will start to experience some repulsion which will peak at the

FIGURE 10.16 Variation in energy of the interaction between two particles as a function of distance

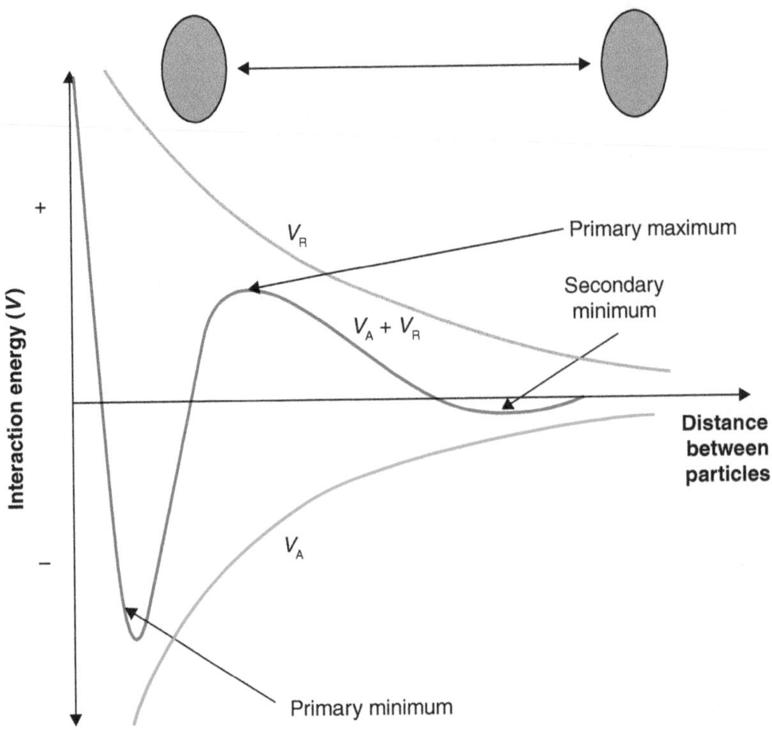

primary maximum. The intensity of this repulsive force is important. If the interaction energy at the primary maximum is high then the particles/droplets cannot get any closer together than the distance at which this separation occurs. In this case, the colloidal particles would be stable and show no tendency to flocculate.

If the energy of interaction at the primary maximum is low then it means that the particles can be forced together. The kinetic energy of the dispersion that results from normal thermal motion may be sufficient to overcome this barrier. Once the particle separation is such that the energy of interaction reaches the primary minimum then the droplets/particles will coalesce/aggregate permanently.

SELF CHECK 10.10

How can DLVO theory be used to explain why a flocculated suspension can be dispersed upon shaking?

KEY POINTS

- Whether or not dispersed particles flocculate will depend on the balance of attractive and repulsive forces between the dispersed particles.
- In order to prepare a stable colloid it is necessary to introduce repulsive interactions between dispersed particles and these may be electrostatic in origin.
- DLVO theory can be used to understand the balance between the attractive and repulsive forces present in a dispersion.
- When the interparticle distance is equal to the secondary minimum, flocculation may occur and this is reversible.
- If the energy of interaction at the primary maximum is low, then particles will readily join together to reach an interparticle separation known as the primary minimum.

CHAPTER SUMMARY

- Disperse systems may be classified as coarse, colloidal, or molecular dispersions according to the size of the domains within the dispersed phase.
- The name used to describe a disperse system depends on the physical state of the dispersed and continuous phases, and whether the dispersion is coarse, colloidal, or molecular.
- Dispersions may be prepared by top-down or bottom-up techniques; each offers specific advantages.
- The surface area, appearance, and viscosity of dispersions can be very different from that of the bulk forms of dispersed and continuous phases.
- Colloids generally have high kinetic stability. Uniquely, microemulsions are thermodynamically stable colloidal dispersions.
- Solid semi-solid, liquid, and gaseous dispersions have a range of applications in topical, enteral, and parenteral dosage forms.
- Whether or not dispersed particles flocculate will depend on the forces between the dispersed particles, and this can be understood using DLVO theory.

FURTHER READING

Florence, A.T. and Attwood, D. *Physicochemical Principles of Pharmacy.* (4th edn). London: Pharmaceutical Press, (2006).

Includes a chapter on disperse systems with an excellent coverage of emulsions and suspensions.

Monynihan, H. and Crean, A. *The Physicochemical Basis of Pharmaceuticals* Oxford: Oxford University Press, (2009).

This text is written in an accessible style and includes two chapters on disperse systems that separate theory and applications in pharmacy.

REFERENCE

Schulman, J.H., Staeckenius, W., and Prince, L.M. Mechanism of formation and structure of micro emulsions by electron microscopy, *Journal of Physical Chemistry* (1959). 63: 1677–80.

11 Colligative properties

PHILIP DENTON

Liquid medicines are commonly prescribed as oral **dosage forms** for young or elderly patients and, more generally, in treatments that rely on topical and parenteral delivery. A liquid dosage form consists of an **active pharmaceutical ingredient (API)**, solvent, and additional **excipients**, for example, to modify the flavour. It is found experimentally that many of the physical characteristics of solutions, such as viscosity, are dependent on the concentration of the solution and nature of the solute and solvent. Some properties, however, are found to be independent of the nature of the solute, being dependent only on the number of solute particles present and the nature of the solvent. These are referred to as the **colligative properties** of the solution.

The term 'colligative' comes from the Latin terms, *co* and *ligatus*, which mean 'together' and 'to tie or bind', respectively. The words 'ligand' and 'ligature' come from the same origin. In the context of this chapter, the word is used because both the observed colligative properties, and the number of solute particles, are 'bound' together.

The principal colligative properties are:

- **Osmotic pressure**.
- Lowering of **vapour pressure**.
- Lowering (or 'depression') of **melting point**.
- Raising (or 'elevation') of **boiling point**.

Of these, osmotic pressure has the most relevance to dosage form design and we will see how this phenomenon must be taken into account when developing liquid dosage forms for topical and parenteral delivery. Moreover, it will be shown how some novel modified-release oral dosage forms and parenteral drug-delivery methods rely on osmotic pressure. The final section of this chapter will discuss the common origin of all colligative properties and how they can be understood quantitatively.

Learning objectives

Having read this chapter you are expected to be able to:

- Define the meaning of the term 'colligative property' and name the principal colligative properties.
- Understand the significance of osmolarity and the van't Hoff factor in relation to osmosis.
- State and use the van't Hoff osmotic pressure equation.
- Define tonicity and how this concept is considered in the design of liquid dosage forms for ophthalmic, nasal, and parenteral delivery.
- Explain how osmotic pressure can be exploited in the design of modified-release tablets and parenteral drug-delivery systems.
- Explain how colligative properties arise in terms of chemical potential.

11.1 The colligative properties of solutions

Colligative properties are evident when we contrast the behaviour of a pure solvent with a solution formed from that solvent. For example, consider a sealed vessel containing water. This represents a closed **system** as no other substances may enter or leave. The water molecules have a range of molecular energies and, even at room temperature and pressure, some molecules of water will have sufficient energy to break free of the liquid surface. The rate of water vaporization will be greater than the rate of vapour condensation until the system reaches equilibrium. The vapour that results will exert a force on the surface of the liquid and the walls of the container and this is called the **vapour pressure**. For water at 298 K, equilibrium is attained when the water vapour pressure is 0.03 bar, around 1/30 of atmospheric pressure.

Medicinal saline is a sterile solution that consists of sodium chloride (the solute) and water (the solvent). It is routinely used to treat dehydrated patients *via* **intravenous** infusion. Standard saline (Figure 11.1) has a concentration of 0.90% (w/v) sodium chloride, equivalent to a molarity of 0.15 mol dm^{-3}. This is an unsaturated solution with a salinity that is roughly one-quarter that of sea water. Sodium chloride is a strong **electrolyte** and fully dissociates upon dissolution to yield solvated sodium and chloride ions. Species such as this, which are molecularly dispersed throughout a continuous solvent phase, are referred to as solute particles.

FIGURE 11.1 Saline solution for intravenous infusion
Source: © dtimiraos/iStockphoto

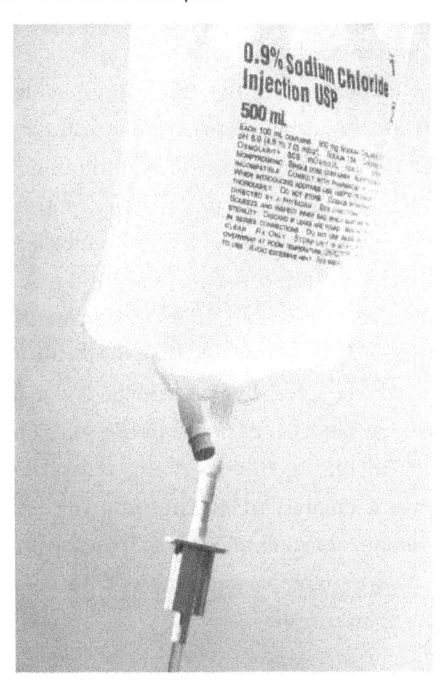

For more information on electrolytes, please refer to 'Strong and weak electrolytes' in Section 6.1.

In a closed system containing saline, a proportion of the water molecules will enter the vapour phase at room temperature. The sodium chloride is not volatile and remains in solution. Experimentally, it is found that the vapour pressure above saline is always less than that above pure water at the same temperature and external pressure (Figure 11.2). **Dissolution** of further sodium chloride causes the vapour pressure to drop still further. The same behaviour is observed when other non-volatile soluble solids are added to water, the phenomenon being independent of the *type* of solute. Only the *number* of solute particles influences the vapour pressure. This phenomenon is therefore referred to as a colligative property.

The addition of sodium chloride to water is also recorded to lower the melting point and raise the boiling point of the liquid. These are further examples of colligative properties, as only the concentration of the solution and nature of the solvent are found to affect the experimentally observed phase transition temperatures.

For more information on phase transitions, please refer to Chapter 7.

Although colligative properties are characteristics of solutions, there must be a physical equilibrium with another phase for any such behaviour to be measurable. In each of the cases above, the colligative property is manifest because the liquid solution phase is in equilibrium with a second phase containing solvent.

FIGURE 11.2 Comparative vapour pressure measurements above (A) pure water and (B) standard saline under standard conditions

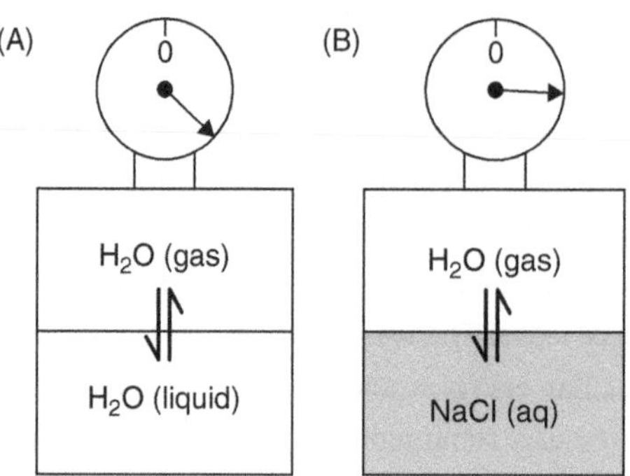

The physical state of this second phase depends on which colligative property is being investigated (Table 11.1). At the boiling point, for example, the liquid solution will be in equilibrium with a second, gaseous phase that will be composed of pure solvent, if the solute is non-volatile.

> **KEY POINT**
>
> The colligative properties of solutions are lowering of vapour pressure, depression of melting point, elevation of boiling point and osmotic pressure. Colligative properties for a particular solution depend only on the number of solute particles in the solution phase, rather than the nature of the solute particles.

> **KEY POINT**
>
> The solution phase must be in physical equilibrium with a second, solvent-containing phase for any colligative properties to be evident.

TABLE 11.1 Physical states of the two phases in equilibrium for systems that exhibit colligative properties

Property	Solution phase	Second phase
Lowering of vapour pressure	Liquid	Gas
Lowering of melting point	Liquid	Solid
Raising of boiling point	Liquid	Gas
Osmotic pressure	Liquid	Liquid

Osmosis

The colligative property that is of most importance when designing dosage forms is **osmosis**. This term describes the spontaneous passage of solvent through a **semipermeable** membrane and into a solution. A semipermeable membrane is a divider through which solvent molecules, but not solute particles, can flow freely. Osmosis is unique among colligative properties as it relates to an equilibrium between two phases that are both liquids (Table 11.1). The effect of this phenomenon is clear when one considers a pair of systems with a permeable and a semipermeable membrane separating the two phases (Figure 11.3).

With a permeable divider, water molecules, sodium ions, and chloride ions will diffuse freely through the membrane over time until an homogeneous saline solution of uniform concentration is obtained. In the presence of a semipermeable membrane, however, osmosis occurs and there is a net flow of solvent into the saline compartment. If no resistance to flow is provided, then osmosis will continue until the solvent compartment is exhausted. However, as the level of liquid in the solution compartment increases, so does the **hydrostatic pressure** that it creates. At equilibrium, the levels of liquid remain constant and the hydrostatic pressure of the solution compartment is said to equal the **osmotic pressure**, Π.

FIGURE 11.3 Behaviour of a water and saline solution system with (A) a permeable divider and (B) a semipermeable membrane

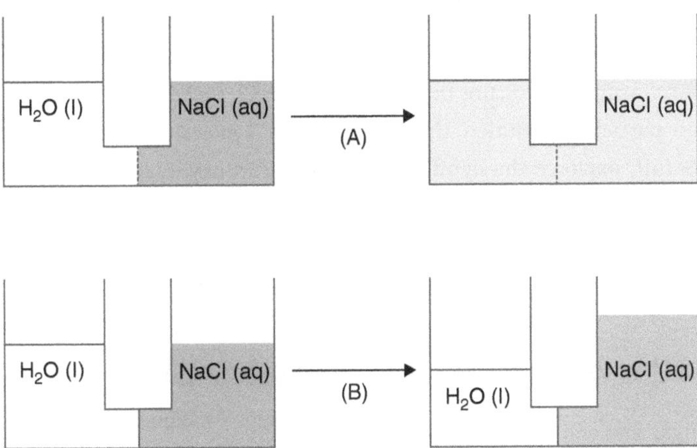

For aqueous systems, the osmotic pressure is found to be dependent only on the difference in the solute concentration on either side of the membrane and it is, therefore, a colligative property. In some circumstances, additional external pressure may be applied to the solution compartment so that the osmotic pressure is exceeded. In this case, the net flow of solvent would then be out of the solution compartment in a process known as **reverse osmosis**. This may be used in the purification of water containing solutes that are unable to pass through the semipermeable membrane.

Osmosis occurs when a system reorganizes itself in order to equalize the solute concentrations on either side of the membrane. On the solvent side, the concentration of solute is zero. Water flows from this compartment into the solution side in order to dilute the solution and reduce the solute concentration closer to zero. In order to understand why this and the other colligative properties occur, we must extend our understanding of **entropy**.

KEY POINT

Osmosis is the most pharmaceutically important colligative property. Osmotic pressure arises through osmosis, when solvent flows into a solution compartment separated from it by a semipermeable membrane.

For more information on entropy, please refer to 'Entropy of a system' in Section 5.4.

All colligative properties ultimately arise because solvent molecules are more thermodynamically stable when in solution, compared to solvent molecules in pure solvent under the same conditions. The reason for this is that a solution is a more disordered system and has a higher entropy. Saline, for example, has a higher entropy than pure water. The water molecules in saline are therefore more stable and are less likely to exit the liquid and enter the vapour phase. This is observed as a lowering of the vapour pressure. In wholly liquid systems, solvent molecules will prefer to reside in a solution phase over a solvent phase and this results in osmotic pressure. A more in-depth discussion of the origin of colligative properties is contained within the final section of this chapter.

SELF CHECK 11.1

Name four colligative properties.

SELF CHECK 11.2

Briefly explain how colligative properties arise in terms of entropy.

11.2 Osmotic pressure

As a colligative property, osmotic pressure depends on the number of solute particles in solution. Up until this point, we have not fully explored the significance of the term 'solute particle' or considered exactly how osmotic pressure and solution concentration are related.

Osmolarity and the van't Hoff factor

Glucose is a soluble sugar that will result in the development of an osmotic pressure when added to one side of a trough of water that is divided by a semipermeable membrane, as in Figure 11.3. Here, the divider is permeable to water but impermeable to glucose. Glucose does not dissociate in solution so a 1 mM solution of glucose will contain 1 mM of solvated glucose molecules.

Solute particles that contribute to osmotic pressure may be molecules or ions and the behaviour of glucose should be contrasted with a solution of 1 mM sodium chloride. As an ionic solid, NaCl electrolytically dissociates in aqueous solution to yield 1 mM of sodium ions and 1 mM of chloride ions. Hence, the total concentration of solvated species is 2 mM. When considering systems where osmotic pressure develops, it is more convenient to measure the effective amount of solute particles present in **osmole** (osmol), rather than mole units. Thus, a 1 mM solution of sodium chloride has **osmolarity** of 2 osmol L^{-1} if we consider that this system behaves as an **ideal solution**.

Molarity and osmolarity can be related using the van't Hoff factor, *i*, where the osmolarity is given by multiplying this factor by the molar concentration. The van't Hoff factor can have a variety of values, depending on the solute studied:

- $i=1$ for solutes that do not dissociate in solution, e.g. glucose.
- $i>1$ for solutes that dissociate in solution, e.g. NaCl.
- $i<1$ for solutes that associate in solution, e.g. benzoic acid.

For NaCl, $i=2$ in dilute solution as each mole of salt yields 2 moles of ionic solute particles. Benzoic, and other carboxylic, acids have van't Hoff factors less than one because they can form complexes. These 'dimers' are formed from the association of two molecules and are held together by hydrogen bonding.

> KEY POINT
>
> Osmotic pressure depends on the effective number of solute particles in solution, and this includes all the discrete molecules and ions that are present.

Osmolarity, osmolality, and non-ideal behaviour

This chapter largely considers dilute solutions that may be assumed to be behaving in an ideal manner. In such systems, osmolarity is equal to the total of the molarities of each different species in solution. In more concentrated systems, the effects of non-ideal behaviour must be considered if the magnitude of osmotic pressure is to be quantitatively understood. Our definition of osmolarity refers to the *effective* molarity of all solute particles in a solution, in recognition of the fact that this might be different to the *actual* molarity. In accurate work, osmolarity cannot be calculated from molarities alone, but must be measured experimentally due to the influence of forces between constituent particles. Osmolarity may be determined using an osmometer which may measure, for example, the depression in vapour pressure or freezing point caused by the addition of the solute.

A standard saline solution that is 0.9% (w/v) sodium chloride contains 9 g of NaCl per litre. Given that the relative formula mass of NaCl is 58.44, we can determine that this solution will have a molarity of 154 mM. This gives an osmolarity of 308 osmol L^{-1} by assuming ideal behaviour and by applying a van't Hoff factor of 2. The actual osmolarity of standard saline has been measured as 286 osmol L^{-1}. This discrepancy can be attributed to non-ideal behaviour.

Like molarities, osmolarities decrease with increasing temperature due the thermal expansion of liquids. For this reason, osmolality is sometimes preferred. Rather than measuring the effective number of moles of solute per *litre* of *solution*, osmolality records the effective number of moles of solute per *kilogram* of *solvent*. As it is temperature independent, osmolality is more suited to accurate measurement. Values for osmolality quoted in clinical settings are invariably those determined by an osmometer. At low aqueous solution concentrations, osmolarities and osmolarities are essentially the same as the mass of the solute is negligible and aqueous solutions have a density very close to 1 kgL^{-1}. When differences in osmolarity and osmolality are recorded, it is often because a comparison is being made between osmolarities calculated by assuming ideal behaviour, and experimentally determined osmolalities.

KEY POINT

Osmolarity is the preferred measure of solution molarity when studying osmotic pressure as it takes into account the behaviour of solutes that dissociate or associate in solution. Osmolarity is the product of the solution molarity and the van't Hoff factor, *i*.

The van't Hoff osmotic pressure equation

The relationship between osmotic pressure and solute concentration may be understood by considering the thermodynamic stability of solvent molecules in solution. Assuming ideal behaviour, this dependence is given by the van't Hoff equation:

$$\Pi = 1000\, i[\mathrm{S}]\, RT \qquad (11.1)$$

where i is the van't Hoff factor and [S] is the molar concentration of solute particles. The term '1000' is required to convert molar units of concentration into equivalent **SI units** of mol m^{-3}.

Equation 11.1 can be rearranged to determine the molar concentration of a solute in solution when both the osmotic pressure and mass of solute are known. This then enables the relative molecular mass of the solute to be determined, a technique known as osmometry. Although any colligative property could be used to determine molecular mass, osmometry is the preferred approach as osmotic pressures are generally very large. Thus, while standard saline ([NaCl]=0.15 M) has a **melting point** and a **boiling point** that are each less than 1 °C different from those of pure water, the saline is calculated to have an osmotic pressure at 298 K of:

$$\Pi = 1000 \times 2 \times 0.15 \times 8.314 \times 298 = 740 \text{ kPa}$$

Such large pressures create problems when using open systems such as that shown in Figure 11.3. To stop the net flow of solvent, the solution would need to rise to a height of around 75 m to generate a hydrostatic pressure equivalent to the osmotic pressure, higher than Westminster Abbey. In practice, sealed systems are used to determine osmotic pressure, with pressure gauges being used to measure the force generated by osmosis.

KEY POINT

The van't Hoff equation relates osmotic pressure, Π, to solute concentration [S] for ideal solutions and can be written as $\Pi = 1000\, i[\mathrm{S}]\, RT$

SELF CHECK 11.3

A soluble organic compound forms dimers in dilute aqueous solution, where each molecule is part of complex formed by the association of two molecules. Based on this information, what will be the van't Hoff factor, *i*, of this solution?

SELF CHECK 11.4

By application of the van't Hoff equation, determine the osmotic pressure created by a solution of NaCl that has a concentration of 0.07 M at 298 K, R=8.314 J K^{-1} mol^{-1}. What will be the osmotic pressure of a solution of 0.07 M NaOH at 298 K?

11.3 Tonicity

The cells that make up our bodies are composed of an aqueous medium, the cytoplasm, surrounded by a semipermeable membrane. We have already established that osmosis will occur whenever a solution and solvent are separated by a semipermeable membrane that is permeable only to the solvent. In practice, it is not necessary for one side of a semipermeable membrane to consist only of pure solvent for osmotic pressure to arise. This effect will also be observed in systems whenever there is a difference in solute concentration on either side of the cell membrane. This is a common scenario in the biological systems targeted by dosage forms.

The cytosol is the liquid phase of the intracellular medium. The precise nature of the cell membrane will determine the type of ions and molecules that are able to pass into the cytosol. Some cell membranes will allow sodium and chloride ions to pass through, for example, and these solute particles would therefore not contribute to any observed osmotic pressure. Cell membranes are permeable to water and it will flow from the less-concentrated side of a cell membrane to the more-concentrated side of the membrane. At equilibrium, osmotic pressure is exerted against the cell membrane surrounding the more concentrated solution.

Whether or not a cell membrane will experience an osmotic pressure will depend on the solute concentrations within both the cytosol and the solution surrounding the cell. It is useful to employ the concept of tonicity to describe the scenarios that can arise due to the effects of osmotic pressure. **Tonicity** is a measure of the osmotic pressure gradient on either side of a semipermeable membrane, normally a cell membrane.

Isotonicity

An isotonic solution is one that has an osmolarity that is the same as that of the cytosol under investigation. A cell bathed in an isotonic solution would experience no osmotic pressure gradient: water molecules will diffuse back and forth across the membrane, but there is no net flow (Figure 11.4A).

The osmolarity of physiological fluids is typically around 0.3 osmol L^{-1}. To minimize osmosis, dosage forms are often designed to be isotonic with the body. Osmosis is not always undesirable, however, and we will see that it can be used to our advantage in treatment of certain ailments and in the design of novel drug delivery systems.

Hypertonicity

A hypertonic solution is one that has a greater osmolarity than the cytosol. When a cell is immersed in a hypertonic solution, water will flow out of the cell and into the solution. Osmosis will continue until equilibrium is attained and the osmotic pressure of the extracellular fluid against the cell membrane stops any further net flow of water (Figure 11.4B). The cell will be observed to shrink.

Hypotonicity

A hypotonic solution is one having a lower osmolarity than the cytosol. When a cell is bathed in a hypotonic

FIGURE 11.4 The three classifications of tonicity, showing the net solvent flow into and out of an example (blood) cell: (A) isotonicity; (B) hypertonicity; (C) hypotonicity

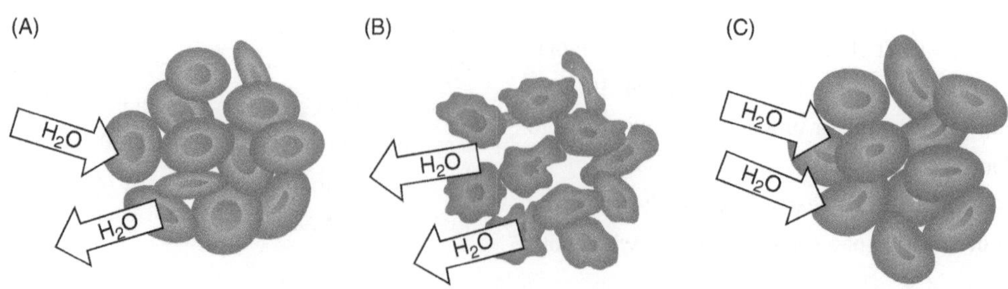

solution, water will flow from the extracellular fluid into the cell. Osmosis will continue until equilibrium is attained and the osmotic pressure of the intracellular fluid against the cell membrane stops the net ingress of water (Figure 11.4C). Alternatively, the cell may rupture before equilibrium is attained, so-called cytolysis (or lysis).

KEY POINT

The osmolarity of physiological fluids is typically around 0.3 osmol L^{-1}. To minimize the potential for osmosis, dosage forms are often designed to be isotonic with the body.

SELF CHECK 11.5

Define the terms isotonic, hypotonic, and hypertonic.

SELF CHECK 11.6

Is standard saline, 0.15 M NaCl(aq), isotonic?

11.4 Osmosis and liquid dosage forms

Both hypertonic and hypotonic solutions will have damaging effects on cells if the body is not able to mitigate against the effects of solutions with osmolarities outside the normal range. The site of administration is a factor, some parts of the body being more sensitive than others. The total volume of solution administered must also be taken into account when designing liquid dosage forms, this being a particular consideration in paediatric medicine.

Topical delivery

Liquid dosage forms designed for direct application to the skin or delivery via the ear will not generally cause harmful effects if they are not isotonic. This is not surprising, given that we know from experience that we are able to bathe our entire bodies in water without suffering due to the effects of osmosis. Seawater, for example, is hypertonic, having an osmolarity that is typically around four times larger than body fluids. Tap water is hypotonic, with the precise osmolarity being dependent on geography. Water from hard-water areas contains dissolved minerals and has a higher osmolarity than 'soft' water. Even freshly distilled water contains H^+ and OH^- ions due to autoprotolysis and the ionic product of water, K_W, is 1.0×10^{-14} $mol^2\,dm^{-6}$. It follows that the osmolarity of freshly distilled water is only 2×10^{-7} osmol L^{-1}, but our skin is sufficiently robust so that laboratory wash bottles need not carry a health and safety warning!

For more information on ionic product of water, please refer to Section 6.3.

Liquids designed for ophthalmic delivery are generally isotonic. Hypertonic eye drops and irrigating solutions will draw water towards the application site, whereas hypotonic liquids will cause water to flow from the site of administration and through the tissues of the eye. In both cases, this could lead to patient discomfort. Hypertonic eye drops may be used in certain instances, however, such as in the treatment of corneal oedema. In this application, a formulation with an osmolarity between two and five times the concentration of the equivalent isotonic solution is used to draw water from the eye and reduce swelling.

The tonicity of nasal formulations will affect both the degree of absorption and whether any irritant effect is produced; isotonic formulations are preferred. Children too young to be prescribed decongestants, for example, may be offered an aqueous nasal spray to soften and unblock mucus. While sterile water could perform this action, these nasal sprays are normally formulated as a 0.90% (w/v) sodium chloride solution to ensure isotonicity. In adults, the nasal mucosa of an adult has a surface area of around 180 cm^2, around one-third the area of this page. This is a consideration as higher surface areas give rise to higher rates of osmosis, giving the body less time to respond to adverse change.

KEY POINT

Liquid dosage forms designed for direct application to the skin or delivery via the ear need not be isotonic with body fluids. Ophthalmic solutions and nasal sprays are generally formulated to be isotonic

Oral delivery

The oral delivery of hypotonic solutions is not hazardous. In other words, drinking tap water is a safe activity (although, too much can be toxic – see Integration Box 11.1). 'Fizzy' soda drinks have osmolarities that are typically double that of normal body fluids and would therefore be classed as hypertonic, yet they can be ingested without harmful effects from osmosis.

Patients who are unable to obtain the nutrients they need from food but have normal gut function may be prescribed enteral nutrition. This is a common form of feeding for those who are weak and struggle to eat normally. It is designed to supplement the patient's diet and is generally preferred over parenteral nutrition as it is less costly and maintains gut action. Those who have difficulty swallowing or are significantly malnourished may be fed enterally *via* a tube. Prescribed drinks typically contain protein and polysaccharides in concentrated amounts, with most patients having no difficulty with isotonic and hypertonic feeds. The same is true for patients taking medicated solutions containing a dissolved API delivered *via* the oral route.

INTEGRATION BOX 11.1

Water intoxication and MDMA

Water intoxication can occur by consuming too much water, overwhelming the regulatory systems of the body. It is for this reason that many 'sports' drinks are isotonic with the body so that they can be safely consumed in large amounts (as much as 10 litres for an endurance athlete during competition). Water intoxication has been the recorded cause of death for some users of the Class A drug MDMA ('Ecstasy') following prolonged exertion. Ecstasy users put themselves in danger by obsessively drinking water to compensate for water lost through perspiration.

Parenteral delivery

Although dipping one's forearm into a bath of water is a harmless activity, the injection of even sterile water is potentially dangerous. Medicinal saline, delivered intravenously, is the preferred way to rehydrate the body. Standard sodium chloride solutions for IV infusion have a concentration of 0.15 M and NaCl has a van't Hoff factor of 2. Thus, standard saline is isotonic with physiological fluids, having an osmolarity of 0.3 osmol L^{-1}.

Tonicity is a particular consideration for IV infusions as they generally use greater volumes of liquids than other types of parenteral delivery. Consequently, they have more potential to interfere with the body's regulatory mechanisms. The body can tolerate hypertonic intravenous liquids, although these must be administered slowly to ensure that the fluid is given time to be diluted to safe levels by the body. Even small variations in the osmolarity of physiological fluids can have critical effects on health. In some patients with diabetes, for example, glucose may build up in the blood (hyperglycaemia), raising the osmolarity of the fluid. An increase in osmolarity of less than 0.1 osmol L^{-1} from the normal level can be sufficient to induce coma.

We saw that in ophthalmic topical applications, the ability of hypertonic liquids to draw out liquids from cells can be used to reduce localized swelling (oedema). In a similar fashion, dosage forms can be used to treat swelling *via* parenteral delivery. The term osmotherapy is used to describe interventions where a hypertonic liquid is administered intravenously to reduce swelling in the brain. This may be due to the accumulation of water in intracellular areas (cerebral oedema), resulting in an increase in intracranial pressure. Solutions of mannitol are traditionally administered to relieve this pressure. However, as osmosis depends only on the number of solute particles, rather

KEY POINT

Solutions for parenteral delivery are generally isotonic, although the body can withstand variations from the normal range if small volumes are delivered over extended periods.

than their type, other hypertonic solutions, including urea and saline, may also be used.

Tonicity agents

If the osmolarity of a liquid dosage form is less than the desired value, then additional excipients may then be added specifically to enhance the tonicity, such as:

- Dextrose.
- Glycerol.
- Urea.
- Mannitol.
- Potassium chloride.
- Sodium chloride.

These will be in addition to any buffers, stabilizers, and anti-microbial agents that are included in the dosage form. All solutes that are non-permeable will contribute to tonicity of the liquid, not just those chemicals listed above. The effect that tonicity agents have on other properties of the liquid must also be considered. Thus, the addition of glycerol to an aqueous solution will increase the viscosity of the liquid and this may or may not be desirable.

KEY POINT

Tonicity agents can be added to a liquid dosage form if the osmolarity is less than the desired value.

SELF CHECK 11.7

Are the following formulations acceptable dosage forms?

(a) A hypotonic solution for oral delivery.

(b) A hypertonic solution for ophthalmic delivery.

(c) A hypertonic solution for IV infusion.

(d) A hypotonic solution for bathing.

SELF CHECK 11.8

Why might sodium chloride be preferred to glycerol as a tonicity agent for eye drops?

11.5 Osmotic pump dosage forms

We saw in the last section how osmosis can be exploited by liquid dosage forms to treat medical conditions, although this was generally restricted to oedemas resulting from the accumulation of water. In recent times, however, osmosis has been harnessed in novel ways to treat a wide range of ailments.

Osmotic pump tablets

In the osmotic-controlled release oral delivery system (OROS®), a water-soluble API is combined with excipients and enclosed by a semipermeable coating in a one-chamber tablet (Figure 11.5). The membrane is not permeable to the API, so a small hole is made in the coating by a laser or drill during tablet production. In the body, water flows into the tablet by osmosis, dissolving the API. The pressure that results causes the API solution to exit via the orifice and this device is therefore described as an osmotic pump dosage form. Eventually, a steady state is reached where the rate of water entering through the membrane is the same as the rate of solution leaving the tablet.

For APIs with limited aqueous solubility, a two-chamber, or push–pull, osmotic pump tablet may be employed. In this tablet, the semipermeable membrane surrounds two layers of material: an upper layer

FIGURE 11.5 Schematic cross section of a one chamber osmotic pump tablet

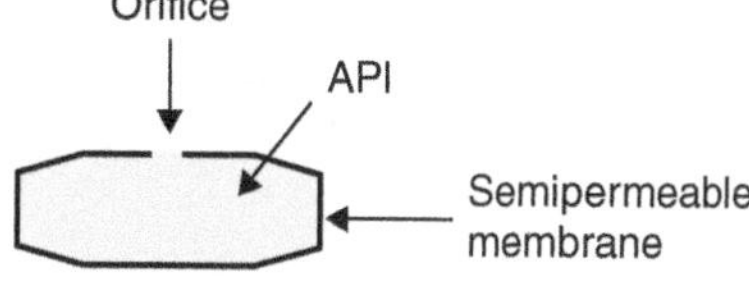

FIGURE 11.6 Mechanism of action of a two-chamber osmotic pump tablet

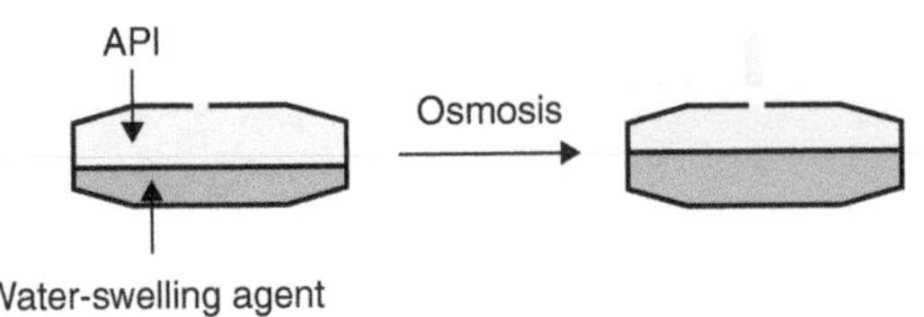

containing the API and a lower layer containing a hydrophilic agent that swells in the presence of water (Figure 11.6). In the body, the device pulls in water by osmosis, and the upper layer creates a suspension containing the API *in situ*. The lower layer expands as the hydrophilic agent takes on water, pushing the suspension out through the orifice.

Osmotic pump tablets are a type of **modified-release** dosage form and this approach may be preferable to diffusion-controlled systems. Once the tablet has been formulated, the rate of release of the API is dependent largely on the tonicity of body fluids. As this remains fairly constant, the API can be delivered at a specific rate with minimal patient-to-patient variability. For the same reason, osmotic pump tablets are also less prone to interference from local physiological conditions, e.g. pH, presence of food, than reservoir or matrix systems.

For more information on modified-release tablets, please refer to 'Modified-release tablets' in Section 2.5.

The desired rate of API release can be controlled during formulation by modification of:

- The nature, surface area, and thickness of the semipermeable coating.
- The nature of medium supporting the API.
- The size of the orifice.
- The nature of the water-swelling osmotic agent (for two chamber tablets).

Using osmotic pump delivery, the majority of the API is released at a constant rate (zero-order kinetics), giving this approach an advantage over modified-release dosage forms. The need for an osmotic pressure to establish itself within the tablet means that there is usually a time delay before the API starts to be released in therapeutic concentrations. This principle can be used in the treatment of arthritis, for example. An analgesic osmotic tablet taken before bed can release its API in time to relieve the 'morning stiffness' that accompanies this condition. A range of osmotic pump tablet types continue to be developed to meet specific needs such as this.

For more information on zero-order kinetics, please refer to 'Zero-order reactions' in Section 12.2.

Parenteral osmotic pump implants

Oral osmotic pump tablets are of particular interest because the API is released with zero-order kinetics. This is also a desirable feature for implanted dosage forms used in the treatment of chronic conditions. Accordingly, parenteral osmotic pump implants may be used for the steady delivery of drugs over extended periods, from a few weeks to one year. The implants of this type with the simplest design have a semipermeable membrane at one end of the device (Figure 11.7). After subcutaneous implantation, water is drawn in from the surrounding tissues due to a hypertonic saline solution on the other side of the membrane. This region of the device is commonly referred to as the 'engine' and the osmotic pressure developed here moves a piston that forces the API out of the implant. In this way, the implant acts like a miniature syringe.

Due to the take-up of water, we would expect that the hypertonic saline solution within the osmotic

FIGURE 11.7 Schematic cross-section of a typical osmotic pump implant

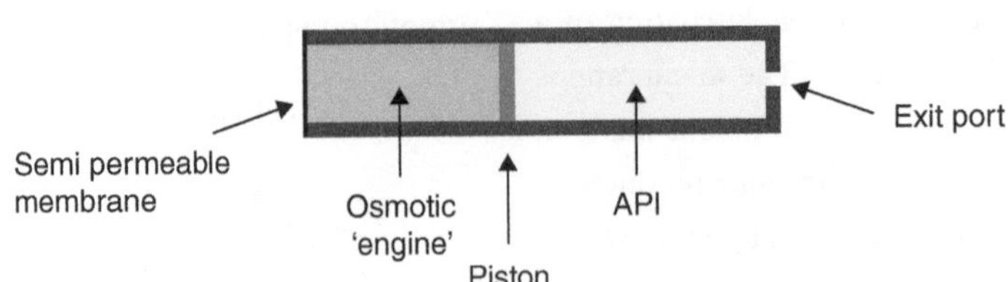

engine would become diluted over the lifetime of the implant. In this case, the osmotic pressure would then drop as it is dependent on the difference in solute concentrations on either side on the membrane. This is undesirable as it would mean that the rate of delivery of the API would also decline over time. An ingenious solution to this problem is to employ a saturated solution of sodium chloride within the osmotic engine. The liquid remains saturated throughout the operation of the device due to presence also of solid NaCl, this solid gradually dissolving as more water enters through the semipermeable membrane. The tonicity of saturated sodium chloride is around 40 times that of the equivalent isotonic solution. It is critical, therefore, that this hypertonic material does not enter the body. The outer casing of the implant, typically 5 mm in diameter, is normally made from a robust titanium alloy. To further minimize the risk of breakage, devices of this type are normally implanted on the inside of the upper arm.

KEY POINT

One- and two-chamber osmotic pump tablets are examples of modified-release tablets. Osmotic pump tablets have advantages as they release the API with largely zero-order kinetics, there being minimal patient-to-patient variability in the rate of release. Osmotic pump implants can release an API over an extended period at a constant rate.

SELF CHECK 11.9

What are the advantages of osmotic pump tablets over matrix and reservoir modified-release tablets?

SELF CHECK 11.10

Why is solid sodium chloride present in the 'engine' of an osmotic pump implant during the lifetime of operation of the device?

11.6 The origin of colligative properties

We noted previously how colligative properties arise due to the influence of entropy, S, and its effects on thermodynamic stability in systems where a solution **phase** is in equilibrium with a second, solvent-containing, phase. We can measure thermodynamic stability in terms of **Gibbs free energy** G, using the standard relationship shown in equation 11.2:

$$G = H - TS \tag{11.2}$$

where H is the enthalpy of the system and T is the **absolute temperature**.

For more information on **Gibbs free energy**, enthalpy, and entropy, please refer to Chapter 5.

To fully understand the origin of colligative properties, it is necessary to employ the concept of **chemical potential**, μ. This is the molar contribution that a component makes to total free energy of a phase. For pure substances, chemical potential is simply equal to the free energy per mole, G.

As it is related to free energy, both enthalpy and entropy contribute to the chemical potential of a component in a system. When a solute is added to water, the enthalpy of the system may increase or decrease, depending on the energies of interaction between the constituent particles. Thus, the addition of NaCl to water at 298 K results in an endothermic change:

$$\Delta H^{\theta} = +3.9 \text{ kJ mol}^{-1}$$

while the dissolution of NaOH is exothermic:

$$\Delta H^{\theta} = -44.5 \text{ kJ mol}^{-1}$$

Regardless of the nature of the solute, however, the addition of a soluble solid to water will always lead to an increase in the entropy of the system. Equation 11.2 indicates that pure substances with higher entropies, S, will generally have lower free energies (chemical potentials). This principle can be extended to mixtures. Thus, the dissolution of NaCl in water leads to an increase in the disorder of the system, raising its entropy, and this may be alternatively expressed as a lowering of the chemical potential of the solvent molecules.

The positive entropy change accompanying dissolution can be understood by considering the number of ways in which a solution can organize itself. Consider a body of solvent that is notionally divided into three sections: left, middle, and right. If one solute particle is present, then at a fixed point in time, the solution can organize itself in three ways: with the particle in either the left, middle, or right sections. We consider a fixed point in time as we understand that configurations can interchange with each other through thermal motion. If two particles are present, then six configurations are possible (Figure 11.8). As the number of solute particles present increases, so does the number of potential configurations. Of course, a real solution would contain many billions of solute particles that could potentially occupy many billions of different positions. The greater the number of potential configurations, or microstates, that are possible, the greater the entropy of the system. Thus, the entropy of a solution will always be greater than the entropy of the solvent alone.

KEY POINT

The addition of solute to a solvent lowers the chemical potential of the solvent molecules in the solution phase due to the associated increase in entropy.

Equilibria and chemical potential

For a system exhibiting colligative properties, the chemical potential of solvent molecules in the solution phase will be the same as the chemical potential of the solvent molecules in the second phase at equilbrium. The associated free energy change, ΔG, is then equal to zero, and this is the general condition for equilibrium.

Equilibria involving two-phase systems are encountered elsewhere in pharmaceutics. Thus, a solute that is soluble in two immiscible solvents will partition between them. At equilibrium, the concentrations of the solute in each phase will remain constant and we may define a partition coefficient. The preference of a solute for one solvent over another during partitioning can also be understood by chemical potential. Thus, a partition equilibrium is attained when the chemical potentials of the *solute* in each of the two phases are equal. Colligative properties arise when a biphasic system changes so that the chemical potential of the *solvent* is the same in the solution and second phase.

For more information on the thermodynamics of partitioning, please refer to Section 8.4.

As solvent molecules have a lower chemical potential when in a solution than when in a pure solvent, the chemical potential of the solvent molecules in the second phase must also decrease to maintain equilibrium. This is manifested as experimentally measurable colligative properties. As chemical potentials, μ, always relates to a particular component, we will identify the chemical concerned by the use of a subscript. Thus, the symbol, $\mu_{H_2O(l)}$, for example, can be used to represent the chemical potential of water molecules in the liquid phase.

KEY POINT

The chemical potential of a pure substance is equal to the molar free energy and chemical potential is related to enthalpy and entropy for all substances.

KEY POINT

At equilibrium, the chemical potential of solvent molecules in the solution phase is the same as that in the second, solvent-containing phase. The chemical potential of the solvent molecules in the second phase lowers to maintain equilibrium when solute is added to the solution phase and this is manifest as the colligative properties.

FIGURE 11.8 Six possible configurations for two solute particles in a body of solvent divided into three notional Sections: left, middle, and right

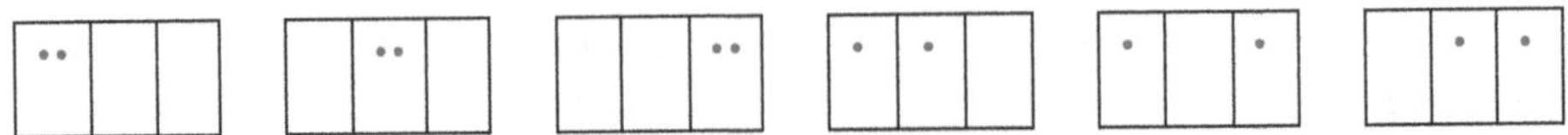

Chemical potential and vapour pressure lowering

The chemical potential of water molecules in a vapour, $\mu_{H_2O(g)}$, is dependent on the vapour pressure. On the basis of ideal gas behaviour and the First and Second Laws of Thermodynamics, it can be shown that:

$$\mu_{H_2O(g)} - \mu^{\theta}_{H_2O(g)} = RT\ln\left(\frac{p}{p^{\theta}}\right) \quad (11.3)$$

where $\mu^{\theta}_{H_2O(g)}$, represents the chemical potential of the vapour at standard pressure, p^{θ} and $\mu_{H_2O(g)}$ is the chemical potential of the same substance at vapour pressure, p.

This relationship is applicable to any vapour phase composed of one component only, such as those that form above water and saline. It predicts that the chemical potential of water decreases with pressure, although in a non-linear fashion (Figure 11.9).

We can now rationalize the observation that the pressure of the water vapour above a solution of sodium chloride in water is less than that above the pure solvent (Figure 11.2). The addition of sodium chloride to water lowers the chemical potential of the solvent. To maintain equilibrium, the molecules of solvent in the second, vapour phase must lower their chemical potential also. Figure 11.9 shows us that this can be accomplished by lowering the vapour pressure, in accord with experimental observation.

FIGURE 11.9 Dependence of the chemical potential of water vapour, $\mu^{\theta}_{H_2O(g)}$ on vapour pressure, p, assuming ideal gas behaviour

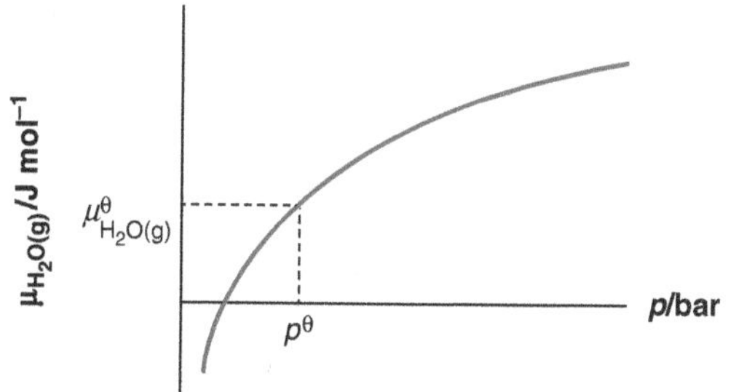

Chemical potential and solute concentration

We can quantitatively understand the effect that the addition of a solute has on the chemical potential of a solvent by assuming that the system behaves as

BOX 11.1

Ideal and non-ideal thermodynamics

Ideal behaviour is rarely seen in practice, but dilute solutions, such as standard saline, approximate to ideal behaviour. Non-ideal thermodynamics provides a more rigorous treatment for real mixtures, although the calculation of the chemical potentials for each component within a real mixture is complex. In saline, for example, the presence of ions affects the strength of attraction between the constituent particles and this will contribute to the overall enthalpy of the system. Compared to solid sodium chloride and pure water, sodium and chloride ions within saline can arrange themselves in innumerable different ways, and the system has a higher entropy. Again, however, attractions between constituent particles will mean that the mixture is not as randomly mixed as it would be if those forces were absent. Oppositely charged sodium and chloride ions will have a tendency to attract each other and stay in the vicinity of each other (Figure 11.10). This effect would be expected to become more significant at higher concentrations as the average inter-ionic distance decreases. As both enthalpy and entropy are affected by concentration, the chemical potential of the solvent is dependent on the composition of the solution.

FIGURE 11.10 A snapshot of solvated ions in an example ideal solution (A) and a typical real mixture (B). The tendency of oppositely charged ions to associate with each other in real solutions, giving rise to deviation from ideal behaviour, is evident

(A)

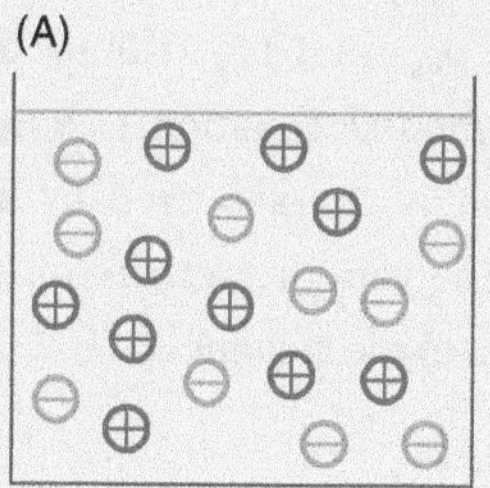

(B)

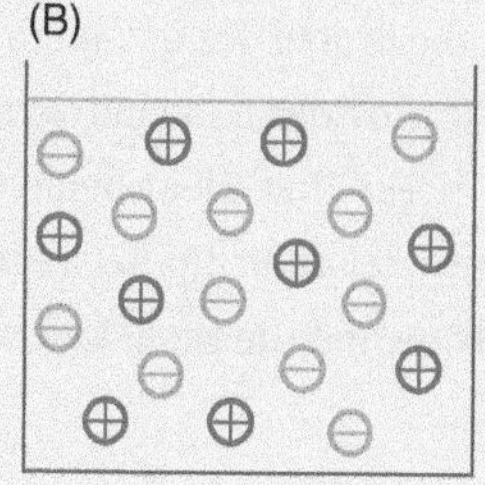

an **ideal solution**. Here, the energies of interaction between all particles (solvent and solute) are assumed to be the same, so that the enthalpy change accompanying **dissolution** is zero. This is not true for concentrated solutions, but is a reasonable approximation for dilute solutions (see Box 11.1).

In equation 11.3, an ideal gas at 1 bar was used as a standard system. The choice of reference system is not critical, however, as long as it remains consistent within a calculation. Thus, while geographers use 'sea-level' as a basis for all altitude measurements, this is an arbitrary (albeit convenient) reference height. Instead of using an ideal gas at 1 bar, we may use the water vapour formed above pure water as a reference system. Under standard conditions this will have an associated pressure, $p^*_{H_2O}$. We will use an asterisk from this point to indicate that reference is being made to a pure substance. We have already noted, for example, that $p^*_{H_2O} = 0.03$ bar at 298 K. Equation 11.3 may be re-written as:

$$\mu_{H_2O(g)} - \mu^*_{H_2O(g)} = RT\ln\left(\frac{p_{H_2O}}{p^*_{H_2O}}\right) \qquad (11.4)$$

This equation relates the chemical potential of water molecules in a vapour above a solution, $\mu_{H_2O(g)}$, to that in the standard system of water molecules in a vapour above pure solvent, $\mu^*_{H_2O(g)}$.

As we have noted, the chemical potential of liquid and vapour phases are the same at equilibrium for a solution, and $\mu_{H_2O(l)} = \mu_{H_2O(g)}$. The same will also be true for the corresponding pure system. If the standard chemical potential of pure water is $\mu^\theta_{H_2O(l)}$ then if follows that at equilibrium that $\mu^\theta_{H_2O(l)} = \mu^*_{H_2O(g)}$. Thus, we may modify equation 11.4 to give:

$$\mu_{H_2O(l)} - \mu^\theta_{H_2O(l)} = RT\ln\left(\frac{p_{H_2O}}{p^*_{H_2O}}\right) \qquad (11.5)$$

This relationship incorporates elements relating to liquids, $\mu_{H_2O(l)}$ and $\mu^\theta_{H_2O(l)}$, alongside parameters that rely on the properties of vapours, p_{H_2O} and $p^*_{H_2O}$. **Raoult's Law** provides a means to harmonize equation 11.5. It proposes that ideal behaviour is characterized by a linear relationship between the vapour pressure of a solvent and the **mole fraction** of the solvent:

$$p_{H_2O} = x_{H_2O}\, p^*_{H_2O}$$

For more information on Raoult's Law, please refer to Section 4.2.

By substitution of Raoult's Law into equation 11.5 we obtain:

$$\mu_{H_2O(l)} - \mu^\theta_{H_2O(l)} = RT\ln x_{H_2O}$$

It is more convenient to consider the mole fraction of the solute, x_S. Given that the sum of the mole fractions of solvent and solute must equal one, we may write:

$$\mu_{H_2O(l)} - \mu^\theta_{H_2O(l)} = RT\ln(1 - x_S)$$

The final term in this expression can be simplified still further as ln $(1 - x_S) \approx -x_S$ when x_S is small. For example, a standard solution of saline has a molarity of 0.15 M. It is reasonable to assume that a litre of this solution contains 1.00 kg of water under standard conditions, equivalent to 55.5 moles. Thus, the negative mole fraction of sodium chloride, $-x_S = -0.15/(0.15+55.5) = -2.695\times10^{-3}$. The equivalent value of ln $(1-x_S)$ is -2.699×10^{-3}. As can be seen, these two values are almost identical and we may write in general that:

$$\mu_{H_2O(l)} - \mu^\theta_{H_2O(l)} = -RTx_S \qquad (11.6)$$

This is a more satisfying form of the equation, as it is immediately apparent that when $x_S > 0$, $\mu_{H_2O(l)}$ will be less than $\mu^\theta_{H_2O(l)}$. In other words, the chemical potential of a solvent will always be lower in solution than in pure solvent. By application of equation 11.6, for example, we find that the chemical potential of water molecules is lowered by 6.6 J mol^{-1} after the addition of NaCl to water to form standard medicinal saline, $x_S = 2.7\times10^{-3}$, at 298 K.

Equation 11.6 also emphasizes the intrinsic link between colligative properties and the number of solute particles, represented by x_S. You will note that terms that relate to the nature of the solute, such as density, molecular mass, and solubility, are absent from this equation.

KEY POINT

The reduction in the chemical potential of a solvent upon addition of a solute to a pure solvent is related to the mole fraction of solute, x_S, and is given by RTx_S. This equation assumes that the solution is behaving ideally.

Chemical potential and transition temperatures

Standard saline has a lower **melting point** (–0.6 °C) and a higher **boiling point** (100.2 °C) than pure water. The presence of salt effectively extends the thermodynamic stability of saline into lower and higher temperature ranges. This can be understood by plotting the variation of the chemical potential of water with temperature for the solvent and saline (Figure 11.11).

The reduction in the chemical potential of water after the addition of sodium chloride is evident from the graph. We can see how the form of pure water with the lowest chemical potential predominates at each temperature, liquid water being most stable at 298 K and 1 atm pressure. The normal melting point of water, T_m=273.15 K, is highlighted on the diagram. At this point, the chemical potential of the pure solid and pure liquid phases is the same and they are in equilibrium, $\mu_{H_2O(s)} = \mu_{H_2O(l)}$. At the normal boiling point of water, T_b=373.15 K, the liquid and gas forms of pure water have equal stabilities, $\mu_{H_2O(l)} = \mu_{H_2O(g)}$.

ΔT_m and ΔT_b show the magnitude of the melting point depression and boiling point elevation (respectively). Notice how the gradients of the correlations for each state of matter vary in Figure 11.11. The relationship between free energy and temperature is linked to entropy. Thus, the correlation for gaseous water has a larger negative gradient than the line for ice as gaseous water has higher entropy. For the purpose of this discussion, it is not necessary to plot an additional line on the graph for solid saline, if we assume that saline freezes to give solid ice. This does not happen in practice, but ultimately this does not affect the general conclusions that we can draw from this diagram.

Chemical potential and osmosis

Consider a trough containing water into which a sample of sodium chloride will be added. The system is subject to a constant external pressure, *p*, and is maintained at fixed temperature. The trough is divided into two sections by a semipermeable membrane. Before NaCl is added, the water molecules will show no preference for one side of the membrane over the other. The chemical potential of pure water, $\mu^{\theta}_{H_2O(l)}$ (*p*), will be the same on both sides of the divider. Here, (*p*) is used to indicate that the chemical potential is for the solvent at an external pressure *p* (Figure 11.12). In an open system, this will normally be atmospheric pressure.

Upon addition of sodium chloride to one side of the divider, the level of liquid in that section rises to a constant level. The total pressure acting on this side of the divider is then $p+\Pi$, where Π is the osmotic pressure. At equilibrium, the chemical potential of the water on each side of the divide is the same:

$$\mu^{\theta}_{H_2O(l)}(p) = \mu_{H_2O(l)}(p+\Pi)$$

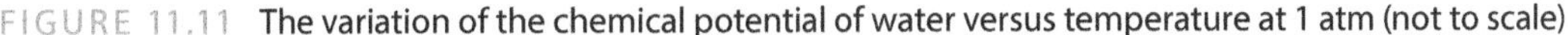

FIGURE 11.11 The variation of the chemical potential of water versus temperature at 1 atm (not to scale)

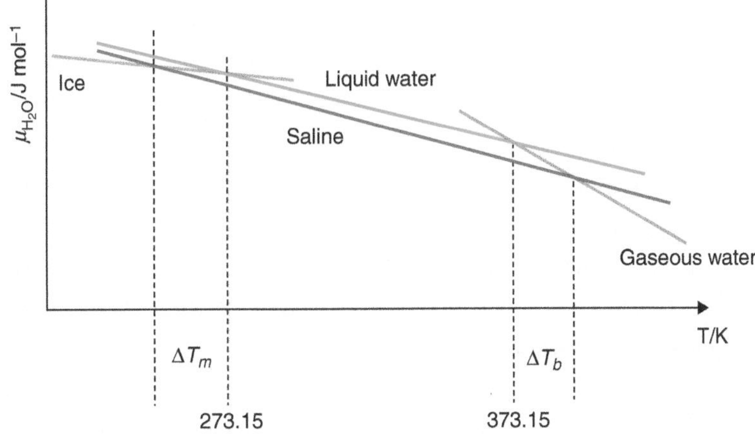

FIGURE 11.12 **The effect of osmosis after the addition of sodium chloride to the right-hand compartment, and the chemical potentials of the solvent in each compartment**

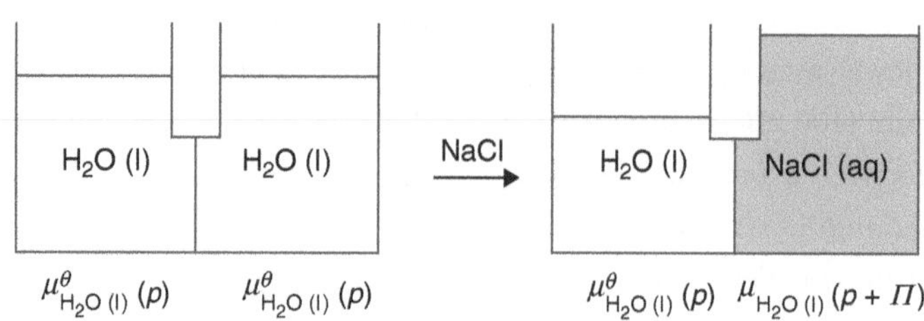

The symbol θ is absent from the chemical potential symbol for water within saline as this is not a pure system. At equal pressures, the chemical potential of solvent molecules in a solution would be lower than those in pure solvent. This can be expressed quantitatively by equation 11.6, assuming ideal behaviour. Crucially here, the pressure on either side of the membrane is not the same.

We established previously that the chemical potential of molecules in a gas is dependent on pressure (equation 11.4). The same is true for solvent molecules in a solution, although changes in pressure have a relatively smaller effect. The chemical potential of solvent molecules in the solution on the right-hand side of the trough is increased by the osmotic pressure, so that it attains the same value that it had before the introduction of NaCl. In this way, the chemical potentials of water on both sides of the divider are equal, as required for equilibrium.

SELF CHECK 11.11

How is the change in the chemical potential of water in solution mathematically related to the amount of solute added for an ideal solution?

SELF CHECK 11.12

Why is salt added to icy roads in winter?

CHAPTER SUMMARY

- The colligative properties of solutions are those dependent only on the number of solute particles present and the nature of the solvent. They are:
  - Osmotic pressure.
  - Vapour pressure lowering.
  - Lowering (or 'depression') of melting point.
  - Raising (or 'elevation') of boiling point.
- Colligative properties are measurable in systems where there is a solution phase in equilibrium with a second phase that is made up of the same solvent as the solution.
- Osmosis is the most important colligative property in pharmaceutics. It arises when a semipermeable membrane is present that is impermeable to solute particles but allows solvent molecules to pass through, generating osmotic pressure.
- Osmolarity is used to measure the effective strength of solutions that generate osmotic pressures, units = osmol L^{-1}. For ideal systems, this is simply the sum of the molarities of the solute particles.
- The van't Hoff osmotic pressure equation can be used to calculate osmotic pressures in ideal systems.
- Tonicity is a measure of the osmotic pressure gradient across a semipermeable membrane, normally a cell membrane.
- An isotonic solution has the same tonicity as body fluids (around 0.3 osmol L^{-1}).

- Liquid dosage forms for oral delivery and for topical application to the skin or ear need not necessarily be isotonic with body fluids.
- Liquid dosage forms for ophthalmic, nasal and parenteral delivery are generally isotonic. Hypertonic solutions may be preferred in the treatment of oedemas, or acceptable when delivered slowly by intravenous infusion.
- Tonicity agents are excipients that may be added to a formulation to attain the desired osmolarity.
- Osmotic pump tablets are a form of modified-release system. They can be used with both soluble and poorly soluble drugs and are characterized by zero-order rates of API release and minimal patient-to-patient variability.
- Osmotic pump implants harness osmotic pressure to release an API slowly and at a near-constant rate over an extended period.
- All colligative properties arise due to the reduction in the chemical potential of solvent molecules upon the addition of solute.
- The decrease in the chemical potential of solvent molecules for an ideal system is given by RTx_S, where x_S is the mole fraction of solute added to a pure solvent.
- To maintain equilibrium, the chemical potential of the solvent molecules in the second phase must be equal to the chemical potential of solvent molecules in the solution phase. This is manifest as the colligative properties of the solution.

FURTHER READING

Atkins, P.W. and de Paula, J. *Physical Chemistry.* (9th edn). Oxford: Oxford University Press (2009).

This book has a section on colligative properties with an associated mathematical treatment. This includes a section on osmosis, including the use of osmometry to determine molar mass.

Florence, A.T. and Attwood, D. *Physicochemical Principles of Pharmacy.* (5th edn). London: Pharmaceutical Press (2011).

This book includes a section on osmosis, including a consideration of systems than behave in a non-ideal manner and the clinical relevance of this phenomenon. Osmotic pump delivery systems are described.

12

Kinetics and drug stability

GARY MOSS

While thermodynamics deals with the tendency for a reaction or process to occur, kinetics deals with the *rate* at which this process *may actually happen*. It therefore differentiates between those processes that are predicted to occur in theory, and those that happen in practice. In the pharmaceutical arena this is vital as it deals with a host of issues, from chemical reaction rates (e.g. for drug decomposition or enzymatic reactions), to physical processes (e.g. drug transport across a membrane).

 For more information on thermodynamics, please refer to Chapter 5.

Kinetic studies can provide information on the mechanism of reactions, and allow the degree of change during a process to be measured against time. This latter point is highly important in pharmaceutics as it is used, for example:

- In studies of drug **dissolution**.
- In developing a formulation for a medicine that ensures it is sufficiently stable, i.e. one that enables it to be stored for a reasonable duration without degradation of the **active pharmaceutical ingredient (API)** to an ineffective or toxic form.
- In establishing the **shelf life** of a drug.

The pharmacist must clearly appreciate potential issues of instability of the medicines that they dispense. This will ensure that the drug is presented in a suitable manner to eventually reach its intended target at an appropriate concentration. Kinetics is also a field that may be applied more broadly to the process of drug absorption, distribution and elimination by, and in, the body.

Learning objectives

Having read this chapter you are expected to be able to:

- To introduce the key concepts of kinetics and how they are applied in pharmaceutical systems.
- To appreciate the different types of reactions relevant to dosage forms, including those in the context of drug stability and how the unwanted reactions may be reduced or eliminated.
- To understand the concept of rate laws, rate constants and reaction order.
- To appreciate the factors that affect reaction rates in pharmaceutical systems.

12.1 Types of reactions

Currently, the vast majority of APIs are small organic chemicals and there are a number of reactions that they commonly undergo. These include chemical degradation of the drug by:

- Hydrolysis.
- Oxidation.
- Photochemical decomposition.
- Polymerization.
- Isomerization.

These reactions can be homogenous or heterogeneous and may happen in various physical states, including solids (e.g. tablets) and liquids (e.g. formulations for injection).

For more information on solids, please refer to Chapter 2.

For more information on liquids, please refer to Chapter 3.

This section will discuss each of these types of reactions and provide examples of the types of chemicals that may be prone to each one. The application of kinetic theories allows stability to be assessed, which is important for determining the **shelf life** of medicines. Formulation strategies used to improve stability will be discussed. The type of packaging used will also affect drug stability. For example, amber bottles are commonly used to store materials that are **photosensitive**.

For more information on pharmaceutical packaging, please refer to Section 13.6.

Hydrolysis

Hydrolysis is the reaction of a chemical with water and it usually results in the molecule splitting into fragments. Certain chemical groups, including esters, amides and lactams, are prone to hydrolysis. It is a process that may be catalysed by the presence of acid or base in solution and this may be defined as either:

- specific acid-base catalysis, where the concentration of reactive species is increased by interaction of reactants with H^+ or OH^-, or
- general acid-base catalysis, where there is an interaction with acidic and basic molecules present in a formulation, such as the components of **buffers**.

Consider a reaction studied at constant **pH**. If it was observed that reaction rate increased with buffer concentration, despite the fixed pH, then this would be indicative of general catalysis. A rate dependant on pH would provide evidence for specific catalysis.

Ester and amide hydrolysis

An example of ester hydrolysis is shown in Figure 12.1, with the local anaesthetic, tetracaine [2-dimethylaminoethyl 4-butylaminobenzoate], the active ingredient in Ametop™ gel.

Hydrolysis of amides involves cleavage of the amide linkage in, for example, lidocaine [2-diethylaminoaceto-2′,6′-xylidide], shown in Figure 12.2. This results in the production of a carboxylic acid and an amine. Other examples of amide-containing drugs that may undergo such reactions include benzylpenicillin sodium, glipizide and atorvastatin calcium.

Oxidation

Oxidative degradation of drugs is a major cause of instability in pharmaceutical **dosage forms**. Compounds affected in this manner include those with phenol groups, such as morphine, adrenaline, steroids, and various vitamins and fats. Oxidation usually occurs via a free radical chain reaction that normally begins with:

- the removal of an electropositive atom, radical, or electron, or,
- the addition of an electronegative species.

These processes happen very slowly over long periods of time. They are usually propagated by the presence

FIGURE 12.1 **Hydrolysis of the amino-ester local anaesthetic tetracaine. Hydrolysis of an ester yields an acid (in the example below, this is *4*-butylaminobenzoic acid) and an alcohol (dimethylaminoethanol). Other examples of APIs containing ester functional groups include enalapril, various esters of testosterone and other amino-ester local anaesthetics, such as procaine and benzocaine**

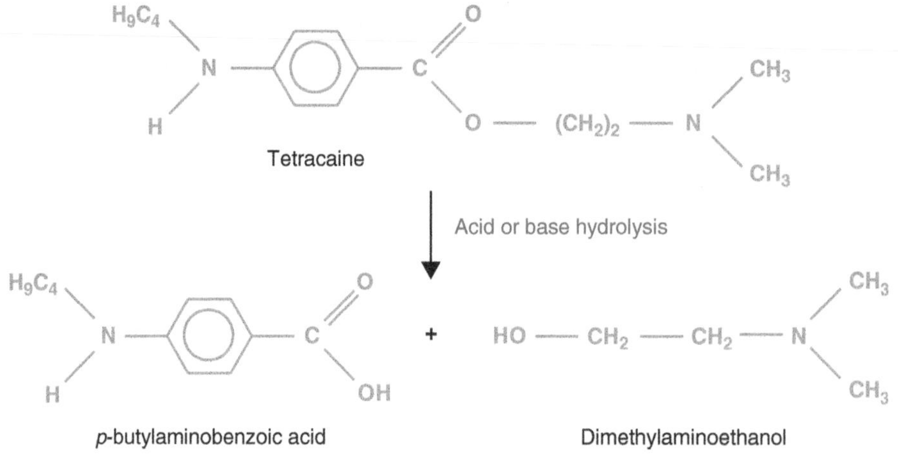

Tetracaine

Acid or base hydrolysis

p-butylaminobenzoic acid + Dimethylaminoethanol

of oxygen in the environment of the formulation, a process called auto-oxidation.

For more information on oxidation, please refer to Chapter 4 'Properties of aliphatic hydrocarbons' and Chapter 5 'Alcohols, phenols, ethers, organic halogen compounds, and amines' of the ***Pharmaceutical Chemistry*** book of this series.

FIGURE 12.2 **General reaction for the hydrolysis of the amino-ester local anaesthetic lidocaine**

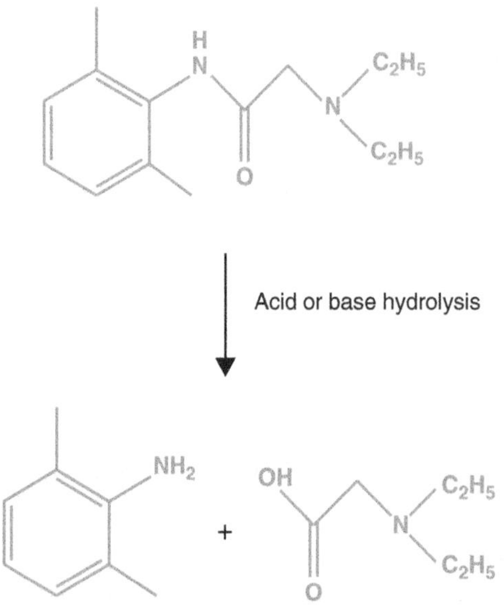

Acid or base hydrolysis

Oxidation reactions may be initiated by the presence of free radicals which are formed by exposure of the dosage form to heat or light. Thus, a chemical prone to oxidative degradation, such as the calcium channel blocker nifedipene, can be stored in an amber bottle to minimize the effects of light. An API that is sensitive to heat may need to be stored below room temperature. Trace metals in the dosage form can also initiate oxidation reactions. In the manufacture of tablets using stainless steel tablet presses, for example, very small amounts of metals may become incorporated. The complete removal of trace metals, or oxygen, is not always possible so formulations may have to be modified to include anti oxidant stabilizers. These work by terminating the propagation steps of the chain reaction. Examples of commonly used anti-oxidants include:

- Butylated hydroxyanisole.
- Butylated hydroxytoluene.
- Various gallates.
- Various tocopherols.
- Various reducing agents.

Sodium metabisulphite is an example of a reducing agent. These work by donating electrons to another species and may be used to reduce the rate of oxidation reactions. Moderating pH, ionic strength (including dielectric and buffering aspects of formulation) and particularly temperature are the most effective ways of controlling hydrolysis and oxidation reactions. The degradation of peptide and protein drugs (such as insulin or calcitonin) can be addressed by reducing the rate of both deamidation (removal of an amide) and oxidation reactions in either the solid state or in solution. Techniques include:

- Conformational control, being the manipulation of structural arrangements in order to prevent sensitive areas of the drug being exposed to potential reactants.
- Lyophilisate formation, being the formation of materials by rapid freezing and dehydration of the frozen product under vacuum.

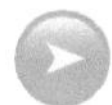
For more information on lyophilization, please refer to 'Drying and lyophilization' in Section 4.3.

Photochemical decomposition

Many pharmaceutical materials are **photosensitive**. Examples of such chemicals include folic acid, prednisolone and hydrocortisone. The reactions of these materials are similar to the oxidation reactions described above, except that they are initiated by exposure to visible or UV light. Reaction proceeds *via* a process of initiation followed by propagation of a chain reaction by free radicals. Modification of a formulation can protect against photochemical decomposition, e.g. by coating tablets with polymeric materials that absorb UV light. Protection from photochemical decomposition is relatively straightforward, as formulations can be stored in amber bottles or kept in the dark away from direct sunlight. Amber glass protects against wavelengths below 470 nm and therefore protects against UV light.

For more information on pharmaceutical packaging, please refer to Section 13.6.

Polymerization

Polymerization is where monomer molecules join together to form large polymer chains consisting of repeating units. In pharmaceutical science, the monomer is normally the API. This type of reaction can occur in solution during long-term storage. Dimerization occurs when two molecules on an API join together to form a complex known as a dimer. Ampicillin shows this type of behaviour and is discussed in Integration Box 12.1.

Isomerization

Isomerization is where an API may be converted into its different isomers, which may be optical isomers or geometric isomers. This is an important process to understand and control as different isomers of an API frequently have altered therapeutic activities or may be toxic. The rearrangement of the active therapeutic agent to its inactive or toxic isomers may be considered as a type of degradation reaction. This results in a reduction of the therapeutic concentration of API provided for the patient or the introduction of toxic substances that may harm the patient (Florence and Attwood, 2005). See Integration Box 12.2 for some examples.

For more information on isomerism, please refer to Chapter 3 'Stereochemistry and drug action' in the *Pharmaceutical Chemistry* book of this series.

Homogenous and heterogeneous reactions

Homogenous reactions are those that occur in a single phase, such as reactions in solutions or gases. Heterogeneous reactions are those that occur in more than one phase, usually as an interfacial phenomenon at the boundary of two phases, perhaps in a disperse

INTEGRATION BOX 12.1

Dimerization of ampicillin

Concentrated solutions of ampicillin undergo concomitant dimerization and hydrolysis. Other β-lactam antibiotics may also undergo this reaction, with the most basic being the most prone to such types of reactions. These reactions are important to understand as they have been shown to be very toxic, being responsible for causing penicilloyl-specific allergic reactions in humans (Florence and Attwood, 2005).

INTEGRATION BOX 12.2

Examples of the isomerization of APIs

The formation of a mixture of enantiomers (racemization) of adrenaline at acidic pH means that the less active form, *L*-adrenaline, increases in concentration. This means that the overall concentration of the active therapeutic agent, *D*-adrenaline, is reduced and the overall therapeutic effect is lessened. Isomerization reactions have also been shown to change the activity of other APIs. The configuration of one of the **stereogenic** centres of tetracycline can change (**epimerization**) in a pH-dependant process (Figure 12.3). It may be possible to stabilize aqueous solutions of both these drugs by the inclusion of buffers which will regulate the pH of the formulation (Florence and Attwood, 2005).

FIGURE 12.3 **The epimerization of tetracycline, showing the transformation between tetracycline (top) and 4-epi-tetracycline (bottom)**

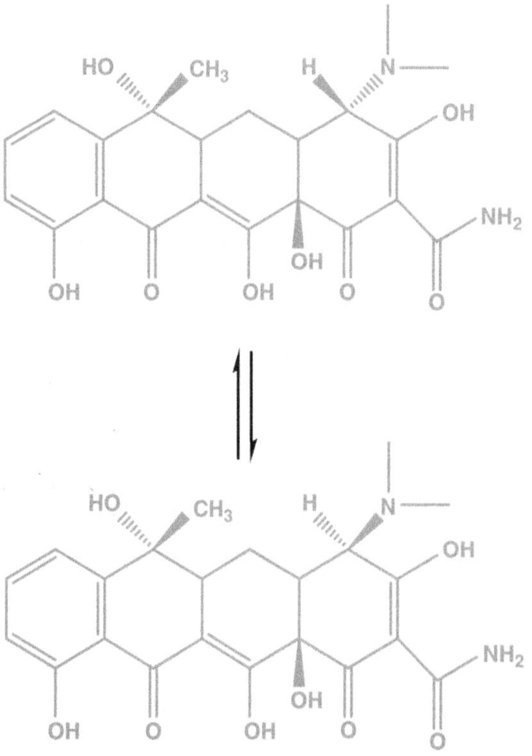

system. In this case the rate of reaction depends on the supply of fresh reactants to the interface. Examples of heterogeneous reactions include the decomposition of APIs in suspension or the dissolution of effervescent dosage forms.

For more information on disperse systems, please refer to Chapter 10.

KEY POINTS

- APIs can degrade through a variety of homogeneous and heterogeneous reaction types.
- Hydrolysis and oxidation are the major causes of instability in pharmaceutical dosage forms.
- Stabilizers may be added to formulations and packaging may be modified to slow the rate of degradation reactions.
- Degradation prior to administration may mean that a medicine delivers less than the therapeutic dose.

SELF CHECK 12.1

The decomposition of an API was studied in pH5, pH7 and pH9 buffer solutions. It was observed that the rate of decomposition increased as pH increased, the concentration of buffer in each solution being constant. On this basis, we may conclude that this reaction is an example of:

(a) Specific acid catalysis.

(b) General acid catalysis.

(c) Specific base catalysis.

(d) General base catalysis.

SELF CHECK 12.2

A cream for topical application can be used to treat minor skin irritations and contains hydrocortisone acetate and sodium metabisulphite. What is the purpose of these two ingredients?

12.2 Reaction rates and reaction orders

Most commonly in pharmaceutical systems, we will be concerned with reactions where a new product is being made, or where a starting material is degrading into unwanted products. The progress of such reactions is followed by measuring the appearance of a product, the disappearance of a starting material, or by the appearance and disappearance of intermediate reactants. To determine the rate of reaction, the change in concentration of the reactant or the product is measured. The units of this process are normally concentration per unit time, i.e. mol dm^{-3} s^{-1}, or mol L^{-1} s^{-1}. The rate of a reaction, v can be represented by the general expressions:

$$v = -\frac{d[Reactant]}{dt} = \frac{d[Product]}{dt} \quad (12.1)$$

BOX 12.1

Converting 'how fast' to 'how far'

While the rate of a reaction tells us *how fast* it is going, it is also important to understand *how far* it has gone i.e. how close to completion the reaction is. In a car, the speedometer tells us how fast we are going, while the odometer (or mileometer) tells us how far we have gone. The distance travelled is obtained by integrating speed in the context of the duration (time) of the journey. Generally the speed is not constant and changes throughout the journey, but this can be dealt with by integration. If a graph of speed versus time is plotted, integration can give the area under the curve between defined starting and finishing points. This area is then equal to the total distance travelled between these limits. In reaction kinetics, we may set the starting time as equal to zero seconds, and the starting concentration as equal to the initial concentration. Integration of rate equations can then yield expressions for the concentration of reactant left after a certain amount of time has passed. Thus, while the rate law tells us how fast a reaction is going, the integrated rate law tells us how far it has gone.

where d is standard mathematical notation that indicates an infinitesimally small change in the quantity shown alongside. Thus, v is the rate of change of concentration with time and, by convention, it is always expressed as a positive value.

The amount of reactant reduces during a reaction and so the rate of change of [reactant] with time always has a negative value. When this is multiplied by the minus sign in Equation 12.1, we obtain a positive value for v, in accord with convention. This tells us how fast a reaction is proceeding, but we are also interested in how close to completion it is, Box 12.1.

The rate determining step

A chemical reaction is always made up of one or more individual, or elementary, reaction steps. Together, these are referred to as the reaction mechanism. Each step involves a fixed number of reactants and products according to the reaction stoichiometry. The number of reacting molecules involved in a specific step is referred to as the **molecularity** of that step.

For example, a unimolecular step is where a single species reacts. Example reaction:

$$N_2O_4 \rightarrow 2NO_2$$

Generic form:

$$A \rightarrow Product(s) \quad (12.2)$$

A bimolecular reaction step is where two species react. Example reaction:

$$HCl + NaOH \rightarrow NaCl + H_2O$$

Generic form:

$$A + B \rightarrow Product(s) \quad (12.3)$$

In a bimolecular process, the two species may be the same. Example reaction:

$$2NO_2 \rightarrow N_2O_4$$

Reactions involving three reactant molecules, so-called termolecular reactions, are rare as the probability of three or more chemicals combining simultaneously is highly unlikely.

The reactions described previously are all clearly defined and could be studied quite easily, but this is not always the case. For example, chlordiazepoxide degrades via hydrolysis to initially form a lactam product. The lactam will then react in acidic condition to yield benzophenone. These kinds of multi-step processes are common in pharmaceutical science. Further complications occur if steps are reversible and pathways branch so that parallel reactions occur. An example is the decomposition of nitrazepam, which decomposes in aqueous solution to form 2-amino-5-nitrobenzophenone or 3-amino-6-nitro-4-phenyl-2(1H)-quinolone. The route taken by the degradation reaction will depend on the conditions, such as the amount of water present. In general, intricate reaction pathways such as this are referred to as complex reactions (see Box 12.2).

The rate-determining step is that part of a chemical reaction that is slowest and which will therefore determine the observed, overall, rate of reaction. For example, consider a patient swallowing a tablet with water. The rate at which the API begins to work in the body depends on:

BOX 12.2

Complex reactions

Most reactions in pharmaceutical systems consist of several steps. These are called complex reactions and the most common types of complex reactions are:

- *Reversible reactions* – where the forward and reverse reaction rates of a reversible process need to be taken into account when determining the overall reaction rate.
- *Parallel reactions* – where one chemical may react in different ways and produce more than one product at the same time.
- *Serial (consecutive) reactions* – where the reaction proceeds from the starting material and produces a product which, in turn, then reacts further to produce another chemical. Usually these reactions happen serially, or one after the other.

- The rate of disintegration of the tablet.
- The rate of dissolution of the API, i.e. the transfer of the solid drug that was in the tablet into solution in the body.

If the rate of dissolution is slow, perhaps because the solubility of the drug is comparatively poor, then the rate-limiting step will be the dissolution of the drug in the body. Similarly, with regard to chemical stability, the rate-limiting step is that one reaction that governs the overall rate of a process. For example, in the discussion of chemical degradation by oxidation (previously), the initiation step is usually the rate-limiting step. The overall order of a reaction is the number of concentrations of the reacting species that determine the rate of reaction. This can be expressed as the rate law; a mathematical relationship that relates the reaction rate to the concentrations of the reactants and their orders. The rate law can only ever be established by performing experiments that investigate the kinetics of the reaction of interest. For example, for a reaction with reactants A, B and C, the rate law may be written as:

$$v = k[\mathrm{A}]^{a}[\mathrm{B}]^{b}[\mathrm{C}]^{c} \tag{12.4}$$

where k is the rate constant for the reaction and this has a fixed value at constant temperature. The exponents a, b, and c represent the order of the reaction in each of the reactants A, B and C, respectively. The sum of the exponents, a + b + c, is the overall reaction order.

While there are many different types of reactions, those overall orders most commonly associated with pharmaceutical systems are zero-, first-, second-, and associated *pseudo* orders. These reactions will be discussed below.

Zero-order reactions

A zero-order reaction is one where the process, such as the degradation of an API in its dosage form or dissolution, proceeds at a constant rate that is not dependent on the concentrations of any of the reactants. The rate of change for a zero-order reaction is given by:

$$-\frac{d[\mathrm{A}]}{dt} = k \tag{12.5}$$

where [A] represents the concentration of reactant remaining (this being the API in drug degradation studies), t is the reaction time, and k is the rate constant.

A negative sign is used as the concentration of A decreases with time. If $[A]_0$ is the concentration of A when time is zero then we may integrate equation (12.5) using:

$$\int_{[A]_0}^{[A]} d[A] = -k\int_0^t dt \qquad (12.6)$$

where the two integration symbols show the starting and finishing limits for concentration and time.

Integration between these limits yields:

$$[A]-[A]_0 = -k(t-0) \qquad (12.7)$$

and this gives:

$$[A] = -kt + [A]_0 \qquad (12.8)$$

This equation has a linear form and a plot of [A] (y-axis), against time, (x-axis), will be linear and have a gradient of $-k$. The units of a zero-order rate constant are the same as those for rate, e.g. concentration time^{-1}. Many pharmaceutical and biological processes follow zero-order kinetics and the rate of degradation does not depend on the concentration. They usually occur at the boundary of two phases where, for example, an API may be dissolving from a solid dosage form into the surrounding solution. This constant rate of drug delivery is important for drug delivery systems as it allows for the delivery of a constant amount of API over a defined time period.

It is also common for drug degradation to occur in some dosage forms (such as suspensions) by zero-order reactions. In a suspension, the drug is usually present as a solid suspended in a liquid medium (usually an aqueous medium). The drug will dissolve in the solution, forming a saturated solution, and excess drug will be present as undissolved particles in suspension. Therefore, the concentration of the drug in solution depends on its solubility. As the drug decomposes in solution it is replaced by suspended drug, ensuring that the concentration of API in solution remains constant despite the degradation that also occurs in solution. This gives rise to *pseudo* (or apparent) zero-order reaction and this will continue until the entire drug in suspension has dissolved and entered solution.

The **half-life** is the time taken for half of the initial concentration to disappear; that is, the time taken for $[A]_0$ to decrease to $[A]_0/2$. To derive an expression for the half-life of a zero-order reaction the term $t_{0.5}$ is used to represent the half-life and is inserted into the rate equation 12.8:

$$\frac{[A]_0}{2} = -kt_{0.5} + [A]_0 \qquad (12.9)$$

which gives:

$$t_{0.5} = \frac{[A]_0}{2k} \qquad (12.10)$$

Example of zero-order kinetics

The amount of drug remaining in a topical ointment after application is shown in Table 12.1. A plot of the amount of drug remaining in the formulation against time is shown in Figure 12.4. According to Equation 12.8, minus gradient is equal to the rate constant, and it follows that $k = 0.63\ \mu g\ h^{-1}$.

First-order reactions

First-order reactions are the most common, and important, in pharmaceutical systems. The rate of a first-order reaction is determined by one concentration term only, and the general rate expression is given by:

$$-\frac{d[A]}{dt} = k[A] \qquad (12.11)$$

TABLE 12.1 **Mass of drug remaining in a topical ointment after application**

Time/h	Mass of drug remaining/µg
0	100.0
12	89.6
24	75.5
48	61.9
96	31.7
144	7.4

FIGURE 12.4 Plot of mass of drug remaining against time for a topically applied ointment

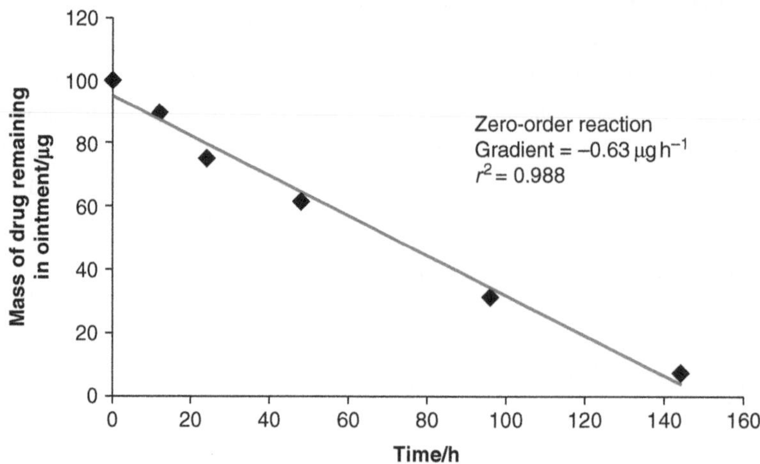

From this expression it is evident that the rate of reaction is dependent on the concentration of reactant that remains. Thus, the rate of a first-order process will be highest at the start of a reaction, when the concentration of reactant is at its highest. To determine the changes that a real dosage form may undergo it is necessary to sum all the changes from the beginning of the process, where the concentration of A is $[A]_0$, to particular point in the reaction at time, t. This is achieved by integrating the rate expression:

$$\int_{[A]_0}^{[A]} \frac{1}{[A]} d[A] = -k \int_0^t dt \qquad (12.12)$$

Integration yields:

$$\ln[A] - \ln[A]_0 = -k(t-0) \qquad (12.13)$$

where ln represents the natural logarithm which is the log to the base e, where e = 2.718.

Rearrangement of equation 12.13 gives:

$$\ln[A] = -kt + \ln[A]_0 \qquad (12.14)$$

Like equation 12.8, this last expression is linear in form, meaning that it takes the general form:

$$y = mx + c$$

A plot of ln [A] (y-axis) against time (x-axis) will result in a straight line, with gradient $-k$. The units of a first-order rate constant are always time^{-1}, e.g. s^{-1}. Equation 12.14 may also be presented in a non-linear form:

$$[A] = [A]_0 e^{-kt} \qquad (12.15)$$

This predicts that the amount of starting material is expected to change exponentially with time for any first-order process. This includes, for example, radioactive decay. Theoretically, the concentration of a reactant in a first-order reaction will asymptotically progress. That is, it will gradually approach the horizontal axis on a graph ([A] = zero) but will never quite reach it.

Both equations 12.14 and 12.15 may be expressed to the base 10, rather than e, by using the correcting factor ln 10 (= 2.303).

$$\log[A] = \frac{-kt}{2.303} + \log[A]_0 \qquad (12.16)$$

where log represents log to base 10. Similarly:

$$[A] = [A]_0 10^{-kt/2.303} \qquad (12.17)$$

As with zero-order kinetics, the half-life of a first-order reaction may be determined if we consider that, when $t = t_{0.5}$, $[A] = [A]_0/2$. Substitution into equation 12.14 gives:

$$\ln\frac{[A]_0}{2} = -kt_{0.5} + \ln[A]_0 \qquad (12.18)$$

Rearrangement and applying the properties of logs gives:

$$kt_{0.5} = \ln[A]_0 - \ln\frac{[A]_0}{2} = \ln\left(\frac{2[A]_0}{[A]_0}\right) \qquad (12.19)$$

which simplifies to yield:

$$t_{0.5} = \frac{\ln(2)}{k} \qquad (12.20)$$

TABLE 12.2 Percentage and log percentage of the drug concentration remaining following hydrolysis of tetracaine

Time/h	Percentage of drug remaining	Log (percentage of drug remaining)
0	100	2.000
2	92.37	1.966
4	80.09	1.904
8	41.33	1.616
16	15.79	1.198
24	8.26	0.917

Expression 12.20 means that the half-life of a first-order reaction is independent of the initial concentration of the reactants. The natural log of 2 has a value of 0.693 and this number can be used in place of ln (2).

Example of first-order kinetics

The hydrolysis of tetracaine in an acidic solution was observed and the data obtained are shown in Table 12.2.

If the reaction follows first-order kinetics then a plot of the log [tetracaine] against time will give a straight line of slope $-k/2.303$. The properties of logarithms mean that we can determine k using any variable that is directly proportional to [A], in this case, the percentage of drug remaining. Thus, a plot of log (percentage of drug remaining) versus time will also give a straight line of slope $-k/2.303$ (Figure 12.5).

$$\text{Slope} = \frac{(y_2 - y_1)}{(x_2 - x_1)} = -\frac{k}{2.303}$$

$$\text{Slope} = (1.198 - 1.966)/(16 - 2) = -0.768/14$$

$$\text{Slope} = -5.48 \times 10^{-2}\ \text{h}^{-1}$$

$$-\frac{k}{2.303} = -5.48 \times 10^{-2}\ \text{h}^{-1}$$

$$k = 0.126\ \text{h}^{-1}$$

We may also calculate the half-life using:

$$t_{0.5} = \frac{\ln(2)}{k} = \frac{\ln(2)}{0.126\ \text{h}^{-1}}$$

Thus, the half-life of the drug in this case is:

$$t_{0.5} = 5.5\ \text{h}$$

Second-order reactions

Second-order reaction equations are used to describe the rates of single-step bimolecular reactions that occur when two molecules react, i.e.:

$$\text{A} + \text{B} \rightarrow \text{Product(s)} \qquad (12.21)$$

In pharmaceutical systems, such reactions include the acid base-catalysed hydrolysis of APIs. The rate of reaction depends on the concentration of *both* reactants, and the rate of decomposition of both A and B will be the same with both being proportional to the product of the concentration of the reactants. The

FIGURE 12.5 A plot of log (percentage tetracaine remaining) against time

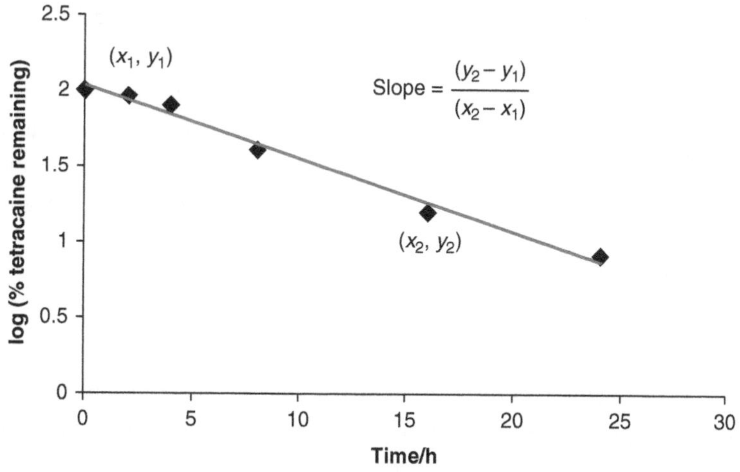

general rate expression for a second-order reaction is given by:

$$-\frac{d[\text{A}]}{dt} = -\frac{d[\text{B}]}{dt} = k[\text{A}][\text{B}] \qquad (12.22)$$

where *A* and *B* are the concentrations of the two reacting species.

As before, a negative sign is used as the concentration of both A and B decreases with time. A single-step bimolecular reaction will always have a second-order rate law, although this principle does not work in reverse. Thus, for example, the reaction of hydrogen and iodine gas has a rate law $v=k\ [H_2]\ [I_2]$. Rather than being a single-step bimolecular reaction, however, experiments indicate a multistep mechanism for this reaction involving reactive free radical intermediates. As always, however, the rate law arises from the slowest, rate-determining step. This need not necessarily require that the species shown in the rate law are actually involved in the slowest step. Multistep reactions and their rate laws can be rationalized by application of the steady state assumption, a topic beyond the scope of this book.

A second-order reaction may occur when two molecules of the same reagent come together in a single step bimolecular reaction.

$$2\text{A} \rightarrow \text{Products} \qquad (12.23)$$

The corresponding rate law is then:

$$-\frac{d[\text{A}]}{dt} = k[\text{A}]^2 \qquad (12.24)$$

Again, integration can be used to determine the concentration of *A* at time, *t*, during the reaction:

$$\int_{[\text{A}]_0}^{[\text{A}]} \frac{1}{[\text{A}]^2} d[\text{A}] = -k\int_0^t dt \qquad (12.25)$$

Integration yields:

$$\left(-\frac{1}{[\text{A}]}\right) - \left(-\frac{1}{[\text{A}]_0}\right) = -k(t-0) \qquad (12.26)$$

You will note that the right-hand side of this expression is the same as for the equivalent expressions for zero- and first-order reactions, equations 12.7 and 12.13, respectively. Rearrangement gives:

$$\frac{1}{[\text{A}]} = kt + \frac{1}{[\text{A}]_0} \qquad (12.27)$$

This expression again has the general form of a straight-line graph: A plot of 1/[A] (y axis) versus time (x axis) is expected to have a slope equal to *k*. As with first-order kinetics, the second-order integrated rate law can be presented non-linearly:

$$[\text{A}] = \frac{[\text{A}]_0}{kt[\text{A}]_0 + 1} \qquad (12.28)$$

These second-order integrated expressions apply to a bimolecular process where two molecules of A combine. However, they can also be applied to the study of bimolecular reactions where A and B combine, but only if the starting concentrations of the two different species are the same, i.e. $[A]_0=[B]_0$. As the stoichiometry of equation 2.21 is 1:1, the concentrations of A and B will also remain the same throughout the entire reaction in this case.

The half-life of a second-order reaction may be determined if we consider that, when $t=t_{0.5}$, $[A]=[A]_0/2$. Substitution into equation 12.27 gives:

$$\frac{2}{[\text{A}]_0} = kt_{0.5} + \frac{1}{[\text{A}]_0} \qquad (12.29)$$

Multiplying throughout by $[A]_0$ gives:

$$2 = [\text{A}]_0\ kt_{0.5} + 1 \qquad (12.30)$$

which simplifies to yield:

$$t_{0.5} = \frac{1}{[\text{A}]_0 k} \qquad (12.31)$$

Unlike the half-life expression for a first-order reaction, the half-life of a second-order reaction depends on the initial concentration of the reactants. Again, for second-order reactions that are first-order in each of A and B, equation 12.31 will be valid only if the initial concentrations of each reactant are the same.

Pseudo first-order reactions

Under certain conditions, single step biomolecular reactions may appear to follow first-order kinetics. This is often observed in pharmaceutical systems where the concentration of one of the reactants is present in a vast excess, compared to the other reactant. In this case, any change in concentration of the reagent in excess is negligible compared to the change in the concentration of the other reactants. This is called a *pseudo* first-order reaction. This type of reaction kinetics is observed in pharmaceutical systems where the API is hydrolysed by water in an aqueous system. For example, tetracaine is an ester (RCO_2R') and is hydrolysed according to the following scheme:

$$RCO_2R' + H_2O \rightarrow RCO_2H + R'OH \qquad (12.32)$$

Experimentally, this reaction is found to have second-order kinetics overall:

$$v = k\left[RCO_2R'\right]\left[H_2O\right] \qquad (12.33)$$

However, as water is the solvent, it is present in a vast excess and any change in its concentration is not significant compared to changes in the concentration of the ester. In such cases $[H_2O]$ is considered to be constant. The reaction is then described as a *pseudo* first-order process, the rate of reaction apparently being proportional to the concentration of the ester only.

Determination of reaction order

The order of a reaction may be determined by several methods,

- Substituting experimental data into integrated forms of the various rate equations.
- Plotting data using linear forms of the various rate equations.
- Analysis of half-lives.
- Method of initial rates.

Examining how [A] varies with time is usually done by determining the amount of API decomposed at different time intervals and substituting the data into the integrated equations for each potential type of reaction: zero-, first- or second-order reactions. The equation that gives the most consistent value of k with all the data, within acceptable bounds of experimental variation, is the one that fits most closely to the order of reaction. In such cases the fit may not be exact and this may be due to experimental errors in the collected data. It may also be indicative of reactions with a fractional order, i.e. reactions where the overall order in not an integer. In some reactions, for example, the reaction rate is found to be dependent on the square root of the reactant concentration. In this case, the reaction order is one-half.

Kinetic data may be plotted using the linear forms of the rate equations described in the previous sections. The aim here is to plot the data until a straight line graph is obtained. For example, if a plot of the amount of API remaining [A] (y-axis) against time (x-axis) is found to be linear, then the reaction would follow zero-order kinetics and the gradient is equivalent to $-k$. If such a plot is non-linear then the reaction cannot be a zero-order process.

The half-life may also be used to determine the order of reaction. The expressions for $t_{0.5}$ in zero-, first- and second-order reaction are shown in equations 12.10, 12.20, and 12.31. A general trend emerges and is shown in equation 12.34:

$$t_{0.5} \; \alpha \; \frac{1}{[A]_0^{n-1}} \qquad (12.34)$$

where $t_{0.5}$ is the half-life, n is the order of the reaction, and $[A]_0$ is the initial concentration.

Taking logs of both sides of this expression and introducing a proportionality constant, C, gives:

$$\log t_{0.5} = \log \frac{C}{[A]_0^{n-1}} \qquad (12.35)$$

Using the properties of logs, we obtain:

$$\log t_{0.5} = (1-n)\log[A]_0 + \log C \qquad (12.36)$$

We can see that whether half-life increases, stays constant, or decrease with $[A]_0$ depends on n.

Equation 12.36 is of a linear form and a plot of log $t_{0.5}$ against log $[A]_0$ will result in a straight line with a slope of $(1 - n)$, allowing the order of reaction to be calculated from the gradient.

Another way to determine the order of reaction is to use the method of initial rates. This involves measuring the rate of a reaction over the initial stages of a reaction lifetime, before any significant changes in concentration occur. The initial rate is then measured for several different sets of starting concentrations and the rate law that best fits the experimental data is selected.

TABLE 12.3 Degradation data for a drug in aqueous solution

Initial concentration, [A]/mM	Half-life,($t_{0.5}$)/ min	log [A]	log $t_{0.5}$
3.793	26.34	0.579	1.42
1.465	80.91	0.166	1.91
0.582	195.67	−0.235	2.29
0.134	534.24	−0.873	2.73
0.056	1134.42	−1.252	3.05

Determination of order of reaction using the half-life method

The degradation of a drug in aqueous solution was measured and the initial concentration and half-life (the time taken for half the initial concentration to disappear, $t_{0.5}$) were determined, and are shown Table 12.3.

To process this data we use equation 12.35; the logs of both terms are required. They are shown in the third and fourth columns of the Table 12.3, and are plotted in Figure 12.6. Using equation 12.35 a plot of log $[A]_0$ against log $t_{0.5}$ will result in a straight line with a gradient of $(1-n)$.

$$\text{Slope} = (y_2 - y_1)/(x_2 - x_1)$$

$$= (1.91 - 3.05)/(0.166 - (-1.252))$$

$$\text{Slope} = -0.80$$

$$(1-n) = -0.80$$

$$n = 1.80$$

This means that the reaction is second-order. Note that the value is not exactly 2 and this may be due to the experimental error associated with the reaction. The resultant scatter may be seen in the quality of the fit of the data to the line in Figure 12.6.

SELF CHECK 12.3

In acid catalysed reaction of iodine and acetone, the reaction rate is found to be dependent on [acetone], but is independent of [iodine]. Suggest an explanation for this observation.

SELF CHECK 12.4

A student studied the reaction between A and B, the starting concentrations of each reagent being 0.02 M and 0.06 M, respectively. A plot of 1/[A] versus time was found to be linear. On the basis of this behaviour, what is the rate law for this reaction?

FIGURE 12.6 A plot of log [A] against log $t_{0.5}$ for the degradation of a drug in aqueous solution

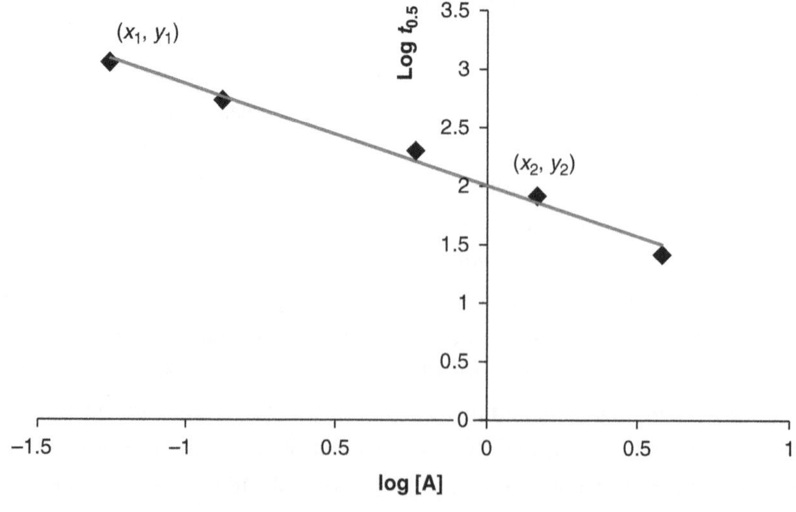

KEY POINTS

- The units of reaction rate are normally concentration per unit time.
- The rate-determining step is the slowest step of a chemical reaction and it will determine the overall rate of reaction.
- The rate law shows how the reaction rate is dependent on both the rate constant and the concentrations of the reactants.
- In a zero-order process, rate is independent of reactant concentration.
- In a first-order process, rate is proportional to reactant concentration.
- In a second-order process, rate is proportional to the square of reactant concentration.

12.3 Factors affecting the rate of reaction of dosage forms

The factors that affect reaction rates in general can be explained by collision theory: In its simplest form this is the notion that reactant particles must collide before reaction is possible. Clearly, the rate at which collisions occur will depend on the frequency of collisions and this, in turn, will depend on three factors:

- The speed of particles.
- The size (specifically, the cross-sectional area) of particles.
- The concentration of particles.

An increase in any of these three factors would be anticipated to increase the rate of collisions.

Not all collisions will lead to a reaction. Consider the hydrolysis of the ester tetracaine, shown in Figure 12.1. During hydrolysis, the water molecule attacks the electrophilic carbonyl carbon. We might imagine that if the water collided with another part of the ester (the leaving group for example) then reaction would not be possible. In quantitative expressions of collision theory it is common to incorporate a steric factor, being a number between 0 and 1 that represents the fraction of collisions with the correct orientation for reaction. There are, for example, four different ways that you can lay your right hand on top of your left hand. Only one of these 'collisions' results in the palms of your hands touching each other. If we imagine that our hands are the reacting molecules, and the palms represent the reactive surface, then we might conclude that the steric factor here is 0.25.

Even collisions that have the correct orientation may not lead to reaction if the energy requirement of the process, the **activation energy** (E_a), is not met. The activation energy is the minimum reactant energy required before reaction is possible and it can be represented by a peak on a plot of an energy diagram for a process (Figure 12.7). The reactants and products appear at the base of energy troughs on this diagram because they are stable chemical species. The transition state is an unstable species and has an extremely short lifetime. It lies at the maximum point of the

FIGURE 12.7 Energy profile for a typical reaction

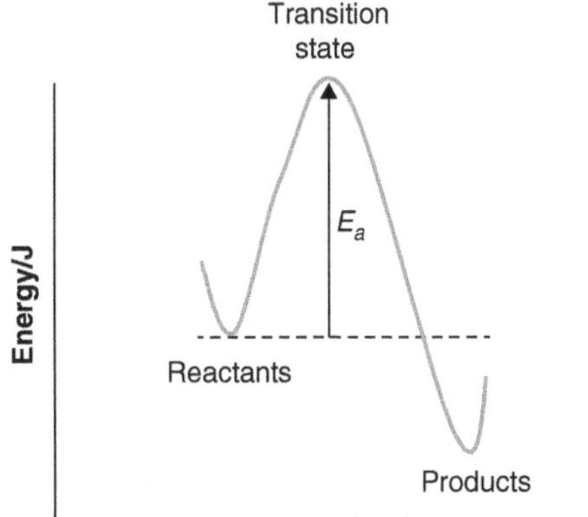

energy barrier and all successful reactions must pass through this point. In a reaction mixture, only a fraction of the collisions between reactant molecules will have an energy greater than E_a and this can be represented on Maxwell-Boltzmann distribution curves (Figure 12.8).

As can be seen, the distribution of molecular energies changes with temperature. The area under each curve is related to the total number of particles and therefore remains constant for a particular sample. As temperature is raised, the peak of the distribution curve shifts to the right reflecting an increase in both energy and the average molecular speed. The curve becomes flatter at higher temperatures, showing that the energies associated with collisions become more evenly distributed at elevated temperature. Notice that, even at low temperatures, some of the molecules have very high kinetic energy. This is in accord with our experience. Thus, water spilt on a desk will evaporate over time. We understand that the water has not reached its **boiling point**, but that some molecules of water within the liquid have sufficient energy to break free of the surface and enter the vapour phase.

A wide range of factors can affect the degradation rates of dosage forms and they can be understood by the application of collision theory, including the principle of activation energy. For example, the particles in liquids are in a state of constant movement and they collide with other frequently. As such, liquid formulations generally have a shorter **shelf life** than solids, such as tablets or capsules, where the particles are held tightly in fixed positions. Such stability issues can influence how drugs are formulated into medicines and administered to patients. For example, some parenteral formulations (i.e. injections) are often prepared shortly before use by a clinician. This means that the solid ingredients (usually the API and excipients) are kept in a solid state, often in an ampoule and reconstituted before injection by the addition of **water for injection**. Thus, the pharmaceutical scientist can improve the stability of certain drugs in dosage forms by selection of a dosage form. This often involves formulating to avoid the presence of water in a medicine.

Dosage forms may be exposed to various types of degradation, including physical, chemical, microbiological and biological. This chapter focuses mainly on chemical degradation of APIs. The factors that affect the rate of these processes will now be considered.

FIGURE 12.8 Maxwell–Boltzmann curves showing the distribution of kinetic energies within a sample of reactant gas at three different temperatures

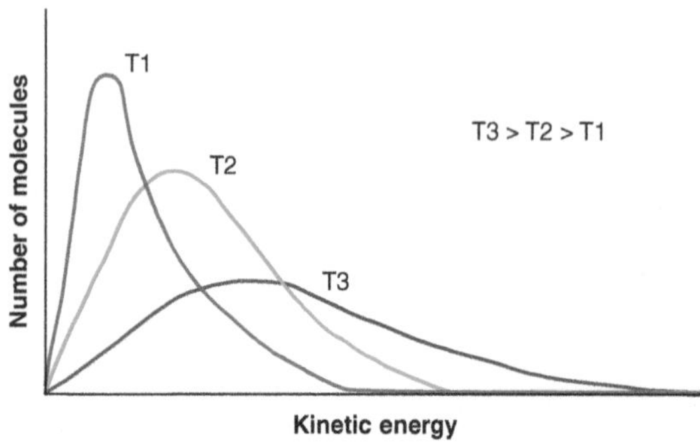

Temperature

Raising the temperature increases the proportion of reactant molecules with an energy greater than the activation energy. Changing the temperature of the reaction is one of the most important factors for pharmaceutical systems as it allows the shelf life of pharmaceutical materials to be determined (Section 12.4).

Concentration

Any reaction that has a non-zero rate law will have a rate that is dependent on concentration. Higher concentrations increase the chance of collision between reactants. For gaseous systems, we may use pressure to measure the amount of reactant particles per unit volume, but the effect of concentration on reaction rate is equivalent. Higher pressures will give a higher rate.

For acidic and basic liquid dosage forms, we may prefer to use **pH** in place of concentration (see Box 12.3). Thus, a reaction that is first-order in H^+ would be expected to proceed faster at lower pH. The hydrolysis of an API in solution may be catalysed in acidic or basic conditions (i.e. specific acid-base catalysis, by H^+ or OH^- ions). Such conditions will affect the aqueous stability of a drug and the local pH can significantly influence the shelf life of a liquid dosage form. The

BOX 12.3

Buffered dosage forms

Control of pH is usually achieved by the use of buffer solutions, but steps must be taken to ensure that the buffer used does not contain chemicals that can catalyse a degradation reaction, such as general acid-base catalysis. The ability of certain buffer components to catalyse acid–base reactions depends on their ability to dissociate. Those chemicals that can dissociate more completely may be more readily able to react and cause acid or base catalysed hydrolysis reactions. The effect that a buffer can have on hydrolysis of a drug can be determined by measuring the reaction rate at a series of different buffer concentrations and then extrapolating back towards the zero buffer concentration. A plot of the extrapolated rate constants against pH can then be used to produce a buffer-independent profile of reactions rates at each pH.

For more information on buffers, please refer to Section 6.7.

relationship between rates of hydrolysis and pH may be complex and non-linear over the pH range examined. This is because different ionized and unionized species present at different pH's may have different reactivities toward water. Changes in pH can also influence the photochemical and oxidative degradation of some drugs by, for example, changing the oxidation–reduction potential of the drug.

Concentration of oxygen and water

As we have seen, the main reaction types that degrade medicines are oxidation and hydrolysis. The concentration of oxygen and water within a dosage form can therefore have a significant impact on its shelf life. The level of oxygen can be reduced in a formulation by manufacturing and packaging within an inert atmosphere such as nitrogen, for example. Other reactive molecules that promote oxidation will also decrease the stability of a medicine if they are present in appreciable amounts.

Solid dosage forms usually offer many stability advantages compared to liquid dosage forms. This is generally due to the absence of large amounts of water or other solvents, as moisture in particular can affect the rate of decomposition. Although a necessary component of many liquid dosage forms, water is generally present as an impurity in solid dosage forms. The absence of moisture is essential in ensuring the stability of these medicines. Even a small amount of moisture means that a water-soluble API may dissolve into solution and thereafter react and degrade.

Moisture may also be present in certain excipients and this may increase degradation. For example, magnesium stearate is used in tablet processing as a lubricant, anti-adherent or **glidant**. As well as potentially being a source of moisture, magnesium stearate itself is a reactive compound that can initiate base-catalysed hydrolysis of the API. In general, reactions between different components of liquid and solid dosage forms (the API and its excipients, including buffers) can occur and might affect the stability of the dosage forms.

Catalysts and enzymes

The presence of a catalyst, including enzymes, lowers the activation energy so that a greater proportion of reactants have an energy greater than E_a, thereby increasing the reaction rate. Although a catalyst facilitates a particular reaction, it remains unchanged at the completion of the reaction. In general, catalysts react in some manner with the reactants, usually through the formation of an intermediate complex. This complex is often unstable and reacts further to yield the products of the reaction and the catalyst in its original form. Alternatively, catalysts may generate free radicals which facilitate the propagation of further reactions, or chain reactions.

Catalysis may be heterogeneous, where the catalyst is in a different phase from the reactants and products of the reaction (such as the catalytic converter of a car exhaust) or homogenous, where the catalyst is in the same phase as the reaction components (such as acids or bases in solution). In a reversible reaction, a catalyst will increase the rate of both the forward and reverse reactions. This can be understood by looking at the energy profile in Figure 12.7. Any decrease in the size of the energy barrier will reduce E_a in both the forward and reverse directions. In the presence of a catalyst, the time that the reaction takes to reach equilibrium is reduced, but the **equilibrium constant**, K, remains unchanged, as does the expected yield of the reaction product(s).

While a range of heterogeneous and homogenous catalysts may be used during the manufacture of APIs, biochemical processes within the body are routinely catalysed by enzymes. These are large proteins and many medicines are designed to inhibit their action.

For more information on enzymes, please refer to Chapter 3 'The biochemistry of cells' of the ***Therapeutics and Human Physiology*** book within this series.

During enzymatic reactions, a reactant molecule (or substrate) binds non-covalently to a reactive portion of the enzyme, the active site. This is a very specific 3D fit, like a hand fitting into a glove, or a key into a lock. The conversion of the bound substrate to products usually requires more than one step. If the concentration of substrate is very much higher than that of the enzyme, all binding sites will be occupied by reactants. In this case, no more enzyme-substrate complexes can be formed and the rate of the enzymatic reaction is as high as it can possibly be. This rate is the maximum rate of reaction, V_{max}. If an enzymatic reaction is proceeding at this limiting rate, increasing the substrate concentration further will not speed up the reaction. The enzyme is described as being saturated with substrate and the kinetics are the same as those for a zero-order reaction. At lower substrate concentrations, where only a fraction of the binding sites are occupied, the rate of the enzyme-catalysed reaction will be dependent on the concentration of the substrate. Enzymatic reactions are observed to be effectively first-order in substrate when the concentration of substrate is very low.

Light

Irradiation by light can cause some molecules to convert into a less stable form, effectively increasing the concentration of reactive particles. This, in turn, will increase the frequency of molecule collisions that can lead to degradation. Photolytic reactions are those initiated by light and they can be significantly reduced if amber bottles are used to store photolabile medicines.

For more information on pharmaceutical packaging, please refer to Section 13.6.

Dissolution medium

For liquid dosage forms, the dissolution medium is composed of a solvent, including any other materials (such as **electrolytes**) that are dissolved within it. Changing the composition of this medium can stabilize the transition state relative to the reactants (Figure 12.7), lowering the activation energy and increasing reaction rate. Generally, the effect that electrolytes have on the rate constant, k, is described by the Bronsted–Bjerrum equation:

$$\log k = \log k_0 + 2Az_Az_B\sqrt{I} \tag{12.37}$$

where k_0 is the rate constant in the absence of electrolytes, A is a temperature- and solvent-dependant constant, z_A and z_B are the charges of the two ions involved in the reaction, and I is the **ionic strength** of the solution.

I is related to the concentration of ions and the magnitude of the charge on those ions. As I increases, the rate of reaction will either increase or decrease, depending on the relative signs of z_A and z_B. Thus if two ions with same charge (positive or negative) react then z_Az_B will be positive and the rate of reaction will increase with ionic strength. However, the reaction of two ions with opposite charges will result in a decrease in the rate of reaction as ionic strength increases. This principle can impact on the design of liquid dosage forms. For example, the addition of sodium chloride to a **parenteral formulation** to adjust the **tonicity** of the solution might result in an increase in hydrolysis, due to an increase in the ionic strength of the solution.

For more information on tonicity, please refer to Section 11.3.

Water is the preferred solvent for liquid dosage forms as it matches the physiological conditions within the body. However, just as we may need to control the level of dissolved ions in a dosage form's dissolution medium, it might be necessary also to use other solvents alongside water. The addition of organic solvents will alter the **dielectric constant** of the dissolution medium and this may influence stability. As with ionic strength, the signs of the two interacting charges will influence whether the reaction rate increases or decreases. For example, the addition of a solvent with a lower dielectric constant will reduce the rate of degradation when the charges of the interacting species (i.e. the drug and the solvent) are the same.

Particle size

Decreasing particle size, by grinding a tablet for example, increases the surface area of the solid and therefore makes collisions with other reactants more likely. Thus, medicines that are intended to be mixed with water before ingestion are generally presented to the patient as a powder to increase the rate of **dissolution**.

Changes in physical state

If an elevated temperature causes a solid dosage form (or one of its components) to melt, then this can lead to problems with physical stability. This will affect semi-solid dosage forms such as pessaries and suppositories. Drugs exhibiting **polymorphism** may change from one form to another, and this can result in significant changes to the rate of dissolution and subsequent **bioavailability** of the drug.

For more information on polymorphism, please refer to Section 2.3.

KEY POINTS

- Collision theory proposes that reaction rate is dependent on the frequency of collisions between reactant particles.
- For reaction to occur, colliding particles must have the correct orientation and have an energy greater than the activation energy.
- A number of factors affect the rate of reactions involving APIs including; temperature, concentration, light, presence of catalysts and reactive molecules, the dissolution medium, particle size and physical state.

SELF CHECK 12.5

According to collision theory, when reactant particles collide, what two factors will determine whether a reaction occurs?

SELF CHECK 12.6

Effervescent tablets release carbon dioxide upon addition to water. Why does this aid dissolution?

12.4 Temperature and reaction rate

In general, it is observed that the rate of reaction of solid, semi-solid and liquid dosage forms increases as temperature is raised. This may be important for dosage forms that require sterile manufacture, as heat sterilization may be unsuitable. As a rule of thumb, an approximate doubling of the reaction rate accompanies every 10 K rise in temperature.

The Arrhenius equation

The Arrhenius equation can be used to determine the activation energy of a reaction. It is more commonly and usefully applied in pharmaceutical systems to determine the shelf life of pharmaceutical products. The equation shows the effect of temperature on the rate of reaction. It is given by the empirical equation:

$$k = Ae^{-\left(\frac{E_a}{RT}\right)} \tag{12.38}$$

where k is the reaction rate constant, A is a constant called the frequency factor, E_a is the activation energy, R is the universal **gas constant** and T is the **absolute temperature**.

The logarithmic form of the Arrhenius equation (12.38) is:

$$\log k = \log A - \frac{E_a}{2.303} \cdot \frac{1}{RT} \quad (12.39)$$

This form of the equation is a linear expression, and a plot of log k (y axis) against $1/T$ (x axis) results in a straight line with a gradient of $-E_a/2.303.R$, and an intercept on the vertical axis of log A. This allows the activation energy, E_a, to be calculated.

TABLE 12.4 Rate constants for the hydrolysis of tetracaine at a range of temperatures

Temperature/°C	Rate constant, k/min^{-1}
80	0.01364
70	0.00448
60	0.00185
50	0.00090

TABLE 12.5 Conversion of the data in Table 12.4 for use in the Arrhenius equation

Temperature/K	$(1/T)$/K^{-1}	log k
353	0.002833	−1.8652
343	0.002915	−2.3487
333	0.003003	−2.7328
323	0.003096	−3.0458

Calculating activation energy

Using the data in Table 12.4, how do you calculate the activation energy, E_a, for the hydrolysis of tetracaine in a weakly acidic solution?

First, the data should be converted into a form that can be used with the linear version of the Arrhenius equation. This means that temperature should be converted from °C to kelvin (k), and that the log of the rate constant should be determined (Table 12.5).

This data now allows us to plot a graph of log k against $1/T$ (Figure 12.9). This graph gives a reasonable straight line, allowing for some variation and error in the experiments that generated the data. The graph also gives us the gradient, or slope, of the line, which is -4.462×10^3 and this has the same units of temperature, K.

$$\text{Slope} = \frac{-E_a}{2.303.R} = -4.462 \times 10^3\,\text{K}$$

The gas constant has a value of 8.314 J K^{-1} mol^{-1} and so this equation may be rearranged to give:

$$-E_a = -4.462 \times 10^3\;.2.303.8.314 = 85435\,\text{J mol}^{-1}$$

Activation energies are always positive and are routinely expressed in kilojoules per mole so in this case:

$$E_a = 85.4\;\text{kJmol}^{-1}$$

This method also allows us to calculate the frequency factor, A, given that the intercept on the y axis = log A.

FIGURE 12.9 Plot of log k against $1/T$ for the hydrolysis of tetracaine in a weakly acidic solution

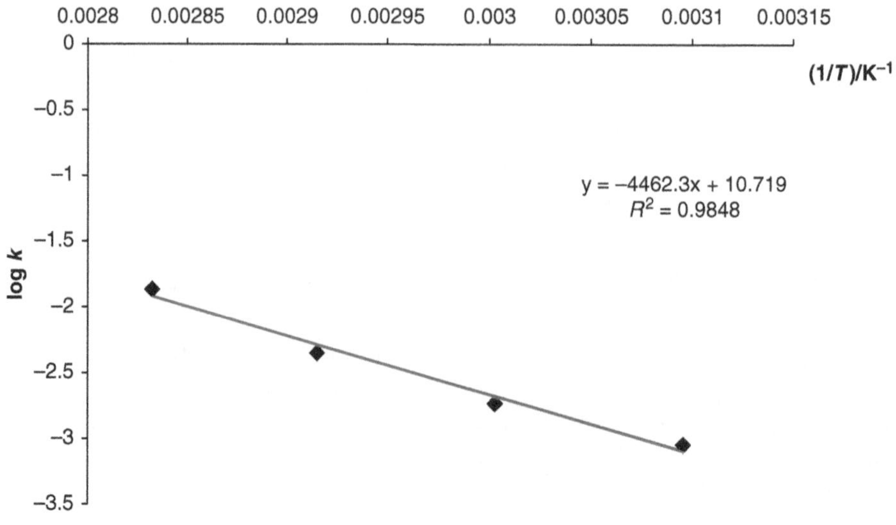

In Figure 12.9, the equation of the best-fit line was determined by computer and the intercept was found to be 10.719. Thus, $A = 5.24 \times 10^{10}\,\text{min}^{-1}$ (same units as k).

Accelerated stability testing and calculation of shelf life

The stability of pharmaceutical dosage forms is measured by a method called accelerated stability testing. This is where the dosage form is stored at a series of higher temperatures and the degradation rate constants at each temperature are determined. The reason for the use of the higher temperatures is that the rate of reaction should be faster and degradation will occur sooner. This data can be measured and plotted, allowing extrapolation back to lower temperatures, such as room temperature. This will provide the pharmaceutical scientist with an estimate of the rate of reaction at room temperature more quickly than allowing the reaction to happen naturally at this temperature. This speed is important in the timeline of pharmaceutical manufacture and allows long-range stability data to be determined relatively quickly.

Once the rate constant is known at a storage temperature for the product then the shelf life may be calculated for this product. The shelf life will be based on an acceptable degree of degradation. For example, a pharmaceutical product may be valid for use if, for example, 90% of the original concentration remains after a given time. This acceptable limit will vary depending on the product type. If a small amount of degradation leads to discolouring of the product then a limit greater than 90% might be appropriate. If a product should be stored in the refrigerator, but is kept at room temperature, then the drug will decompose more rapidly. The product will then have a shorter half-life than would be expected if the storage instructions were adhered to.

Calculating shelf life: example one

Using the data (shown in Tables 12.4 and 12.6) we can extrapolate the plot from the higher temperatures to lower temperatures and therefore obtain information that is relevant for storage at room temperature, or whatever other chosen temperature we might want to consider (for example, we might consider 4 °C if the product was to be stored in the refrigerator). We are able to do this as we know the equation of the line of best fit, and that line of best fit has a reasonable accuracy given the value of its correlation coefficient, r^2, was close to 1, Figure 12.9. When log k (y axis) was plotted against $1/T$ (x axis) the equation of this best straight line was found to be $y = -4462.3x + 10.719$. As the plot is a straight line then it may be used to extrapolate the data to, for example, room temperature, 25 °C. Alternatively, the values could be substituted into the equation and the unknown value, the rate constant at 25 °C, can be calculated by solving the equation. This would allow the rate constant at this temperature to be calculated as approximately $5.6 \times 10^{-5}\,\text{min}^{-1}$. This data relates to decomposition by first-order kinetics and will therefore obey the equation:

$$\ln[\text{A}] = -kt + \ln[\text{A}]_0 \qquad (12.14)$$

If the shelf life is dependent upon having greater than 90% of the drug in the dosage form then we need to calculate the time taken for 10% of the reactant to degrade, $t_{10\%}$. When $t = t_{10\%}$, it follows that $[\text{A}] = 0.9[\text{A}]_0$. These terms can be added into the above equation:

$$t_{10\%} = \frac{\ln \frac{[\text{A}]_0}{0.9[\text{A}]_0}}{k} = \frac{\ln(1.11)}{k} \qquad (12.40)$$

Thus, just as with half-life, the $t_{10\%}$ for a first-order process is independent of the starting concentration of A. In this example,

$$t_{10\%} = \frac{\ln(1.11)}{5.6 \times 10^{-5}} = 1.9 \times 10^3\,\text{min}$$

which is approximately 31 hours.

Calculating shelf life: example two

A drug has an initial concentration of $2.50 \times 10^{-3}\,\text{g cm}^{-3}$ in aqueous solution. After 24 months it is known that the concentration has dropped to $1.16 \times 10^{-3}\,\text{g cm}^{-3}$. The drug is ineffective at 90% or less of its initial concentration. The degradation of the drug in aqueous solution follows first-order kinetics.

Determine the shelf life of this formulation.

Step one: as the process follows first-order kinetics, we can substitute the information above into the first-order rate equation (equation 12.13):

$$\ln(1.16 \times 10^{-3}) = -k.24 + \ln(2.50 \times 10^{3})$$

Rearrangement gives $k=3.2\times10^{-2}$ month^{-1}.

Step two: we have been told that the drug is ineffective at less than 90% of its initial concentration so we need to calculate the $t_{10\%}$.

$$t_{10\%} = \ln 1.11 / 3.2\times10^{-2}$$

Working through this calculation and taking care to consider the units (which should be time, in this case, months) $t_{10\%}=3.3$ months. This means that the shelf life of the product is 3.3 months. This figure might be rounded down to give a more meaningful and common-sense shelf life of three months.

KEY POINTS

- As a general rule of thumb, the reaction rate doubles for every 10-degree rise in temperature.
- The Arrhenius equation relates the value of the rate constant, k, to the absolute temperature, T, and is given by $k=Ae^{-\left(\frac{E_a}{RT}\right)}$
- Activation energy, E_a, may be determined from the slope of an Arrhenius plot of log k versus $1/T$.
- Accelerated stability testing is where the degradation rate of a dosage form is determined at elevated temperature. Data is then extrapolated to a lower temperature of interest.

SELF CHECK 12.7

A student studied the decomposition of hydrogen peroxide at various temperatures in aqueous solutions containing catalase. It was noted that the rate of reaction decreased as the temperature was raised from 40 °C to 60 °C. Suggest a reason for this observation.

SELF CHECK 12.8

For chemical reactions, Arrhenius plots of ln k versus $1/T$ are generally linear. Why do they always have a negative slope?

CHAPTER SUMMARY

- APIs can degrade through a variety of reaction types, hydrolysis and oxidation being major causes of instability in pharmaceutical dosage forms.
- Stabilizers may be added to formulations and packaging may be modified to slow the rate of degradation reactions.
- The rate-determining step is the slowest step of a chemical reaction and it will determine the overall rate of reaction.
- The rate law shows how the reaction rate is dependent on both the rate constant and the concentrations of the reactants.
- Most processes of interest in pharmaceutics are either zero-, first- or second-order.
- Collision theory proposes that reaction rate is dependent on the frequency of collisions between reactant particles, their orientation, and the activation energy.
- A number of factors affect the rate of reactions involving APIs including; temperature, concentration, light, presence of catalysts and reactive molecules, the dissolution medium, particle size and physical state.
- The Arrhenius equation may be used to model the relationship between rate constants and temperature.
- The expected shelf life of a drug at its normal storage temperature can be estimated by using accelerated stability testing and applying the Arrhenius equation.

FURTHER READING

Florence, A.T. and Attwood, D. *Physicochemical Principles of Pharmacy*. (5th edn). London: Pharmaceutical Press (2011).

Includes a chapter on drug stability that containing numerous examples.

Sinko, P.J. *Martin's Physical Pharmacy and Pharmaceutical Sciences*. (6th edn). Lippincott Williams and Wilkins (2010).

Includes a chapter on chemical kinetics and stability and an introduction to the steady state approximation.

Jones, D.S. *FASTtrack: Pharmaceutics – Dosage Form and Design*. London: Pharmaceutical Press (2008).

Each chapter of this book considers related dosage forms and information is provided in a succinct and accessible style.

Attwood, D. and Florence, A.T. *FASTtrack: Physical Pharmacy*. London: Pharmaceutical Press (2007).

A revision guide that includes a section on drug stability.

Woolfson, A.D. and McCafferty, D.F. *Percutaneous Local Anaesthesia*. London: Taylor & Francis (1993).

Discusses how formulations may be developed that penetrate the skin and induce local anaesthesia.

Manning, M.C., Chou, D.K., Murphy, B.M., Payne, R.W. and Katayama, D.S. (2010). Stability of protein pharmaceuticals: An update. *Pharm. Res.* 27: 544–75.

Schersch, K., Betz, O., Garidel, P., Muehlau, S., Bassarab, S. and Winter, G. (2010). Systematic investigation of the effect of lyophilizate collapse on pharmaceutically relevant proteins 1: Stability after freeze-drying. *J. Pharm. Sci.* 99: 2256–78.

Waterman, K.C. and Adami, R.C. (2006). Accelerated aging: Prediction of chemical stability of pharmaceuticals. *Int. J. Pharm.* 293: 101–25.

REFERENCE

Florence, A.T. and Attwood, D. *Physicochemical Principles of Pharmacy*. (4th edn). London: Pharmaceutical Press (2005).

13

Drug discovery, development, and delivery

CRAIG A. RUSSELL AND AFZAL R. MOHAMMED

Drug discovery, development, and delivery are important areas of the pharmaceutical industry. The scale of investment into the research and development of new drug substances and their subsequent **dosage forms** is now higher than ever. The first stage in any medicine's life is the identification of the **active pharmaceutical ingredient (API)** at the heart of the medicine. The first part of this chapter explains how, from millions of molecules, a relative few of interest are identified and selected for further investigation. With the likely molecules identified, the focus turns to making these molecules as effective as possible. Optimized compounds are subject to preformulation investigations to learn as much as possible about the molecule to ensure there are no underlying reasons as to why the molecule may prove unsuitable. These tests also prevent any snags during the formulation process, which are costly both in terms of time and money.

The formulation process itself is just as important as the identification and optimization of a molecule in the first place. There is no point in having a 'wonder drug' if there is no means of getting it to its site of action and in an active form. Fortunately, there are many dosage forms to choose from, which are described within this chapter, each with their own advantages. With all of the developmental work completed, the final hurdles that medications are required to clear are clinical trials. Here, the dosage form is scrutinized to ensure its safety and efficacy over long periods of time and in large patient populations. All being well, the medicine will prove itself to be suitable and will find its way onto the shelves, or behind the counter of pharmacies everywhere.

Learning objectives

Having read this chapter you are expected to be able to:

- Describe methods involved with the identification of new candidate compounds.
- Understand the methods and reasons behind the optimization of candidate compounds.
- Understand the relevance of the relationship between molecular structure and biological activity and how this is applied in drug development.
- Describe considerations which are taken into account prior to the formulation of a dosage form.
- State the various routes of administration, their associated dosage forms and how they are used.
- Describe the available packaging for dosage forms and understand the benefits of each.
- Understand and describe the four stages of clinical trials.

13.1 Identification of candidate compounds

Following the identification and validation of a biological target by molecular biologists, the next hurdle to be overcome is the identification of molecules that are predicted to interact with the target to produce a therapeutic effect. These molecules are referred to as candidate compounds and they may also be referred to as new chemical entities (NCEs). The term NCE is commonly used to describe novel pharmacologically active substances that have not yet been approved for use within medicines. The term API is generally used to describe the pharmacologically active agent within a commercially available medicine. A 'drug' is defined as a pharmacologically active substance, and so this term includes both APIs and NCEs.

The identification of candidate compounds normally involves the screening of huge numbers of molecules. Computerized systems are used to identify a handful of likely looking molecules, which will be taken on for further study. Methods involved in this process commonly include:

- **High-throughput screening (HTS).**
- Modification of an existing molecule.
- Rational drug design.

High-throughput screening

In the area of drug development, the identification of candidate compounds most often involves the use of **high-throughput screening (HTS)** in order to identify the compounds that will most likely be of use. In the process of HTS, databases containing information on large numbers of chemical compounds are assessed to determine their usefulness at targeting the cause of a particular disease or symptom. The implementation of HTS also acts to identify the specificity of a candidate compound. This is necessary, in order to identify a compound that is active only against the intended target and not against other similar targets. This is known as **cross-screening** and is used to identify all of the targets that will be affected by a chosen candidate compound. This is an important procedure in the identification of candidate compounds, as APIs acting at targets other than that intended can often lead to off-target toxicity. The likelihood of a candidate being identified that fits all of the desired criteria is very low. In most cases, there are multiple compounds identified that exhibit some level of activity against the target.

For more information on high throughput screening, please refer to Chapter 10 'Origins of drug molecules' of the ***Pharmaceutical Chemistry*** book within this series.

Modification of an existing molecule

Although HTS is a widely implemented method in the identification of new drugs, it is not the only method available. It is possible to produce NCEs by modifying an existing molecule that displays some of the characteristics that would be desirable in the final drug (see Integration Box 13.1). The existing molecules can be found in previously developed medicines or alternatively come from natural sources. Methods such as virtual HTS (vHTS) are also implemented by using large computer databases and computer-modelling techniques. The advantage of vHTS over conventional HTS is that the huge costs involved with performing the millions of biochemical assays in HTS are replaced with an efficient computational screening method in vHTS.

Rational drug design

In rational drug design, the biological target is studied with both its biological and physical properties being investigated. From this, a list of candidate compounds is drawn up that display properties that suggest possible activity; for example, a structure that may allow a chemical to act as an analogue for a receptor site. This is achieved through two major forms of drug discovery: structure based and ligand based. From developmental procedures such as this, new drug discoveries can be made quickly; one such example of this methodology is fragment-based lead discovery (FBLD), which is described in Box 13.1.

INTEGRATION BOX 13.1

Angiotensin-converting enzyme (ACE) inhibitors

Following the identification of angiotensin-converting enzyme (ACE) and its effects on blood volume and vasoconstriction, it was very soon realized that a means of inhibiting its effect would provide a useful means of reducing high blood pressure (or hypertension).

It was identified that peptides found in the venom of a South American snake, *Bothrops jararaca*, prevented the formation of angiotensin II from angiotensin I in the renin–angiotensin aldosterone system (RAAS), whilst also increasing the activity of bradykinin (a potent vasodilator) on smooth muscle and blocking the inactivation of bradykinin. These peptides were assessed for their usefulness as a drug and it was found that it was possible to suppress the formation of angiotensin II by inhibiting ACE and in doing so effectively treat hypertension and heart failure.

From these peptides, captopril was developed following the study of the structure of ACE using peptide analogues and carboxypeptidase A as a model. It was developed via quantitative structure–activity relationship (QSAR) based modification, which suggested that the terminal sulphhydryl moiety of the peptide bradykinin potentiating factor (BPF) provided a high potency of ACE Inhibition. This was amongst the earliest successes of a revolutionary concept of structure-based drug design.

Following the identification of captopril, further ACE inhibitors were developed from the same basic structure to improve their taste by removing the foul tasting sulphhydryl moiety. These include benazepril, enalapril, fosinopril, lisinopril, moexipril, ramipril, quinapril, and trandolapril. All of the ACE inhibitors are only slightly different to captopril in the main aspects of their structure, with the active moiety of fosinopril being a phosphinyl group and the active moiety of nalapril, lisinopril, benazepril, quinapril, ramipril, trandolapril, and moexipril being a carboxyl group. In most cases further modification of the molecule was necessary to maintain or improve the potency of the API. Pro-drugs (ramipril and enalapril) were developed to protect the ACE inhibitors from first pass metabolism and also to improve the drug permeability.

For more information on 'first pass' metabolism, please refer to Chapter 1 'The scientific basis of therapeutics' of the ***Therapeutics and Human Physiology*** book within this series.

BOX 13.1

Fragment-based lead discovery (FBLD)

Fragment-based lead discovery (FBLD) involves the identification of the small fragments of a molecule that allow its interaction with a biological target of interest. HTS methods are then employed to scan large numbers of molecules that possess this fragment. Further development of the molecules, e.g. combining them, allows for the production of molecules with improved affinity for their target. In this way a lead compound is produced to be taken further into the drug development procedure (Carr *et al.*, 2005). FBLD and HTS methods are not mutually exclusive and are likely to be used in combination with each other.

SELF CHECK 13.1

How is high-throughput screening (HTS) used in drug discovery?

SELF CHECK 13.2

What advantage does vHTS have over conventional HTS?

KEY POINTS

- Candidate compounds are predicted to interact with the biological target to produce a therapeutic effect. Novel candidate compounds may be referred to as new chemical entities (NCEs).
- In high-throughput screening (HTS), databases of information regarding chemical compounds are assessed to identify candidate compounds.
- Candidate compounds may also be created by the modification of existing APIs.
- In rational drug design, candidate compounds are identified by studying the biological and physical properties of the therapeutic target.

13.2 Optimization of lead compounds

The candidate compound that is considered the best prospect is termed the **lead compound**. The group of candidate compounds are assessed for any shared features from which pharmacophores can be developed. **Pharmacophores** are molecular frameworks that contain the essential features responsible for a drug's biological activity. The identification of pharmacophores allows for the computational analysis of millions of molecules to screen for those possessing the same molecular frame work. Typical features of a molecule that can contribute to a pharmacophore include: hydrophobic regions, aromatic properties, hydrogen bonding ability, and charged centres.

With the NCEs that display activity against the target identified, medicinal chemists use structure–activity relationships in order to improve the lead compound. The compound's activity and specificity to the target, and also its absorption, distribution, metabolism, and excretion (ADME) properties, are analysed. This involves many screening runs of the compounds by which the above properties will be improved following modification.

With the lead compound optimized, it will progress into ***in vitro*** and ***in vivo*** testing specific to the condition that the drug is intended to treat. The physiochemical properties of the NCE are assessed, including its **permeability**, **acid dissociation constant**, and **solubility**. Methods such as parallel artificial membrane permeability assay (PAMPA) and tissue culture are used for the determination of a compound's permeability. PAMPA is preferred as an early screening technique due to its close correlation to the behaviour of the gastrointestinal tract (GIT) and blood–brain barrier (BBB). PAMPA also requires only small amounts of compound and costs relatively little when compared to tissue culture methods.

A compound or indeed a series of compounds can be assessed by analysing a range of parameters, as described by Lipinski's Rule of Five (Box 13.2). Included in this are parameters that are calculated and those that are determined using laboratory-based analysis. Quantities such as the **partition coefficient (*P*)** are used to predict properties such as:

- Molecular weight.
- Polar surface area.
- Lipophilicity.

Laboratory-based analysis is carried out to investigate parameters such as the enzymatic clearance or potency, for example. In some instances, mathematical and laboratory-based analysis is performed to assess a compound, or series of compounds', ADME characteristics. This is the case for ligand efficiency (LE) and lipophilic efficiency (LiPE).

For more information on Log *P*, please refer to Section 8.2.

Following the identification of a selection of possible compounds, the final lead compound is identified by comparing the target potency, the selectivity, and other favourable properties that the compounds may display.

BOX 13.2

Lipinski's Rule of Five

In the late 1990s, Christopher Lipinski developed a simple list of parameters that were useful in predicting the possibility of poor absorption or permeability of new drug molecules. The parameters are as follows:

A molecule is expected to show poor absorption/permeability when:

- There are more than five hydrogen bond donors.
- The molecular weight is over 500.
- The Log *P* is over 5.
- The sum of nitrogen and oxygen atoms is higher than 10.

The collective name for the parameters is the rule of five. This is not because there are five rules, as in fact there are only four, but instead it refers to the parameter limits all being multiples of five (Lipinski *et al.*, 1997). The rule of five is good as a general guideline; however, it must be noted that it is a very basic check and some of the major APIs available today do not fit the pattern. For example, substrates for transporter proteins and other natural products are exceptions to these rules.

For more information about Lipinski's rule of five, please refer to Chapter 12 'The molecular characteristics of good drugs' of the **Pharmaceutical Chemistry** book within this series.

This lead compound will then be continued through drug development and the other, less ideal, compounds will be maintained as backup compounds should the lead compound prove unsuitable at any stage.

SELF CHECK 13.3

Explain what is meant by the term 'pharmacophore'.

SELF CHECK 13.4

An NCE contains three oxygen atoms, four nitrogen atoms, and five hydrogen bond donors. If the log *P* is 0.3 and the molecular weight is 314, does Lipinski's rule of five predict that this compound will have poor absorption and permeability?

KEY POINTS

- The candidate compound that is considered the best prospect for development is termed the lead compound.
- After optimization, the lead compound will progress into *in vitro* and *in vivo* testing specific to the medical condition of interest.
- Lipinski's rule of five is a set of four rules that act as a rough guide as to whether a compound is expected to show poor absorption and permeability, based on molecular structure and log *P*.
- Candidate compounds not selected as the lead are maintained as backup should the lead compound prove unsuitable at any stage.

13.3 Introduction to QSAR: optimization of lead compounds

Quantitative structure–activity relationships (QSAR) are mathematical models based on the correlation between chemical compounds' biological activity and physiochemical descriptors. These descriptors are numbers that quantify specific properties of molecules. QSARs allow for the prediction of an NCE's biological activity based on relevant properties of structurally related compounds. **Log *P*** is used in QSAR for the determination of a compound's absorption, distribution, metabolism, excretion, and toxicology (ADMET) characteristics and is a physiochemical descriptor for lipophilicity. Thus, compounds with a low log *P* are **lipophobic**, while compounds with a high log *P* are **lipophilic**.

In most cases, the biological activity of an NCE is investigated using inhibition assays, which quantitatively identify the level of decreased functionality of either a signalling or a metabolic pathway. Also, the level of non-specificity and toxicity of a compound can be compared using QSAR, allowing for the identification of highly specific, highly active, non-toxic drug compounds.

There are three components to any QSAR model:

- A dataset for the biological activity.
- A knowledge of the molecular structure of each NCE investigated.
- A suitable statistical method to determine any correlation.

The limiting factor of any QSAR is the quality and the quantity of the experimental data.

In modern QSAR techniques it is becoming common to implement the use of theoretical molecular descriptors, which cover a wide range of descriptor types. This allows all of the structural factors of an NCE to be represented numerically and also allows predictions to be made based on three-dimensional structure models. Understandably this type of modelling requires complex computer software and some of the most commonly used include ADAPT, OASIS, CODESSA, MolConnZ, and DRAGON.

SELF CHECK 13.5

What does QSAR stand for? Log *P* is used a physiochemical descriptor for which property of molecules?

SELF CHECK 13.6

What three factors are essential for the production of a QSAR model and what is the limiting factor of any QSAR model?

KEY POINTS

- Quantitative structure–activity relationships (QSARs) are mathematical models that correlate the biological activity of compounds with physiochemical descriptors.
- Physiochemical descriptors are numbers that quantify specific properties of molecules.
- Log *P* is used widely as a physiochemical descriptor for lipophilicity
- The limiting factor of any QSAR is the quantity and quality of the experimental data used in the development of the QSAR.

13.4 Preformulation considerations

Having discussed the different routes for the development of NCEs, the development of a potential lead compound enters into the next stage involving extensive deciphering of its physicochemical properties, structural determination, and assay methods. Information generated at this stage of drug development is vital to inform the formulation of a suitable drug-delivery system. The various studies that are carried out in the next phase of drug discovery include:

- The determination of the fundamental physical and chemical properties.
- The analysis of **powder** characteristics (micromeritics).
- **Excipient** compatibility studies.
- The development of assays to identify and quantify the NCE.

Studies that are carried out during this stage, called **preformulation**, are aimed at assessing the properties of NCEs in order to accumulate substantial information on the NCE's properties. This will equip the formulation scientist with the necessary information required to select a suitable drug dosage form.

TABLE 13.1 Areas for investigation during preformulation studies

Drug Profiling	Analytical Characterization
Solubility	Structural Assessment
Acid dissociation constant	Purity determination
Partition Coefficient	Assay Development
Drug Stability	
Excipient Compatibility	

FIGURE 13.1 A spectrophotometer is used in the analytical characterization of NCEs

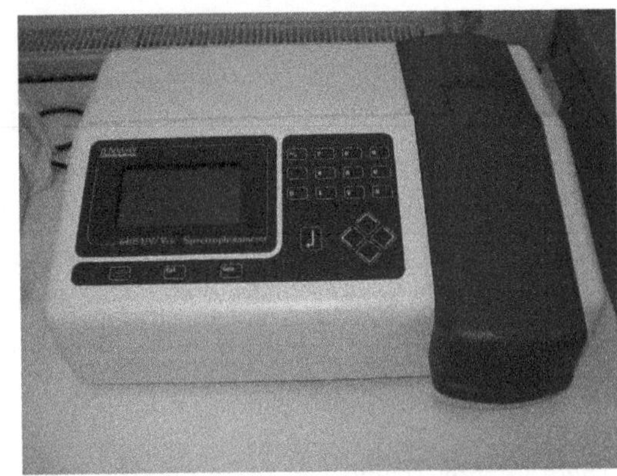

Preformulation studies consist of two sets of studies and can be broadly classified into **drug profiling** and **analytical characterization** (Table 13.1). Data generated from analytical studies is also used to help understand the pharmaceutical development of the NCE. For instance, the development of an assay such as high-pressure liquid chromatography (HPLC) to identify and quantitatively determine the NCE can be used to study the oxidative or photolytic stability, as well as excipient compatibility.

Assay via UV spectroscopy is one of the first stages during preformulation studies. It includes the determination of the specific wavelength at which the NCE exhibits maximum absorption using a spectrophotometer (Figure 13.1). The development of a UV assay is vital as it provides a rapid method to enable quantitative measurements of the NCE. This is achieved by running a broad-wave scan in the UV region (approx 200–400 nm) and choosing the wavelength with the highest associated absorbance (λ_{max}) for the drug in question.

Once a wavelength has been decided upon, the next phase involves the development of a calibration curve to assess unknown drug concentrations for any future experiments. However, utmost care should be taken when developing the calibration curve due to the limitations of the Beer–Lambert Law (Box 13.3).

BOX 13.3

Beer–Lambert Law

The Beer–Lambert Law is represented by:

$$A = \log_{10}(I_0 / I) = \varepsilon.c.L$$

where A is the absorbance, I_0 is the intensity of light at a given wavelength, I is the transmitted intensity, L is the path length through the sample in decimetres (dm), c is the concentration of the absorbing species in mol dm^{-3}, and ε is the extinction coefficient in dm^2 mol^{-1}.

This equation relates the absorption of light to the nature of the material through which it is passing. The most common path length used in UV assays is 1 cm and this is equivalent to 0.1 dm.

When developing a calibration curve for a spectrophotometric assay, the calibration can only be assumed to be linear between the lowest and highest standard absorbance values (if the calibration is linear). Above the highest standard concentration, linearity cannot be guaranteed as at higher concentrations the absorption coefficient of the molecules can deviate as a result of electrostatic interactions between the molecules. Also, changes in the refractive index of the sample at high analyte concentrations can result in non-linear absorbance readings.

Other factors, such as light scattering due to particles in the system or the fluorescence or phosphorescence of a sample, can contribute to non-linear behaviour.

For more information, please refer to Chapter 11 'Introduction to pharmaceutical analysis' of the *Pharmaceutical Chemistry* book of this series.

Solubility is one of the critical parameters that will have an influence on the amount of API that will be absorbed into the systemic circulation (**bioavailability**) after administration. APIs with solubility values below 1% (w/v) over the pH range of 1–7 at 37°C can pose potential problems with drug absorption. Also, a dissolution rate of less than 0.1 mg min^{-1} for each square centimetre of exposed surface can result in dissolution rate limited absorption. This is where the absorption is controlled by the rate at which the API is released from the formulation.

Another important parameter for ionizable APIs is the pK_a. As a rule of thumb for acidic drugs, two pH units below pK_a will result in the formation of unionized form of the API and two units above will result in complete ionization. The Henderson–Hasselbalch equation can be used to calculate the extent of API ionization upon changes in pH and, predict solubility profiles for ionizable drugs. If the dosage form is a tablet, a capsule, or novel drug-delivery system (such as liposomes or polymer-based nanoparticles) an API solubility of less than 1 mg mL^{-1} is not normally acceptable. Solubility can be improved by using a salt formed from an acidic or basic API.

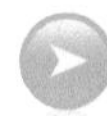

For more information on the Henderson–Hasselbalch equation, please refer to 'Acidic buffers' in Section 6.7.

The determination of the solubility and pK_a of an ionizable NCE can help in choosing the right pH to ensure sufficient drug solubility and in deciding on the type of counter ion for salt formation. An increase in drug solubility in acidic media is indicative of basic nature of the drug molecule and *vice versa*. However, an increase in solubility in both acidic, as well as basic, media suggests either an **amphoteric** molecule or **zwitterion** comprising of two ionizable groups. During preformulation studies, the intrinsic solubility (C_o) of the NCE is determined, this being the solubility of unionized form. This is done by measuring solubility in an acid medium for an acidic NCE, and in an alkaline medium for a basic NCE. Solubility measurements are taken at 4°C, as water exhibits anomalous expansion at this temperature: The consequent high **density** results in low solubility. Studies for solubility are also undertaken at 37°C and would be indicative of the drug solubility profile in humans.

For more information on acids, bases, salt formation, amphoteric molecules and zwitterions, please refer to Chapter 6.

Solvents

The solubility of an NCE is assessed in various solvents, including water and co-solvent mixtures such as methanol–water and ethanol–water. The choice of appropriate solvent or mixtures of solvents is important to facilitate drug extraction and separation in chromatography, improve solubility, and formulation development (for example, injection for initial pre-clinical evaluation of the drug). When a suitable aqueous solvent or mixture of aqueous solvents cannot be found due to drug instability or insufficient solubility, oils such as castor oil or liquid paraffin are used (see Box 13.4).

BOX 13.4

Solvent components used in drug solubility profiling

- Water.
- Polyethylene glycol.
- Propylene glycol.
- Glycerin.
- Sorbitol.
- Ethyl alcohol.
- Methanol.
- Benzyl alcohol.
- Isopropyl alcohol.
- Tweens.
- Polysorbates.
- Castor oil.
- Peanut oil.
- Sesame oil.
- Various buffers.

The choice of the solvent is influenced by drug properties. When the log P of the candidate compound is greater than 2, it results in poor aqueous solubility, which necessitates the use of water-miscible solvents to improve solubility and stability. The choice of the exact composition of the solvent mixtures can be determined using a phase diagram, which measures the effect of increasing/changing the ratio of solvent mixtures on drug solubility. The most suitable solvent/mixtures of solvents is the one where polarity of the solvent matches that of the solute.

For more information on phase diagrams, please refer to Chapter 7.

Data from these experiments can be used for both formulation development in the future as well as choosing the right combination of solvents for chromatography (e.g. HPLC) during assay development.

Partition coefficient

The extent of distribution of an NCE between water and an organic phase (usually octanol) is termed partition coefficient (P). It can be determined in a variety of ways, the shake flask method being most common. Determination of partition coefficient has a wide range of applications in drug development, such as:

- Identification of the NCE's solubility and hydrophilic/lipophilic nature.
- Prediction of the NCE permeability *in vivo*.
- Selection of mobile phase and stationary phase for chromatography techniques, such as HPLC and TLC, for assay development.

For more information on the shake flask method, please refer to Section 8.5.

Melting point

The determination of the **melting point** of an NCE provides information on purity and **polymorphism** and it may be determined using dedicated apparatus (Figure 13.2). A pure compound is characterized by a well-defined melting temperature and the existence of polymorphism is detected by multiple melting temperatures. Understanding of the melting point of an API allows for decisions to be made with regard to the developmental procedure. For example, an API with a low melting point may be unsuitable to undergo processes such as high-speed rotary pressing, as this produces significant heat due to friction. Implementing encapsulation of the API would be a more suitable option for the dosage form production in this case.

FIGURE 13.2 Typical melting point apparatus. As temperature is increased by the heating element, the physical state of the sample can be viewed through the observation window

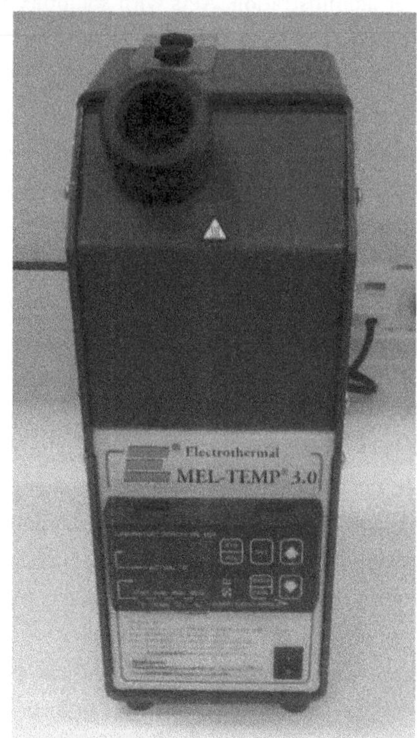

For more information on polymorphism, please refer to Section 2.3.

Micromeritics

Micromeritics is the science and technology of small particles and is used during investigations into:

- Particle size and size distribution.
- Identification of particle shape and surface area.
- Pore size.

In pharmaceutical formulations, the size, shape, and surface area of the drug particles play a large role in the physical stability of that formulation and also the rate of release of an API from the formulation. Generally, reducing the particle size increases the rate of **dissolution** and this enhances absorption. The flow properties of granules and powders are also linked with particle size. This is of particular relevance during the production of tablets where the uniformity of the tablets produced can be compromised if there are large variations in particle sizes and flow properties. The main methods of particle size analysis include:

- Microscopy.
- Sieving.
- Sedimentation methods.
- Coulter counter method.
- Laser light-scattering methods.

KEY POINTS

- Preformulation is a stage of drug development that consists of the physicochemical profiling of an NCE and its analytical characterization.
- Drug profiling includes the investigation of solubility, pK_a, partition coefficient, stability, and excipient compatibility of the NCE.
- Analytical characterization involves the assessment of purity and molecular structure, and assay development.
- The flow properties of granules and powders are linked to particle sizes and shapes and this is of particular relevance during the production of tablets.

SELF CHECK 13.7

During preformulation studies, what drug profiling and analytical characterization areas are investigated?

SELF CHECK 13.8

The melting point of two crystals of the same NCE were determined. The first was found to have a melting range of 129 °C to 137 °C, while the second crystal had a melting range from 191 °C to 198 °C. What conclusions might we draw?

13.5 Routes of administration and associated dosage forms

The body is made up of a variety of complex structures and fluids. Each of these presents a potential pathway through which a dosage form can be given to the patient, called the **route of administration**. A solid dosage form placed in the mouth, for example, may be intended for delivery via the oral cavity, perhaps through the **buccal** mucosa or **sublingual** membrane. More often, it is designed to be swallowed and the term 'oral administration' is often used, without qualification, to refer to this type of delivery.

This section will summarize and detail the main routes of administration (Figure 13.3), and will include cross-references to chapters that cover the associated dosage forms in more detail. Many of the terms used to describe the routes of administration are not exclusive. Thus, nasal delivery includes decongestant sprays and these are also an example of **topical delivery**, the nasal mucosa being an external surface of the body. Here, the decongestant is intended to produce a local effect. Some apparently distinct routes ultimately represent the same type of delivery. Thus, both oral and rectal administration can produce a systemic effect *via* absorption of the API through the gastrointestinal tract (GIT). They are both, therefore, examples of **enteral delivery**. The definition of **parenteral delivery** is perhaps the most clear-cut, literally, given that it always involves the piercing of the skin or **mucous membranes**.

FIGURE 13.3 The main routes of administration. For the routes next to the brackets, the site of administration of the dosage form is not restricted to a particular body location; those on the left involving the piercing of the skin (parenteral delivery)

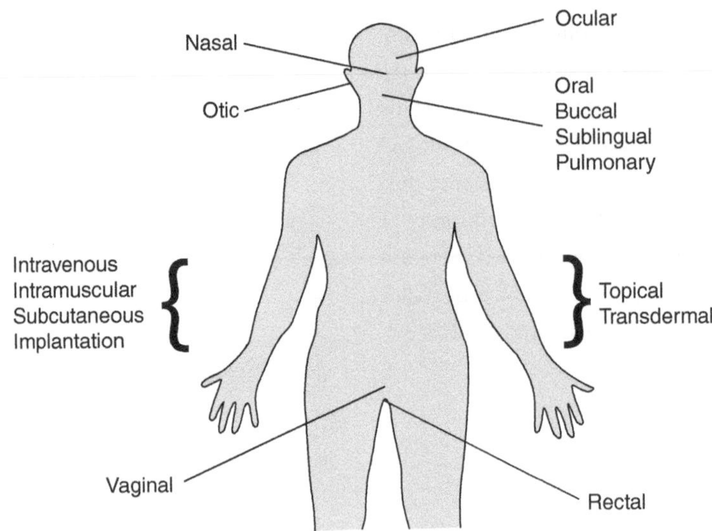

For more information on enteral, parenteral, and topical delivery, and systemic and local effects, please refer to Chapter 1.

Oral administration

The delivery of API's via the oral route can be achieved in a variety of ways depending upon the limitations of the drug in question. Oral dosage forms may be liquid or solid. Solutions, suspensions, and emulsions account for the liquid dosage forms, while tablets, capsules, and powders make up the solid dosage forms that are used in oral administration.

Various types of liquid medicine are designed to be swallowed and delivered enterally:

- Solutions.
- Elixirs.
- Syrups.
- Linctuses (Figure 13.4).

FIGURE 13.4 A typical oral liquid medicine designed for delivery to the GIT
Source: Copyright Alice Mumford

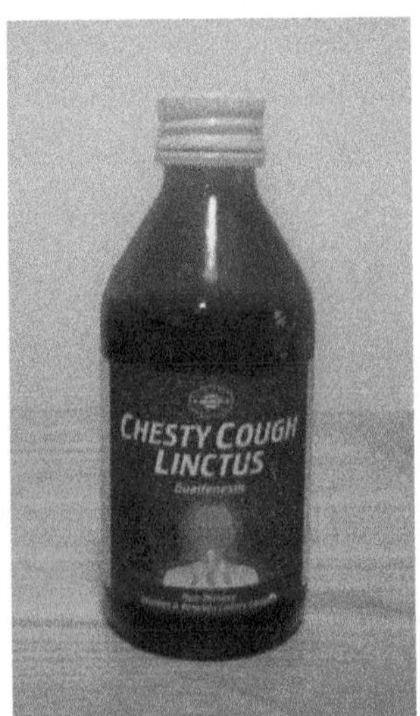

Mouthwashes fall into the category of orally administered solutions, although these are not designed to swallowed, being classified as oropharyngeal formulations (Figure 13.5).

Tablets (Figure 13.6A), capsules (Figure 13.6B), and powders (Figure 13.6C) account for the solid dosage forms which may be orally administered. There are many sub-classes of tablet, including:

- Compressed and layered.
- Coated.
- Modified release.
- Oral disintegrating.
- Chewable.

FIGURE 13.5 A typical mouthwash, an oral liquid product that is not to be swallowed
Source: Copyright colematt/iStock

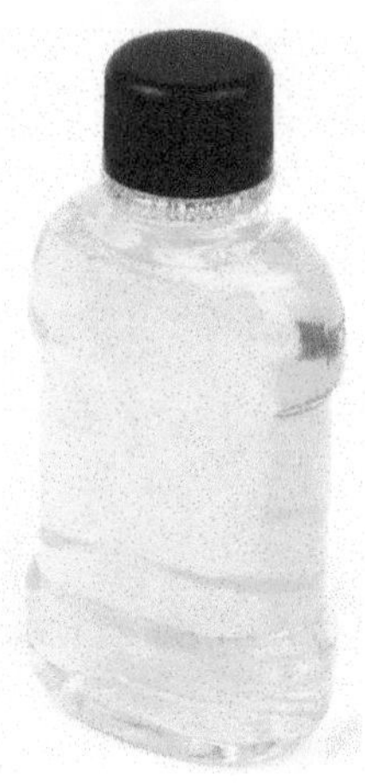

- Effervescent.
- Lozenges.
- Buccal and sublingual.

Capsules normally fall into one of two categories:

- Hard gelatin capsules.
- Soft gelatin capsules.

In each case, the instructions for use will indicate when these solid forms should be taken. Some medicines, for example, may need to be taken on an empty stomach or immediately after eating.

For more information on tablets, capsules, and powder, please refer to Chapter 2.

For more information on solutions, elixirs, syrups, linctuses, and mouthwashes, please refer to Chapter 3.

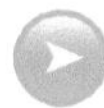

For more information on emulsions and suspensions, please refer to Chapter 10.

Ocular administration

Ocular administration involves the treatment of conditions affecting the eyes using either:

- Solutions.
- Suspensions.
- Ointments.

Liquid dosage forms used for ocular administration most commonly include eye-drops (Figure 13.7). There are also some intraocular ailments that can be treated in the same manner, although for most intraocular conditions, and more serious conditions,

FIGURE 13.6 Solid oral dosage forms (A) tablet, (B) capsule, (C) powder

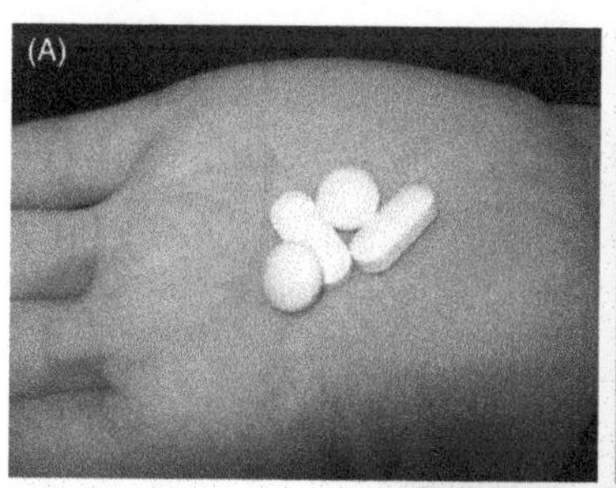

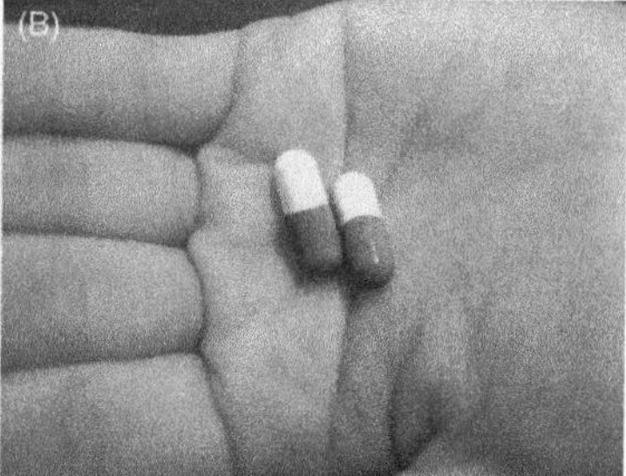

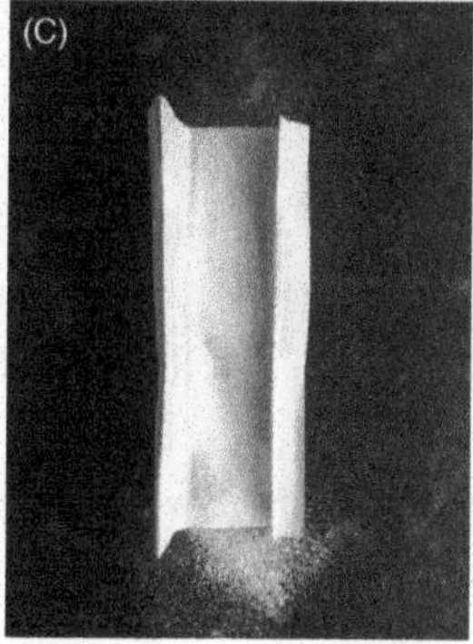

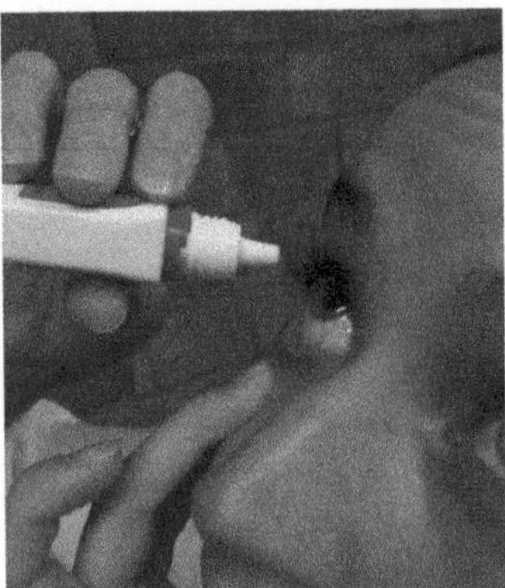

FIGURE 13.7 The administration of eye-drops, a dosage form for ocular delivery

intraocular injections are preferred. There are many disadvantages of ocular treatment, including blurring of vision and local irritation. The main advantages of ocular drops are that they are applied directly to the problem site and, with practice, they can be administered effectively by the patient.

For more information on solutions, please refer to 'Solutions' in Chapter 3.

For more information on suspensions and ointments, please refer to Chapter 10.

Nasal administration

Nasal delivery generally involves the delivery of an API via a non-inhalation aerosol spray and is most commonly used in the relief of congestion (Figure 13.8). When the spray is used for the first time, it may be necessary for the patient to prime the pump by activating the device several times until spray is released. The patient may be instructed to tilt their head after administration is complete.

For more information on non-inhalation aerosols, please refer to Chapter 4.

Otic administration

Otic administration is necessary for the treatment of infection, inflammation, and earache or more severe pain. Similarly to ocular administration, the following dosage forms are used in the treatment of ear conditions:

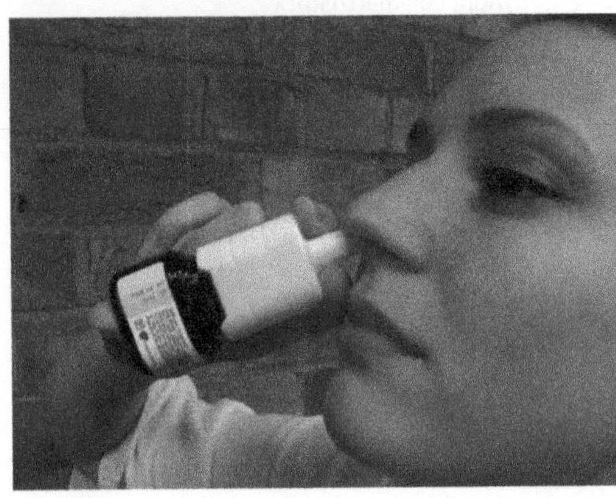

FIGURE 13.8 The administration of a nasal spray, a dosage form for nasal delivery

- Suspensions.
- Solutions.
- Ointments.

For liquid medications, patients may be instructed to lie on their side during administration and for a short time afterwards. The patient may also be guided to plug their ear loosely with cotton wool to prevent leakage.

Vaginal administration

There are many types of dosage form that are suitable for vaginal administration, including:

- Creams.
- Ointments.
- Gels.
- Tablets.
- Capsules.
- Pessaries.

These may require the use of an applicator and the patient will require teaching on how to use it correctly. Vaginal implants may also be used and are excellent in the controlled release of the API and the fixed nature of the dosage form ensures accurate delivery.

For more information on creams, ointments, and gels, please refer to Chapter 10.

For more information on tablets, pessaries, capsules, and implants, please refer to Chapter 2.

Rectal administration

Suppositories are the main mode of rectal administration, although lotions, liniments, ointments, pastes, and gels are also used. Suppositories are solid dosage forms, which undergo melting, softening, or dissolution upon administration and have the advantage that they can be suitably administered to patients who are unconscious or vomiting. Drugs that are liable to degradation in the upper areas of the GIT can also be administered rectally to avoid this problem. The main disadvantages of rectal administration are slow absorption, the patient-to-patient variation in the rate of rectal absorption, and also the patient acceptability of the dosage form.

For more information on lotions and liniments please refer to Chapter 3.

For more information on ointments, pastes, and gels, please refer to Chapter 10.

For more information on suppositories, please refer to 'Depots and implants' in Chapter 2.

Pulmonary administration

The administration of APIs via the respiratory system is predominantly for the treatment of pulmonary disorders. Due to the physiology of the lungs and their optimization for the exchange of substances, drug absorption is highly efficient. This has been exploited as a route of drug delivery using dry powder inhalers (DPIs), pressurized metered dose inhalers (pMDIs) (Figure 13.9), nebulizers, and aerosols. DPIs and pMDIs differ in that DPIs administer dry powders containing the API, whereas pMDIs administer a suspension or a solution much in the same way. Nebulizers involve the administration of solutions to the respiratory tract.

For more information on pMDIs, DPIs, and nebulizers, please refer Chapter 4.

FIGURE 13.9 A patient using a metered dose inhaler (MDI), a method of pulmonary administration

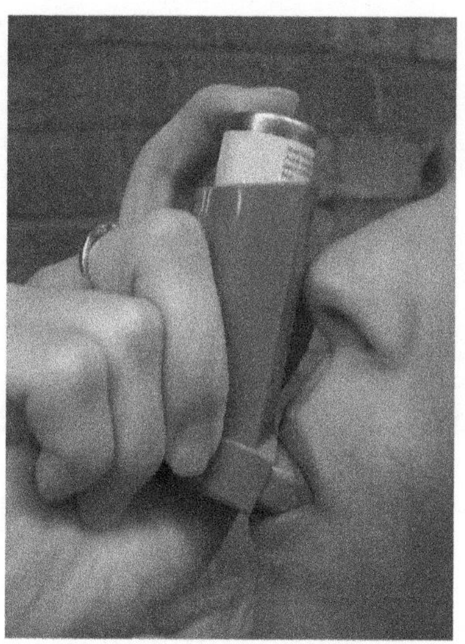

Topical and transdermal administration

Topical administration can involve a variety of liquid and semi-solid dosage forms:

- Gels.
- Pastes.
- Ointments.
- Collodions.
- Liniments.
- Lotions.

These are applied externally to the area in need of treatment and are intended to produce primarily a local effect (Figure 13.10). Collodions, liniments, and lotions all fall into the categories of either solutions or suspensions and are often applied for the treatment of parasitic, bacterial, fungal, and viral infections. Transdermal is a route of administration where the API is delivered across the skin to produce a systemic effect. This includes transdermal patches and drug absorption across skin can be understood through the principles of partitioning.

For more information on collodions, liniments, and lotions, please refer to Chapter 3.

FIGURE 13.10 The administration of a topical formulation to the skin

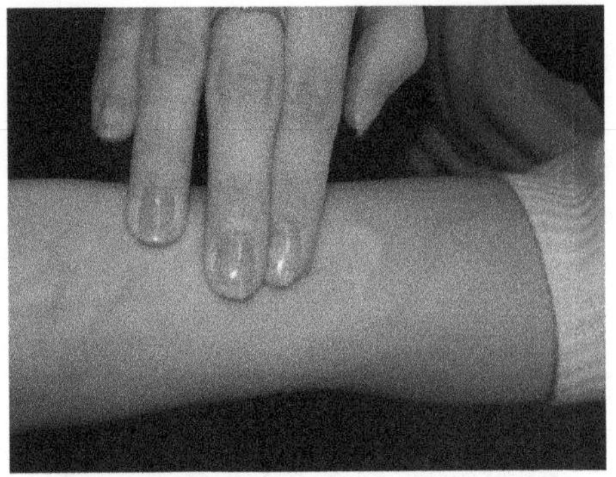

 For more information on gels, pastes, and ointments, please refer to Chapter 10.

Parenteral administration

Parenteral administration involves the administration of the dosage form by piercing the skin. It is used extensively for liquid medicines and there are numerous routes of administration:

- **Intravenous** (IV) administration is used widely and has many advantages. Relatively large amounts of parenteral preparations, up to 500 ml, may be delivered. The IV route also allows for the administration of APIs directly into a vein, which would otherwise result in irritation if administered via another method. The **bioavailability** of IV administrated drugs is such that 100% of the administered dose is available for action. The main drawback of IV administration is the need for training to ensure correct targeting of the injection and that the drug is administered to the vein at the correct rate.
- Intramuscular (IM) administration is usually delivered to the muscles in the buttocks, the thigh, or the upper arm. The maximum volume for administration via IM is lower than IV and the time from delivery to response is slower than the IV method of administration. Response is also slower for suspensions than it is for solutions. Bruising and soreness at the site of administration can often result if the injection technique is poor.
- Subcutaneous (SC) administration involves the administration of the preparation to the fat layer directly below the skin. One of the most common uses for SC administration is in the self-delivery of insulin in the treatment of diabetes. This method of administration is also used when there are problems accessing a vein for IV delivery. The time for the drug to be available at its active site is slower when administered subcutaneously when compared with IV and IM administration. Normally, the volume of an SC preparation administered is low, around 1 ml.

IV, IM, and SC are the three most common routes of administration with the remaining routes of intradermal (ID), intra-arterial (IA), intrathecal (IT), intradural/extradural, and intracardiac (IC) being used less frequently and reserved for specialist treatments.

Solid parenteral implants are also used as a means of drug delivery and these involve the subcutaneous insertion of a sterile solid preparation of a suitable shape and size. This may be placed inside the upper arm to minimize the risk of the implant breaking and includes devices that rely on an osmotic pump to deliver the API. In general, implants have the advantage of being able to deliver an API over a long period of time, which is not possible with other parenteral methods.

 For more information on osmotic pump implants, please refer to Chapter 11.

 For more information on implants, please refer to Chapter 2.

 For more information on liquids for parenteral delivery, please refer to Chapter 3.

SELF CHECK 13.9

In the administration of APIs via the oral route the dosage form can take six main forms (three liquid and three solid). What are these?

SELF CHECK 13.10

Name nine routes of administration where the site of administration of the dosage form is at a particular body location.

KEY POINTS

- Oral administration may use liquid or solid dosage forms.
- Ocular conditions are most commonly external and can be treated via the application of eye drops.
- Nasal administration generally involves the delivery of an API via a non-inhalation aerosol spray.
- Otic formulations are generally used to treat local ear infections.
- Vaginal formulations may be applied via the use of a specially designed applicator.
- Suppositories include rectally administered solid dosage forms that undergo melting, softening or dissolution during use.
- The administration of APIs via the respiratory system is predominantly for the treatment of pulmonary disorders.
- Topical formulations are applied externally to the area in need of treatment and primarily have a local effect. Transdermal delivery is designed to produce a systemic effect.
- IV, IM, and SC are the three most common routes of parenteral administration.

13.6 Packaging considerations for pharmaceutical dosage forms

In pharmaceutics, the packaging of a dosage form is more than just a means of delivering the drug to the consumer in a neat and presentable fashion. Much more important is the role of the packaging in the preservation of the formulation and protection of the product from tampering and spoilage as a result of microbial contamination. Modern dosage forms are more complicated to package than may be first anticipated as interactions between the API, excipients, and packaging are a real concern and careful consideration of the packaging form and material is necessary.

A suitable packaging form must:

- Protect the API from damage as a result of mechanical stress, such as during transport or if accidentally dropped.
- Prevent microbial infiltration of the product during transport and storage.
- Protect the product from physical factors, such as light, moisture, and oxygen, to prevent the degradation of a formulation.
- Carry the relevant product information.

A suitable packaging form must not:

- Bring about an undesirable change in the product following interaction between the product and package.
- Be itself altered in an undesirable way following interaction between product and package.

The general requirements for packaging of pharmaceutical products are listed in the **pharmacopoeiae**; however, the actual packaging requirements of each new product will need thorough investigation.

There are numerous forms of packaging and each has its purpose (Table 13.2). The packaging materials used for the production of each package form are used for specific reasons and are divided into two classes: primary and secondary packaging. Primary packaging is in contact with the pharmaceutical product, while secondary packaging is often present to improve the appearance of the product. For example, a glass bottle which contains the medication packaged inside a cardboard box. The three main materials used in the

TABLE 13.2 **Packaging forms found in the pharmaceutical industry**

Packaging Form	Description
Ampoule	Package containing a single use medication opened by breaking.
Bag	Formed from a flexible material and sealed on at least three sides.
Blister	Twin-layer package with one layer acting as a housing for the dose and the second acting as a sealed cover.
Bottle	Plastic or glass bottle for containing solid or liquid dosage forms.
Cartridge	Cylindrical container used in specialist equipment, e.g. pre-filled syringe.
Gas cylinder	Container for the controllable release of a gas.
Injection needle	Hollow needle for administration of liquid dosages.
Injection syringe	Cylindrical design for holding/measuring a liquid dose before administration.
Pressurized container	Container for the controllable release of a gas.
Single-dose container	Container for solid, semi-solid, or liquid single dosages.
Strip	Multi-dose container often consisting of multiple blisters.
Tube	Semi-solid dosage container where contents in released upon squeezing.
Vial	Small container for parenteral dosage.

production of primary packaging containers are glass, plastic, and metal. Table 13.3 highlights the range of materials used within pharmaceutical products and their example uses.

Glass is most often the favoured choice and is used extensively for the packaging of pharmaceuticals, especially for medicines that are administered orally or locally where tablets or liquid dosage are used. The glass type is important and dependent upon the formulation contained. Classifications of types of glass are given in the European and United States pharmacopoeiae.

Increasingly, containers are being made of plastics. When compared with glass, plastic containers have several advantages including the fact that:

- They are almost unbreakable.
- They can be collapsible.
- They are much lighter than glass containers of the same size.

The European, Japanese, and United States pharmacopoeiae all describe the plastics suitable for use; however, it should be noted that there is variation in the entries of each pharmacopoeia. It must also be noted that plastic containers are incompatible with some organic solvents.

Metal containers are used solely for medicinal products designed for non-parenteral administration. Aluminium and stainless steel are the metals used and they have many positive attributes. They are ideal for producing tamper-evident containers that are also strong, shatterproof, and impermeable to gases. Used widely in aerosol and gas cylinders, they are also implemented as the seal for blister-type packaging and in cans. Requirements are not given in pharmacopoeiae; the suitability of a particular material for a container is normally established by conducting stability studies in which the material is in contact with the drug in question.

In addition to the materials used for the packaging container, the material used for the packaging closure is also of importance. Closures have the task of sealing the dosage form inside the container to protect it from outside elements. At the same time, however, the closures must be easily and safely removed to allow for the administration of the product. Where possible, the use of closures is avoided but when used, involve the use of rubber closures and caps/overseals (WHO, 2002).

TABLE 13.3 Summary of the materials and their uses in the production of pharmaceutical packaging (WHO, 2002)

Material	Use
Cardboard	Boxes
	Display Units
Paper	Labels
	Instruction leaflets
Glass	Ampoules
	Bottles
	Vials
	Syringes
	Cartridges
Plastic	Closures
	Bottles
	Bags
	Tubes
	Laminates with paper or foil
Metal	Collapsible tubes
	Rigid cans
	Foils
	Needles
	Gas cylinders
	Pressurized containers
Rubber	Closures
	Plungers

Caps or overseals are used to secure the rubber closure to the container in order to maintain the integrity of the seal under normal conditions of transport, handling, and storage during the intended **shelf life** of the product. Such caps are usually made of aluminium and can be equipped with a plastic top to facilitate opening. Caps also provide evidence of tampering: once opened or removed they cannot be repositioned. This is especially true for caps with a plastic top.

Modern rubber compounds used in the production of closures for the packaging of pharmaceuticals contain only a limited number of ingredients. Closures made from such materials generally do not pose any problems, and can be used in contact with a large number of drug preparations. Rubber closures for pharmaceutical use must meet the relevant requirements of the European, Japanese, and United States pharmacopoeiae.

KEY POINTS

- Packaging helps to preserve the formulation and protect the product from tampering and spoilage as a result of microbial contamination.
- The materials used for the production of pharmaceutical packages are divided into two classes: primary and secondary.
- The three main materials used in the production of primary packaging are: glass, plastic, and metal.
- Closures are used to seal the dosage form inside the container to protect it from outside elements.

SELF CHECK 13.11

Name four attributes of appropriate pharmaceutical packaging.

SELF CHECK 13.12

Where are the general requirements relating to pharmaceutical packaging readily available?

13.7 Clinical trials for new medications

Clinical trials are carried out on all new medications as a means of determining the effectiveness of the medication on the target population. The group of individuals selected for the clinical trials are often volunteers and are intended to replicate on a small scale the patient population (or 'segment') for the target medication. These volunteers are subjected to the new medication for predetermined time periods. A medication's performance is normally measured against a control group who receive a pharmacologically inert substance or placebo. This has similar organoleptic properties to the active dosage form, including appearance, taste, and smell. Clinical trials of this type are described as 'blind', as those involved do not know who received the placebo and who was given the medication.

There are four phases involved in the clinical trials of new medications. The first, phase I, includes pharmacological studies aimed at providing information on the safety of a drug. The effect of dosage and other therapeutic effect studies make up the majority of the phase II trials. Phase III trials are used to develop the safety profile for the drug at the same time as being used to reinforce the findings in the phase II trials. Elements of the phase III trials are often integrated into phase II or phase IV trials. The fourth stage of the clinical trials process is almost always used to investigate the effect of the drug over a range of patient segments. Any unusual side effects which had not been previously seen in the trial process may be recorded at this stage. This is summarized in Table 13.4.

Phase I trials

Although laboratory based analysis can provide detailed information following ***in vitro*** and ***in vivo*** animal trials, information derived from human studies is also necessary. It is in the first phase of clinical trials that the human-based investigations are first carried out. Volunteer groups totalling around 100 healthy participants are monitored closely, following the administration of the medication, in order to provide information on the safety, tolerance, **pharmacokinetics (PK)**, and **pharmacodynamics (PD)** of the drug. Dose escalation (dose-ranging) is also carried out during the phase I testing stage in order to identify the correct dose for use. In rare cases there is a need to enlist volunteers and patients who are not healthy; for example, HIV or cancer sufferers, who have not responded to any currently available treatments. The phase I clinical trials fall into three categories: single ascending dose studies (SAD), multiple ascending dose studies (MAD), and food-effect studies.

SAD studies involve the administration of a single dose of the medication to a small subject group, who are then observed for their response over a period of time. So long as the group does not show signs of any side-effects and also that the group responds to the medication in the expected manner as predicted by the pharmacokinetic data, the dose is then increased and this higher dose is given to a separate group of subjects. This process is repeated until either the predetermined safety level is reached or until side-effects that are severe are observed. This point is termed the MTD, which is the maximum tolerated dose.

MAD studies are conducted to investigate the effect of multiple doses of the medication on subjects in order to further understand the pharmacokinetics and pharmacodynamics of the drug. To undertake the MAD studies, small groups of subjects are given

TABLE 13.4 **Summary of the phases of clinical trials (*n* = number of participants)**

Phase	Aim	Subjects	Data	*n*	Time
IA	Exploratory safety	Healthy Single dose	Adverse effects PK/PD	40–60	6 months
IB	Exploratory safety	Healthy Repeat dose	Adverse effects PK/PD	30–50	6 months
IIA	Preliminary safety and efficacy	Patients Intended clinical dose	Adverse effects PK Efficacy data	50–200	9 months to 2 years
IIB	Confirm dose	Patients	Dose-response	200–500	2–3 years
III	Efficacy and safety	Patients in target indication	Safety, efficacy Economics	500–1000+	2–5+ years
IV	Post-marketing	Treated patients	Adverse effects	10000+	2–4+ years

multiple doses of the drug at a level that is known to be safe and they are then monitored in much the same way as for SAD studies. If no side-effects or changes in the pharmacokinetics and pharmacodynamics of the drug are seen then the dose is increased.

Food-effect studies are usually quick and easy to perform but provide vital information on the effect of eating on the absorption of the API into the body. The drug is given to subjects in a fasted state and the level of absorption is measured The investigation is then repeated at a later date with the subjects having recently eaten. The results from the two studies are compared and recommendations such as 'take with or after food' can be included in the administration instructions on the packaging.

Phase II trials

If the completion of phase I trials results in the acquisition of satisfactory results, then the medication can progress into phase II trials. These are a means of testing the drug's efficacy at the safe dose determined following the phase I trials. The phase II trials also act as a scaled-up version of the phase I trials where similar criteria are assessed. The phase II trials normally involve up to three times the number of subjects used in the phase I trials, Table 13.4. The entry requirements for a subject into the test group are much more controlled for phase II trials. During phase II trials there are a number of tests performed and these are carried out over a range of dosage levels. The quality and scope of the phase II trials are limited in the main by the data derived from the phase I testing. The second phase of the clinical trials is also the stage at which most new medications fail the testing procedure due to the emergence of toxic effects or evidence indicating that the drug is not acting in the desired way. As with phase I trials, there are sub sections to phase II trials and these are referred to as phase II A and phase II B trials. The former (Phase IIA) relates to the assessment of the dosage requirements, i.e. how much drug should be given, and the latter (Phase IIB) relates to investigation of the medicine's efficacy. Many case studies are designed to investigate phase I and phase II at the same time and in doing so investigate efficacy and toxicity.

Phase III trials

Phase III trials are carried out at various locations and involve the use of randomized controlled groups. These groups can be as much as ten times larger than phase II trials, with as many as 3000 subjects being used. These trials are designed to act as an ultimate confirmation of the medication's effectiveness and allow for accurate comparison of a medication's value with other currently marketed products.

As a result of the scale of phase III trials, and the complexity involved in the studies themselves, the cost of phase III trials is the highest of all the stages. More often than not, the third phase of the clinical trials' process will continue throughout the time period in which regulatory approval will be gained. This has the advantage that the producer of the medicine can identify any further uses for the product for which it was not initially intended. They can also collect further evidence on which to base safety information and also continue to provide the medication to patients before the medication is actually available for purchase. For approval to be given by the EMA in the EU and the FDA in the United States, it is common that two phase III trials are carried out in order to confirm a medications safety and efficacy.

Phase IV trials

The fourth phase of the clinical trials process is described as pharmacovigilance; this is the monitoring of a medicine's performance following its approval for marketing. The main aim of these phase IV trials is to identify any undesired effects of the drug, which may develop as a result of long term use. Any undesired effects that may present themselves may have the impact of removing the medication's right to be sold, or alternatively its use may be limited to specific patient segments. Post-marketing surveillance trials are at times required by the regulatory authorities; however, they are commonly carried out by the development company as a method of identifying new indications and also drug–drug interactions. The effect of the drugs on pregnant females is also monitored as it is unlikely that pregnant women would take part in the clinical trial of a new medication.

KEY POINTS

- Clinical trials are carried out on all new medications as a means of determining the effectiveness of the medication on the target population.
- There are four phases involved in the clinical trials of new medications.
- In phase I clinical trials, the first human-based investigations of a drug are carried out.
- Phase II trials involve more test subjects than phase I trials. It is this stage at which most new medications fail the testing procedure.
- Phase III trials involve the use of large randomized controlled groups and are the most costly of all the phases.
- Phase IV trials involve the monitoring of a medicine's performance following its approval for marketing.

SELF CHECK 13.13

Briefly describe the areas covered by each stage of the clinical trials process.

SELF CHECK 13.14

In Phase I, trials fall into three categories. Describe each category in brief.

CHAPTER SUMMARY

- Candidate compounds are those predicted to interact with the biological target of interest to produce a therapeutic effect. They may be referred to as new chemical entities (NCEs).
- Candidate compounds may be identified by high-throughput screening, modification of existing APIs or rational drug design.
- The candidate compound that is considered the best prospect for development is termed the lead compound.
- Quantitative structure–activity relationships (QSARs) are mathematical models that correlate the biological activity of compounds against physiochemical descriptors.
- Preformulation is a stage of drug development that consists of the physicochemical profiling of an NCE and its analytical characterization.
- The main routes of administration where the site of administration is at a particular location on the body are: nasal, otic, ocular, oral, sublingual, buccal, rectal, vaginal, and pulmonary.
- The main routes of administration where the site of administration can be in a variety of locations are IV, IM, SC, topical, and transdermal.
- Packaging helps to preserve the formulation and protect the product from tampering and spoilage as a result of microbial contamination.
- There are four phases involved in the clinical trials of new medications.

FURTHER READING

Aulton, M.E. (ed.) *Aulton's Pharmaceutics: The Design and Manufacture of Medicines.* (3rd edn). Edinburgh: Churchill Livingstone (2007).

A comprehensive text that includes sections devoted to powder processing and the control of microorganisms.

Monynihan, H. and Crean, A. *The Physicochemical Basis of Pharmaceuticals.* Oxford: Oxford University Press (2009).

Includes comprehensive list of all the routes of administration.

REFERENCES

Lipinski, C.A., Lombardo, F., Dominy, B.W., and Feeney, P.J. Experimental and computiational approaches to estimate solubility and permeability in drug discovery and development settings, *Advanced Drug Delivery Reviews* (1997). 23, 1–3: 3–25.

World Health Organization. Guidelines on packaging for pharmaceutical products, *World Health Organization technical report series*, No. 902, Annex 9. Geneva (2002).

Glossary

Absolute Temperature, T The absolute temperature scale expresses temperature in units of kelvin, K.

Acid dissociation constant, K_a The acid dissociation constant is a modified equilibrium constant for the acid ionization equilibrium. By definition, $pK_a=-\log K_a$.

Activation energy The activation energy is the minimum energy that molecules must have before a chemical reaction or physical process is possible.

Active Pharmaceutical Ingredient (API) The active pharmaceutical ingredient is the drug; that part of a medicine that provokes the desired pharmacological effect.

Active transport Active transport is where the body uses cellular energy to move a substance across a cell membrane against a concentration gradient.

Activity Activity is the effective concentration of solute in solution that contributes to the chemical potential of that solute.

Adhesive force An adhesive force is the attraction between entities of a different kind, such as between water and oil, or between water and the walls of a capillary tube.

Adsorption Adsorption refers to the process of molecules (adsorbate) binding to the surface (adsorbent) of solids and liquids.

Aerosols An aerosol is an example of a dispersed system where fine solid particles or liquid droplets are dispersed throughout a carrier gas.

Agglomeration Agglomeration, or flocculation, is when colloidal particles aggregate (join together) to form clusters.

Aggregation Aggregation is when particles join together to form larger particles, losing their individual identity.

Agonist An agonist is a molecule that binds to a receptor causing a biological response.

Amorphous Amorphous substances are those lacking a crystal structure.

Amphiphilic Amphiphilic materials have an affinity for both polar and non-polar media

Amphiprotic Amphiprotic substances can donate or accept protons.

Amphoteric An amphoteric substance is able to act as an acid or a base

Analgesic An analgesic is a drug that relieves pain.

Analytical characterization Analytical characterization includes studies undertaken during preformulation to establish analytical techniques that may be used to determine a new chemical entity.

Anion An anion is a negatively charged ion.

Antisolvent An antisolvent is one that does not have any affinity for the solute.

Aprotic Aprotic solvents neither accept nor donate protons.

Autoprotolysis Autoprotolysis is the process by which a proton is transferred between two identical molecules.

Bacteriostatic agents Bacteriostatic agents stop bacteria from reproducing and multiplying, inhibiting the growth of bacteria without killing them.

Bernoulli's equation Bernoulli's equation predicts that an increase in the speed of a fluid is accompanied by a decrease in fluid pressure.

Bioavailability Bioavailability is the fraction or percentage of an administered dose of an unchanged API that reaches the systemic circulation. This may be less than 100% due to, for example, low solubility, poor permeability, and pre-systemic metabolism.

Boiling point, T_b The normal boiling point is the temperature at which the liquid and vapour phases of a substance are in equilibrium at an external pressure of 1 atmosphere.

Boyle's Law Boyle's Law states that, at fixed temperature, the pressure of a sample of gas will be inversely proportional to its volume.

Brönsted acid A Brönsted acid is a proton donor.

Brönsted base A Brönsted base is a proton acceptor

Bubble point The bubble point is the temperature at which the first bubble of vapour evaporates from the liquid phase as the temperature is raised.

Buccal Buccal delivery is the absorption of a drug through the oral mucosa, specifically the cheek.

Buffer capacity, β Buffer capacity is defined as the amount of acid or base that must be added to a buffer so that the pH changes by 1 unit.

Buffer A buffer is an aqueous solution of a weak acid and its conjugate base, or a weak base and its conjugate acid, which undergoes little change in its pH when small amounts of acid or base are added to the solution.

Calorimeter A calorimeter is a device used for measuring the heat changes associated with chemical reactions or physical processes.

Cannula In general, a cannula is a tube that is inserted into the body. A nasal cannula ends with two tubes that are placed in each nostril.

Capsules Capsules are dosage forms in which the API is contained within a shell, normally made of gelatin.

Catheter A catheter is a sterile tube that is inserted into a fluid-containing vessel within the body, e.g. a vein, most commonly to assist in the delivery of an API.

Cation A cation is a positively charged ion.

Centrifugation Centrifugation is the separation of molecules by size or density using the force generated by a spinning rotor.

Charles' Law Charles' Law states that, at fixed pressure, the volume of a sample of gas will be inversely proportional to its absolute temperature.

Chemical potential, μ The chemical potential of a component within a phase is the molar contribution that the component makes to total free energy of that phase.

Chemisorption Chemisorption is a type of adsorption where strong covalent or ionic bonds form between the adsorbate and adsorbent, resulting in monolayer adsorption.

Chewable tablets Chewable tablets are designed to be broken up mechanically in the mouth before swallowing.

Clinical trials Clinical trials are a series of investigations that are undertaken during drug development to investigate the efficacy and safety of a new chemical entity and associated dosage forms.

Closed system A closed system can exchange heat but not matter with the surroundings.

Coalescence Coalescence is where domains join together to form larger domains, losing their individual identity. It is generally preferred to the term aggregation when the domains are liquid.

Cohesive force A cohesive force is the force of attraction between molecules of the same type, such as water molecules.

Colligative property A colligative property is a physical property of a solution that depends only on the number of solute particles present.

Colloid A colloid consists of one substance dispersed throughout another. Colloidal domains have sizes in the range 1 to 1000 nanometres.

Component A component is a chemically independent constituent of a mixture.

Compression When a material is reduced in volume by compressive stress

Condensation point, T_b The normal condensation (or boiling) point is the temperature at which the liquid and vapour phases of a substance are in equilibrium at an external pressure of 1 atmosphere..

Contact angle, θ The contact angle of a liquid droplet resting on a solid surface is the angle between the liquid/air interface and solid surface.

Contrast matching Contrast matching occurs in dispersions where the dispersed and continuous phases have comparable refractive indices.

Critical Micelle Concentration (CMC) The critical micelle concentration is the concentration of surfactant at which micelles first start to form.

Critical pressure, T_p The critical pressure of a closed fluid system is the minimum pressure at which the boundary between liquid and vapour disappears and the substance becomes a single phase supercritical fluid.

Critical temperature, T_c The critical temperature of a closed fluid system is the minimum temperature at which the boundary between liquid and vapour disappears and the substance becomes a supercritical fluid.

Cross-screening Cross-screening is the process used to identify all of the biological targets which will be affected by a chosen candidate compound. Ideally, the compound is active only against the intended target.

Crystal habit Crystal habit is the visible external shape of a crystalline material. The term can be applied to individual, or clusters of, crystals.

Crystalline Crystalline solids or crystals are composed of particles that are arranged in an orderly, repeating pattern that extends in all three dimensions.

Dalton's Law Dalton's Law states that the total pressure of a mixture of gases is equal to the sum of the respective partial pressure of each gas. It applies to both ideal and real gases.

Decimetre cubed (dm^3) A decimetre cubed has a volume equivalent to a cube with side length 1 dm (10 cm). 1 dm^3 has the same volume as 1 litre, 1000 millilitres, 1000 centimetre cubed, or one-thousandth of a metre cubed.

Deliquescence Deliquescence is when a solid absorbs moisture from the atmosphere until a solution is formed.

Density, ρ Density is the mass of a substance per unit volume.

Dew point The dew point of a fluid system is the temperature at which the first droplet of liquid forms from the vapour phase as the temperature is lowered.

Dielectric constant, ε The dielectric constant of a material is a measure of the resistance that is encountered to the formation of an electric field across that material.

Diffuse Particles diffuse when they move randomly through a fluid as a result of thermal energy. Net particle movement will occur until the fluid has an homogenous composition throughout.

Diffusion-controlled release In diffusion-controlled release systems, the release of the API from the tablet is achieved by molecular diffusion. This arises due to the concentration gradient, the API having a lower concentration outside the tablet.

Dilatant liquids Dilatant liquids become more viscous as the rate of shear increases.

Diprotic acids Diprotic acids possess two hydrogen atoms that can be donated by each molecule.

Direct compression (DC) Direct compression involves the formation of tablets by applying or compressing the powdered API and excipients without the prior physical modification of this material.

Disperse system A disperse system consists of one component, the dispersed phase, that is distributed in discrete domains throughout a second component, known as the continuous phase. Disperse systems may also be referred to as dispersions.

Dispersion A dispersion consists of one component, the dispersed phase, that is distributed in discrete domains throughout a second component, known as the continuous phase. Dispersions may also be referred to as disperse systems.

Dissolution The process by which a solid, liquid or gas forms a solution in a solvent. The maximum amount of material that can be dissolved at equilibrium is known as the solubility of that substance.

Dissolution-controlled release In dissolution-controlled release systems, the release of the API from the tablet is achieved by dissolution. The API is embedded within a slowly dissolving matrix.

Distillation Distillation is a technique that can be used to separate thermally stable liquids by successive vaporization and condensation. The liquid obtained is known as the distillate.

Distribution coefficient, D The distribution coefficient is the ratio of the concentration of a chemical species (regardless of its chemical form) in two identified phases, e.g. octanol–water.

Domains Domains are discrete units of matter that are dispersed throughout another medium. They may be solid particles, liquid droplets, or gas bubbles.

Dosage form A dosage form is the physical form of a drug that is presented to the patient.

Drug profiling Drug profiling includes studies undertaken during preformulation to establish the physical properties of a new chemical entity.

Drug The term drug refers to a pharmacologically active compound that acts within the body to prevent, alleviate or treat a medical condition.

Dry powder inhaler (DPI) Dry powder inhaler devices employ solid excipients as carrier particles to deliver an API through breath actuation.

Dusting powders Dusting powders are fine medicinal powders intended to be dusted on the skin by means of a container with a perforated lid.

Dynamic equilibrium A dynamic equilibrium exists when the concentration of reactants and products remain constant in a chemical or physical process with on-going forward and reverse reactions.

Dynamic viscosity, η Dynamic viscosity is the measure of the resistance to flow of liquid under an applied force.

Effervescent tablets Effervescent tablets are those which release carbon dioxide when in contact with water.

Electrolyte An electrolyte is a substance that ionizes or dissociates into ions when in solution.

Emulsification Emulsification is the process of dispersing one liquid in a second immiscible liquid.

Emulsifier An emulsifier is a substance that can stabilise an emulsion e.g. surfactants.

Emulsion An emulsion is formed from two immiscible liquids where droplets of one liquid are dispersed throughout the other liquid.

Enantiotropic Enantiotropic systems are polymorphic solids where each polymorph has a specific temperature and pressure range where it is the most stable form. The polymorphs may reversibly change between the different forms as conditions alter.

Endothermic An endothermic reaction or process absorbs heat from the surroundings.

Enteral delivery Enteral delivery occurs when the drug is absorbed through the gastrointestinal tract.

Enthalpy, H Enthalpy is a state function that measures the heat absorbed by a system at constant pressure. It has units of J mol^{-1}.

Entropy, S Entropy is a state function that measures the disorder within a system and has units of J K^{-1} mol^{-1}.

Epimers Epimers are diastereomers that differ only in their configuration around one asymmetric carbon atom.

Epimerization Epimerization is an interchange between epimers.

Equilibrium constant, K The equilibrium constant is a ratio that describes the composition of a chemically reversible reaction at equilibrium.

Eutectic mixture A eutectic mixture is a mixture of chemical compounds or elements with a single chemical composition that solidifies at a lower temperature than any other composition made up of the same ingredients. This mixture has the eutectic composition and the temperature is known as the eutectic temperature.

Eutectic point The eutectic point represents a composition of a mixture that has the lowest melting point and that will freeze without previously depositing any of the components in the mixture.

Excipient An excipient is generally a pharmacologically inactive substance used as a carrier for the active ingredients of a medication. Any component of a dosage form, other than the API, is an excipient.

Exothermic An exothermic reaction or process releases heat to the surroundings.

Extemporaneously prepared medicines Extemporaneously prepared medicines are generally formulated for immediate use by a specific patient where an equivalent medicine is not commercially available.

First-pass metabolism First-pass metabolism is when the concentration of an API absorbed in the gastrointestinal tract is reduced by the action of the liver before it enters the main circulatory system.

Flocculation Flocculation is a process by which two or more domains in the disperse phase aggregate to form clusters without losing their individual identity.

Foaming agent A foaming agent is used with gas-in-liquid dispersions to stabilise a foam by lowering the interfacial surface tension.

Formulation Formulation describes the process of transforming a drug into a medicine.

Freezing point, T_m The normal freezing (or melting) point is the temperature at which the solid and liquid phases of a substance are in equilibrium at an external pressure of 1 atm.

Fusion Fusion is the phase change from solid to liquid.

Gas constant, R The gas constant is the ratio of the product of pressure and volume to the product of the absolute temperature and the amount of substance for an ideal gas. $R = 8.314\,JK^{-1}\,mol^{-1}$.

General acid or base catalysis Acid or base catalysis in solution is general when catalysis is observed from species other than the ions formed from the solvent itself, e.g. those from an added buffer.

Gibbs free energy, G The Gibbs free energy is related to the maximum amount of non-expansion work that a system can do and it is measured in J mol^{-1}. Spontaneous processes are able to do work and the associated free energy change, ΔG, is less than zero.

Glidant A glidant is a substance added to a powder to improve its flow properties.

Graham's Law Graham's Law states that the rate of diffusion of a gas is inversely proportional to the square root of its density.

Granules Granules are formed when fine powder particles adhere together to form larger aggregates, a process called granulation.

Half maximal inhibitory concentration (IC_{50}) The half maximal inhibitory concentration is the concentration of a specified API needed to inhibit a particular biological process (e.g. an enzymatic reaction) by half.

Half-life, $t_{½}$ The drug half-life is the period of time required for the concentration of an API to be reduced by one-half. This may be used to express drug stability prior to administration or when the API is dissolved in a physiological fluid.

Heat, q Heat is the amount of energy flowing from one object or substance to another due to a difference in temperature and through chaotic molecular motion.

Heat capacity, C_p The heat capacity of a substance is a measure of how much heat a substance must absorb in order to bring about temperature rise of 1 K at constant pressure. It has units of J K^{-1}.

Henry's Law Henry's Law predicts a proportionate relationship between gas solubility and external pressure.

High-throughput screening (HTS) High-throughput screening is the scanning of huge numbers of candidate compounds in order to identify a compound or group of compounds which appear to be of use as a drug substance.

Hydrate The term hydrate is used to indicate that water is contained in a crystal structure.

Hydroethanolic A hydroethanolic solvent is a mixture of water and ethanol.

Hydrophilic A hydrophilic material has an affinity for polar media, such as water.

Hydrophobic A hydrophobic material has negligible affinity for polar media. It includes materials that have an affinity for non-polar media, such as oil.

Hydrophobicity Hydrophobicity is a physicochemical property that expresses a substances affinity for non-polar media, such as oil.

Hydrostatic pressure Hydrostatic pressure is the pressure exerted by a fluid due to the force of gravity. For liquids, hydrostatic pressure is directly proportional to the height of liquid.

Hygroscopic A hygroscopic substance is one that can absorb moisture from the surrounding environment.

Hyperdiscriminating A hyperdiscriminating solvent is less polar than octanol and, when used with water, can normally be used to distinguish between the partition coefficients of a series of structurally analogous compounds.

Hypodiscriminating A hypodiscriminating solvent is more polar than octanol and, when used with water, cannot normally be used to distinguish between the partition coefficients of a series of structurally analogous compounds.

Hypoxia Hypoxia is a condition in which the body, or part of it, is deprived of an adequate oxygen supply.

Ideal gases An ideal gas is a theoretical model in which the particles of gas occupy negligible volume, exert no forces on each other, and experience elastic collisions with each other and the walls of the container. The physical properties of ideal gases conform to the ideal gas equation.

Ideal solution An ideal solution is one in which the energies of interaction between all component particles, including those of the solute and solvent, are equivalent.

Immediate-release In an immediate-release tablet the API is released rapidly after administration.

Immiscible Immiscible liquids do not form a homogenous mixture upon mixing or shaking. Instead, the liquid components separate into distinct layers.

Implants Implants are solid dosage forms that are delivered parenterally, often subcutaneously, and are designed to release an API over an extended period.

In vitro *In vitro* refers to the study of the isolated components of an organism, e.g. cells, typically within a laboratory environment in order to closely model the *in vivo* scenario.

In vivo *In vivo* refers to study in a living organism.

Inductive effect The inductive effect is the transmission of electronic charge through the sigma bonds of a molecule.

Internal energy, U Internal energy is a state function that is the sum of kinetic and potential energy contained in a substance, measured in J mol^{-1}.

Intravenous (IV) A medicine administered through intravenous delivery is injected directly into a vein.

Ionic product of water, K_W The Ionic product of water is obtained by multiplying the molar concentrations of protons and hydroxide ions in an aqueous solution. $K_W = [H^+][OH^-]$.

Ionic strength, I The ionic strength of a solution is a measure of both the molar ion concentrations and the magnitude of the charges of all ions present.

Isobar An isobar is a function that defines a region of constant pressure.

Isolated system An isolated system cannot exchange matter or heat with the surroundings.

Isopleth An isopleth is a function that defines a region of constant composition.

Isotherm An isotherm is a function that defines a region of constant temperature.

Isotonic An isotonic solution is one that contains the same effective concentration of dissolved solutes as the physiological fluid of interest.

Kinematic viscosity, v Kinematic viscosity is the ratio of a liquid's dynamic viscosity to its density.

Kinetic energy Kinetic energy is the energy associated with movement.

Kinetic theory Kinetic theory states that the particles that make up solids, liquids and gases are in constant, random motion.

Lamellar flow Lamellar flow is where a fluid flows in parallel layers in the same direction, with no fluid movement perpendicular to the direction of flow.

Le Chatelier's principle Le Chatelier's principle states that a system at equilibrium experiencing a change will respond to counteract the imposed change.

Lead compound During drug development, the lead compound is selected following screening and is the compound that looks the most promising for development.

Lewis acid A Lewis acid is an electron pair acceptor.

Lewis base A Lewis base is an electron pair donor.

Lipophilic A lipophilic material has an affinity for non-polar media, such as oil.

Lipophobic A lipophobic material has no affinity for non-polar media, such as oil.

Liquidus The liquidus is a line on a phase diagram that can be used to determine the composition of the liquid phase at a particular composition and temperature.

Local action Local action is where a medical condition is addressed by a drug whose biological target is close to the site of application.

Local delivery Local delivery is where the biological target of a drug is located at the site of administration.

Log *D* Log D is the common logarithm of the distribution coefficient, being the ratio of the concentration of a chemical species (regardless of its chemical form) in two identified phases, e.g. octanol–water.

Log *P* Log P is the common logarithm of the partition coefficient, being the ratio of the concentration of a unique chemical species in two identified phases, e.g. octanol–water.

Lozenges Lozenges are designed to dissolve or disintegrate slowly in the mouth.

Lyophilization Lyophilization, or freeze-drying, is where a material is frozen before the external pressure is reduced so that ice sublimates, carrying water out of the sample.

Melting point, T_m The normal melting point is the temperature at which the solid and liquid phases of a substance are in equilibrium at an external pressure of 1 atm.

Meniscus The meniscus is the curved surface produced at the upper surface of a liquid when in a capillary. It is either concave or convex.

Mesomeric effect The mesomeric effect is the transmission of electronic charge by delocalized electrons through the overlapping p orbitals of a molecule, such as those within conjugated π bonds.

Metastable Metastable systems are those with a state of apparent equilibrium that are nevertheless capable of changing to a more thermodynamically stable state.

Micelle A micelle is a colloidal particle formed through self-assembly.

Milling Milling includes any methods where there is an input force to a particle system that results in a reduction of the particle size.

Miscibility Miscibility is the capacity of one liquid to dissolve in another liquid.

Miscible Miscible liquids will form a homogenous mixture upon mixing or shaking.

Modified-release (MR) In a modified-release or sustained-release tablet the API is released slowly over time. This has advantages over immediate-release formulations because MR dosage forms can be taken less frequently and maintain a steadier concentration of the API in the bloodstream.

Molecularity Molecularity is the number of reactant particles involved in an elementary step of a chemical reaction.

Mole fraction, x The mole fraction of a component in a mixture is the fraction of the total number of moles that the component contributes to the mixture.

Monodisperse Monodisperse describes dispersions where the dispersed domains are of uniform size throughout the system.

Monolayer A monolayer is a film (e.g. of gas) that has a thickness of one molecule.

Monoprotic acids Monoprotic acids possess one hydrogen atom that can be donated by each molecule.

Monotropic Monotropic systems are those where one polymorph is the most stable, regardless of conditions. Over time, other polymorphs will irreversibly transform into the most stable form.

Mouth-feel The mouth-feel is the tactile sensation of a substance placed in the mouth.

Mucous membranes The mucous membranes are moist, mucus-secreting tissues that line the entrances to the body.

Multilayer A multilayer is a film (e.g. of gas) that has a thickness of more than one molecule.

Nebulizers Nebulizers use high velocity gas flows or ultrasound to generate mists that can be used to delivery an API to the respiratory system.

Neutral solution A neutral solution is one in which $[H_3O^+] = [OH^-]$. At 25 °C, the pH of a neutral solution is 7.0.

New chemical entity (NCE) The term new chemical entity is generally used to describe novel pharmacologically active substances that may ultimately form the API of a commercially available medicine.

Newtonian Newtonian fluids obey the relationship where the rate of flow is directly proportional to the applied stress.

Non-Newtonian Non-Newtonian fluids exhibit a non-linear relationship between the rate of flow and the applied stress.

Non-polar solvents Non-polar solvents are composed of molecules with minimal charge separation. They have the ability to dissolve non-polar materials.

Non-terminal sterilization In non-terminal sterilization, the dosage from and container are sterilized separately and brought together in the final form in a sterile environment during aseptic preparation.

Open system An open system can exchange heat and matter with the surroundings.

Ophthalmic Ophthalmic formulations are administered to the eye.

Orally disintegrating An orally disintegrating or orodispersible tablet is one that disintegrates rapidly in the mouth and may be taken without the need for water.

Osmolarity The osmolarity of a solution is the effective molarity of a solute in a solution that contributes to the osmotic pressure. It has units of osmol L^{-1}.

Osmole The osmole is a measure of an amount of substance. It equals the effective number of solute particles, in moles, that contribute to osmotic pressure. It has units of osmol.

Osmosis Osmosis describes the spontaneous passage of solvent into a solution separated from it by a semipermeable membrane

Osmotic pressure, Π Osmotic pressure is the additional pressure that must be applied to a solution to stop osmosis.

Ostwald ripening Ostwald ripening occurs in polydisperse systems where two domains of the dispersed phase combine to yield a larger and smaller domain. Eventually, small domains become so small that they dissolve in the continuous phase.

Otic Otic formulations are administered to the ear.

Parenteral delivery Parenteral delivery is a route of administration that involves the piercing the skin or mucous membranes.

Parenteral formulation A parenteral formulation is a medicine intended for parenteral delivery, i.e. via piercing of the skin or mucous membranes.

Partition coefficient, P The partition coefficient is the ratio of the concentration of a unique chemical species in two identified phases, e.g. octanol and water.

Partitioning Partitioning occurs when an API distributes itself, or 'partitions', between two phases. The two phases may be two immiscible liquids at equilibrium.

Passive diffusion Passive diffusion is where a substance moves across a cell membrane due to the associated concentration gradient. It does not require cellular energy.

Path function A path function is a physical quantity that depends on the path taken to reach one state from another.

Patient compliance Patient compliance is a measure of whether a patient takes a medication as intended. This means the correct number of doses, at the correct time and in the correct manner, including the correct deployment of medical devices such as inhalers and syringes. It may also be referred to as patient adherence, concordance, or capacitance.

Permeability Permeability measures a compound's ability to pass through a defined barrier e.g. an API through a biological membrane.

Pessary A pessary is a small plastic or silicone suppository used to deliver APIs that are readily absorbed via the rectum or vagina.

pH The pH scale is used to indicate the relative acidity or alkalinity of a solution; typically solutions have a range of pH 0 to 14.

Pharmaceutical care Pharmaceutical care is a term used to describe the responsible provision of medicines that are intended to improve a patient's quality of life.

Pharmacodynamics (PD) Pharmacodynamics is the study of the interaction of APIs with target receptors.

Pharmacokinetics (PK) Pharmacokinetics is a branch of pharmacology that studies the fate of substances, including APIs, after administration.

Pharmacology Pharmacology is the study of the biochemical and/or physiological effect of drugs within organisms.

Pharmacophores Pharmacophores are the structural aspect of a molecule that results in biological activity.

Pharmacopoeiae Pharmacopoeiae contain monographs that describe drug substances, their associated formulations, and the required quality of these formulations according to local regulatory requirements e.g. the British Pharmacopoeia (BP).

Phase transition A phase transition occurs when one or more phases change physically and/or chemically to produce a new phase or phases.

Phase A phase is a form of matter that is uniform throughout in both its physical state and chemical composition.

Photosensitive Chemicals that react and/or degrade in the presence of light.

pH-partition hypothesis The pH-partition hypothesis states that weakly acidic APIs will be preferentially absorbed in acidic regions of the gastrointestinal tract, while weakly basic APIs will be preferentially absorbed in alkaline regions.

Physisorption Physisorption, or physical adsorption, is reversible and involves weak van der Waals forces between the adsorbent and adsorbate that can lead to multilayer adsorption.

Physicochemical Physicochemical properties are those relating the physical and chemical behaviour of a compound.

Polar solvents Polar solvents are composed of molecules where there is charge separation, e.g. due to ionic charges or polar covalent bonds. They have the ability to dissolve other polar materials.

Polydisperse Polydisperse describes dispersions where the dispersed domains are of varying sizes throughout the system.

Polymorphism Polymorphism ('many forms') is the occurrence of different physical forms of the same material. In pharmaceutical terms solid materials may exist in different physical forms (polymorphs) which may have different physical properties, such as solubility and dissolution rates.

Polyprotic acids Polyprotic acids possess more than one hydrogen atom that can be donated by each molecule.

Potential energy Potential energy is the energy associated with position.

Powder A powder contains very fine particles that are not cemented together and will flow freely when shaken.

Powders for reconstitution Powders for reconstitution are solid sterile powders that must be mixed with liquid, normally water, before use.

Preformulation Preformulation is a stage of drug development that consists of the physicochemical profiling of a new chemical entity and its analytical characterization.

Pressurized metered dose inhaler (pMDI) A pressurized metered dose inhaler is a drug delivery device that is actuated mechanically by the user and releases the API in the dispersed liquid phase on an aerosol.

Protogenic Protogenic solvents can donate protons.

Protophilic Protophilic solvents can accept protons.

Pseudoplastic liquids Pseudoplastic liquids become less viscous as the rate of shear increases.

Pseudopolymorphs Pseudopolymorphs are solvated forms of a compound that differ in their crystal structures and/or the nature of the included solvent. They have different physical properties to the anhydrous form.

Quantitative structure-activity relationships (QSAR) A quantitative structure-activity relationship is a correlation between a molecule's structure and the biological activity that results from the presence of that structure.

Raoult's Law Raoult's Law states that the partial vapour pressure of a volatile solvent in a multicomponent closed system will directly proportional to the mole fraction of the solvent in the liquid phase.

Reaction step A reaction step is a unique elementary reaction that occurs during the conversion of reactants to products. The number of reactant particles involved in a specific step is referred to as the molecularity.

Real gases Real gases are those that exhibit properties that cannot be fully explained by the ideal gas law.

Receptor A receptor is a molecular structure that can bind to specific substances, such as APIs and hormones, bringing about a specific physiological effect. The API is said to bind to the 'target receptor'.

Reduction (redox) potential The reduction, or redox, potential of a chemical is a measure of its tendency to acquire electrons and be reduced.

Respiratory tract The respiratory tract is that part of the human anatomy comprising the nasal passages, throat and lungs.

Reverse osmosis Reverse osmosis occurs when the pressure applied to a solution exceeds the osmotic pressure so that there is a net flow of solvent through the semipermeable membrane and out of the solution.

Reynolds number The Reynolds number is a unitless parameter that takes into account the properties of a fluid, and the dimensions of the tube through which it flows. It can be used to predict whether fluid flow will be laminar or turbulent.

Rheopectic liquid Rheopectic liquids become more viscous over time when a constant shear stress is applied.

Route of administration The route of administration of a medicine is the path by which it is taken into the body.

Saturated solution A saturated solution contains the maximum amount of material that can be dissolved under equilibrium conditions.

Sedimentation Sedimentation occurs when dense particles settle under the influence of gravity.

Semipermeable membrane A semipermeable membrane is one that is permeable to solvent molecules but not to solute particles.

Shear stress Shear stress is the force applied per unit area that results in deformation of a material along a plane or planes parallel to the applied force.

Shelf life The shelf life of a pharmaceutical product is the total period of time, from when the product is manufactured, to its expiry date. It is based on the chemical, physical, biological and microbiological stability of the product and is the period of time when the product can be safely used.

SI units SI units are an internationally agreed system of units for physical quantities.

Solidus The solidus is a line on a phase diagram that can be used to determine the composition of the solid phase at a particular composition and temperature.

Solubility The solubility of a substance is the maximum amount of material that can be dissolved at equilibrium.

Solvate The term solvate is used to describe crystalline solids where solvent molecules are contained within the crystal structure.

Specific acid or base catalysis Acid or base catalysis in solution is specific when the only catalytic effects observed are those due to the ions formed from the solvent itself, e.g. H^+ and OH^- for water.

Standard enthalpy of combustion, ΔH_c^θ The standard enthalpy of combustion is the enthalpy change when one mole of a reactant completely reacts with oxygen at 1 bar pressure and fixed temperature.

Standard enthalpy of formation, ΔH_f^θ The standard enthalpy of formation is the change in enthalpy that accompanies the formation of one mole of a compound from its elements in their standard state at 1 bar pressure and fixed temperature.

Standard enthalpy of fusion, ΔH_{fus}^θ The standard enthalpy of fusion is the enthalpy change which occurs when 1 mol of solid is converted to 1 mol of liquid at 1 bar pressure and fixed temperature.

Standard enthalpy of sublimation, ΔH_{sub}^θ The standard enthalpy of sublimation is the enthalpy change which occurs when 1 mol of pure solid is converted to 1 mol of vapour at 1 bar pressure and fixed temperature.

Standard enthalpy of vaporization, ΔH_{vap}^θ The standard enthalpy of vaporization is the enthalpy change which occurs when 1 mol of a pure liquid is converted to 1 mol of vapour at 1 bar pressure and fixed temperature.

Standard temperature and pressure (STP) Standard temperature and pressure is 273.15 K and 1 bar, respectively. This is equivalent to a temperature of 0 °C and a pressure of around 1 atmosphere.

State function A state function is a property of a system that depends only on the current state of the system, not on the path the system took to reach that state.

Stereogenic A stereogenic centre is an atom that has different groups bound to it such that its mirror image is non-superimposable. It is also known as chiral centre.

Strain Strain is deformation that arises as a result of shear stress. In fluids, strain can be measured as the change in velocity between layers in a liquid and it may therefore be also referred to as the shear rate.

Strong electrolytes Strong electrolytes are substances that completely ionize or dissociate into ions in solution.

Subcutaneous implant A subcutaneous implant is a solid medicine that is inserted under the surface of the skin and is normally designed to release an API over an extended period.

Sublimation Sublimation is the direct phase transition of a solid to a gas without passing through the liquid state.

Sublingual Sublingual delivery is when a dosage form absorbed through the oral mucosa, specifically under the tongue.

Supercritical fluid A supercritical fluid is a fluid that exists at temperatures and pressures where separate liquid and gas phases do not exist.

Supersaturated solution A supersaturated solution contains more dissolved material than can be dissolved under equilibrium conditions. It is a thermodynamically unstable system.

Suppositories Suppositories are solid dosage forms designed to melt or dissolve in the rectum, vagina or, less commonly, the urethra. They are used to delivery drugs both locally and systemically.

Surface area The extent of a two-dimensional surface enclosed within a boundary.

Surface tension, γ_{LV} The surface tension of a liquid is the contracting force that develops across a liquid-vapour (LV) interface per unit length of the interface's perimeter.

Surfactants Surfactants are surface active agents. They are amphiphilic molecules that have a hydrophilic 'head' and a hydrophobic 'tail'.

Surroundings The surroundings is the environment outside the system. Together, the system and surrounding make up the Universe.

Suspending agent A suspending agent is used with solid-in-liquid dispersions to stabilise suspensions and inhibit agglomeration.

Suspension A suspension consists of fine solid particles suspended in a liquid phase.

System The system is that part of the Universe in which we have a special interest e.g. a beaker of water.

Systemic action Systemic action is where a medical condition is addressed by a drug that is transported to the biological target by the body's circulatory system.

Systemic delivery Systemic delivery is where the body's circulatory system is used to transport an API from the site of administration to the biological target.

Terminal sterilization Terminal sterilization is process of sterilizing dosage forms and their containers with the dosage form within the container.

Thaw point The thaw point is the temperature at which a heated solid mixture is observed to start melting.

Therapeutic Index (TI) The therapeutic index is the ratio between the toxic dose and the therapeutic dose of an API. It is used as a measure of drug safety, APIs with high TIs being preferable.

Therapeutic window The therapeutic window of a drug is the range of dosages that can effectively address a medical condition without significant adverse effects.

Thermal contact Objects are in thermal contact if they can exchange energy with each other through heat flow.

Thermal equilibrium Thermal equilibrium occurs when two or more objects or substances in thermal contact have attained an equal temperature and there is no flow of heat between them.

Thermodynamics Thermodynamics is the study of energy changes in chemical processes. It considers the bulk energy of substances, rather than energies of individual atoms or molecules.

Thixotropic liquids Thixotropic liquids become less viscous over time when a constant shear stress is applied.

Tonicity Tonicity is a measure of the osmotic pressure gradient on either side of a semipermeable membrane, normally a cell membrane. This gradient may be negative, zero, or positive.

Topical application A topical application is a medicine applied to the external surfaces of the body, including the skin, mucous membranes and respiratory tract.

Topical delivery Topical delivery is where a medicine is applied to the external surfaces of the body, including the skin, mucous membranes and respiratory tract.

Transdermal patch A transdermal patch is an adhesive patch that is placed on the skin and delivers an API through the skin and into the bloodstream.

Triple point The triple point is the temperature and pressure at which all the phases of a pure substance; solid, liquid and vapour, can co-exist in equilibrium.

Turbulent flow Turbulent flow is chaotic and there is movement, or mixing, of fluids between adjacent layers.

Unit cell The unit cell is the simplest repeating structure in a crystal.

Vaporization Vaporization is the phase transition from the liquid phase to the gas phase.

Vaporus The vaporus is a line on a phase diagram that can be used to determine the composition of the vapour phase at a particular composition and temperature.

Vapour pressure The vapour pressure is the pressure of a vapour that is in thermodynamic equilibrium with its condensed phase in a closed system.

Vapour A vapour is the gaseous form of a substance that exists below the critical temperature. A vapour can be converted to a liquid by increasing the pressure.

Venturi tube A Venturi tube contains a constriction and a fluid will flow faster through the constriction. According to Bernoulli's equation, the fluid will have a lower pressure within the constriction and this is known as the Venturi effect.

Viscosity Viscosity is the measure of the resistance to flow of liquid under an applied force.

Water for injection Water for injection is a term used to describe sterile purified water that is reserved for the preparation of some aqueous medicines. It is used in the reconstitution of powders for parenteral administration.

Weak electrolytes Weak electrolytes are substances that only partially ionize or dissociate into ions in solution.

Wet granulation In wet granulation, the powder is mixed with a liquid, such as water or ethanol, to form a paste that can be processed to the yield the required granule size.

Wettability Wettability is a property of solids that describes the degree of wetting by a specified liquid. It can be estimated from the contact angle forming between the solid and liquid.

Work, w Work is the flow of energy from one body to another through uniform molecular motion. A system that does work is able to raise a weight.

Zeta potential, ζ The potential difference across phase boundaries between solids and liquids.

Zwitterion A zwitterion is a molecule that contains both positive and negative ionic charges.

Answers to self-check questions

Chapter 1

1.1

- It might be unstable and decompose before it is administered.
- It might be acidic and irritate the body.
- It might be so potent that some kind of dilution is essential before it can be administered safely.

1.2 For a drug with a high therapeutic index, the patient would have to take a much higher dose to reach the toxic level. Thus, drugs with a high therapeutic index lower the risk of adverse side effects.

1.3

1. B
2. D
3. A
4. C

1.4 An elderly patient may have difficulty swallowing tablets or have insufficient motor skills to use an inhaler.

1.5 There are 1 million cm^3 in 1 m^3. Thus, $1 \times 10^6\,cm^3 = 1\,m^3$.

A cube with dimensions $1\,m \times 1\,m \times 1\,m$ will have a volume of $1\,m^3$

The dimensions of the cube can also be expressed in cm, where 100 cm = 1 m. Thus, we can calculate the volume as:

$$1\ m^3 = 100\ cm \times 100\ cm \times 100\ cm = 1 \times 10^6\ cm^3$$

1.6

$$1\ g = 1 \times 10^{-3}\ kg \text{ so } 81.25\ g = 81.25 \times 10^{-3}\ kg = 0.08125\ kg$$

$$1\ g = 1 \times 10^{3}\ mg \text{ so } 81.25\ g = 81.25 \times 10^{3}\ mg = 81250\ mg$$

Chapter 2

2.1 (c) Definite colour.

2.2 (d) The molecules lose freedom.

2.3 Any four from: cubic, tetragonal, orthorhombic, hexagonal, trigonal (rhombohedral), triclinic, and monoclinic.

2.4 (a) A is actually the more stable polymorph.

2.5 0.79.

2.6 Mix the powder with a little water and stir before drinking.

Look up the Summary of Product Characteristics (SPC) for Beechams Powders and find the list of other excipients. Identify the likely main role for each of these in the formulation.

- Lactose-diluent
- Maize starch (dried)-disintegrant
- Colloidal anhydrous silica-anti-caking agent, glidant
- sodium lauryl sulphate-wetting agent
- saccharin sodium-sweetener
- spice flavour blend 17.42.5890-flavour

2.7 Sugar coated, film coated, gelatin coated, enteric coated.

2.8 Diffusion-controlled, dissolution-controlled, osmotic pump.

Chapter 3

3.1

(a) Two types of forces associated with molecules within a liquid are van der Waals interactions and hydrogen bonds.

(b) (i) Molecules within the liquid lock into very specific order, the bonds between them become rigid and the liquid undergoes a phase change into a solid. (ii) The cohesive forces that bind the liquid molecules closely together break and the liquid undergoes a phase change to a gas.

3.2

(a) 0.025 L

(b) 0.250 L

(c) 2.5 L

3.3

$$\rho = m/V \text{ rearranges to give } V = m/\rho$$

$$V = m/\rho = 27\ g / 1.35\ g\ cm^{-3} = 20\ cm^3$$

3.4 A Newtonian liquid has a linear relationship between shear stress and strain and therefore maintains the same dynamic viscosity regardless of what forces are applied to it. A non-Newtonian liquid has a non-linear relationship between sheer stress and strain and therefore has a viscosity which changes depending on the force applied to it.

3.5 First, the values for density and dynamic viscosity must be converted into comparable units:

$$\rho = 1.5\ g\ cm^{-3} = 1500\ kg\ m^{-3}$$

$$\eta = 2.3\,cP = 0.0023\,kg\,m\,s^{-1}$$

$$v = \eta/\rho = 0.0023\ kg\ m^{-1}\ s^{-1}/1500\ kg\ m^{-3} = 1.53 \times 10^{-6}\,m^2\,s^{-1}$$

3.6

(a) $C = \nu/t = 2\,mm^2\,s^{-1} / 300\,s = 0.0067\,mm^2\,s^{-2}$.

(b) $\nu = Ct = 0.0067\,mm^2\,s^{-2} \times 450\,s = 3\,mm^2\,s^{-1}$.

3.7

(a) $F = 1 - (2.1\ (d/D)) = 1 - (2.1(0.2/4)) = 0.895$.

(b) First, calculate the terminal velocity. $u = s/t = 15\text{ cm}/30\text{ s} = 0.5\text{ cm s}^{-1}$.

All units are now expressed in g, cm and s, so no conversion is necessary before we calculate v.

$$v = [d^2 g\ (\rho_s - \rho_l)\ F]/[0.18\ u\rho_l]$$

$$= (0.2^2 \times 981 \times (8 - 1.4) \times 0.895)/(0.18 \times 0.5 \times 1.4)$$

$$v = 1840\ \text{cm}^2\text{s}^{-1}$$

3.8 A 0.9 %w/v sodium chloride solution contains 0.9 g of NaCl in 100 mL (0.1 dm³). The number of moles, n, can be calculated from the relative molecular mass.

$$n = 0.9/58.5 = 0.015\ \text{mol}$$

The concentration of sodium chloride is then given by:

$$[S] = n/V = 0.15/0.1 = 0.15\ \text{M}$$

3.9 The solubility of drug A is 50 mg mL^{-1}.

The solubility of B is 500 g L^{-1} which is equivalent to 500 mg mL^{-1}.

The solubility of drug C is 500 µg mL^{-1} which is equivalent to 0.5 mg mL^{-1}.

Therefore, the drugs in order of decreasing solubility is B>A>C.

3.10

(a) Methyl paraben.

(b) Sodium saccharin.

(c) Methyl cellulose.

(d) Ethanol.

(e) Sodium metabisulphite.

3.11 Parenteral and ocular routes require solutions to be sterile

Chapter 4

4.1 A: The pressure of the gas will quadruple as volume and pressure are inversely related.

4.2

$$V = nRT/p$$

At STP,

$$T = 273.15\ \text{K}$$

$$p = 100\ 000\ \text{Pa}$$

Thus,

$$V = 2.60 \times 10^{-2} \times 8.314 \times 273.15/100\ 000 = 5.90 \times 10^{-4}\ \text{m}^3$$

$$1\ \text{m}^3 = 1\ \text{m} \times 1\ \text{m} \times 1\ \text{m} = 100\ \text{cm} \times 100\ \text{cm} \times 100\ \text{cm}$$

$$= 1 \times 10^6\ \text{cm}^3$$

It follows that:

$$V = 590\ \text{cm}^3$$

4.3 A: Using Raoult's law: $p = x_A p_A^* = 0.680 \times 46.1 = 31.3\ \text{kPa}$

This is slightly higher than the experimentally recorded value, 27.1 kPa, and so this system does not precisely conform to Raoult's law. We can conclude that molecules of acetone in this system are less likely to enter the vapour phase than would be expected on the basis of ideal behaviour.

4.4 A vacuum pump is used to reduce pressure so that frozen solvent sublimes directly to the gas phase. At normal atmospheric pressure, many solvents transform from the solid to gas phase through the liquid state.

4.5 The storage temperature is less than the pseudocritical temperature and the nitrous oxide in the mixture can liquefy. Warming before use ensures that a mixture of 50% N_2O and 50% oxygen is provided to the patient.

4.6 In a pressurized metered dose inhaler (pMDI) the API is present in a liquid dispersed phase of an aerosol, either as a solution or suspension. The device is mechanically actuated by the user.

In a dry powder inhaler (PDI), the API is present as fine solid particles within a gaseous continuous phase. The device is breath actuated.

Chapter 5

5.1 Temperature is how we perceive the thermal motion of the atoms in a substance; heat is a flow of energy from one substance to another.

5.2 To convert a temperature from kelvin to degrees Celsius, subtract 273.15.

5.3 A path function has a value that depends on the path taken between two states. Work (w) and heat (q) are examples of path functions.

5.4 The standard enthalpy of fusion is the enthalpy change that occurs when 1 mol of solid is converted to 1 mol of liquid at 1 bar pressure and constant temperature.

5.5 Hess's Law states that if a reaction takes place in a series of steps, the overall enthalpy change is the same as if it takes place in one chemical step. Hess's Law allows us to determine enthalpy changes for reactions which cannot be measured directly.

5.6 The Second Law of Thermodynamics states that the entropy of an isolated system increases during spontaneous change.

5.7 Entropy is a measure of disorder.

5.8 $\Delta G^\theta < 0$

5.9 Expansion work, electrical work, osmotic pressure work and surface tension work.

5.10 By using the equation

$$T = -\left(\frac{\Delta H^\theta}{\Delta S^\theta}\right)$$

we can determine the temperature at which $\Delta G^\theta = 0$. This is the temperature at which the reaction will become spontaneous.

5.11 $\Delta G = 0$

Chapter 6

6.1 The equilibrium lies to the right.

6.2 Acid strength depends on the nature of the acid and the equilibrium position for electrolytic dissociation. This is not dependent on concentration.

6.3 Trifluoroacetic acid, because flourine is a stronger electron-withdrawing group than hydrogen.

6.4 pH=7.47.

6.5 pH=1.70.

6.6 Concentration of H_3O^+ ions=1.6×10^{-4} mol dm^{-3}.

6.7 pH=5.7.

6.8 0.79% aspirin would be ionized.

6.9 1.2% morphine remains unionized.

6.10 The isoelectric point=5.98.

6.11 pH=−log (0.008)=2.1. The pH therefore changes by 4.9 units.

6.12 [acetate]=0.015/0.1=0.15 M.

$C=0.1+0.15=0.25$.

$\beta_{max}=0.144$ mols L^{-1} pH unit^{-1}.

Chapter 7

7.1 Define the terms phase and phase transition.

A phase is a form of matter that is uniform throughout in both its physical state and chemical composition. A phase transition occurs when one or more phases change physically and/or chemically to produce a new phase or phases.

7.2 Briefly define vaporization and melting. In each case, give one example of a dosage form that relies on these phase transitions.

- Vaporization – solid to vapour phase transition. This is important in medicines such as chest rubs.
- Melting – solid to liquid phase transition. This is important in medicines applied topically to the skin and those taken as suppositories.

7.3 State the phase rule, clearly outlining the meaning of each term.

- For a closed system the phase rule is: $F=C-P+2$.
- F=the number of degrees of freedom.
- C=the number of chemical components.
- P=the number of phases in the system.

7.4 Define the terms critical temperature and critical pressure.

- In a closed system the critical temperature is the temperature at which the density of the liquid and density of the vapour are equal.
- The pressure at the density of the liquid and the density of the vapour are equal is known as the critical pressure.

7.5

- The triple point is the point on a temperature-pressure phase diagram at which all three phase (solid, liquid and vapour) co-exist.

How many degrees of freedom are there at the triple point for water?

- At the triple point there are three phases present (solid, liquid and vapour) $\therefore P=3$.
- The system only contains a single component (water) $\therefore C=1$.
- Using the phase rule: $F=C-P+2$.
- $F=1-3+2=0$.

What does this mean in terms of the allowed temperature and pressure values at which the triple point can exist?

Recall that in a single component phase diagram there are two independent factors that can be varied – temperature and pressure (represented by the variables on the axis in Figure 7.4). Given that the phase rule indicates there to be zero degrees of freedom at the triple point this means that it exist only at a single temperature and pressure value. If either the temperature or the pressure was altered then the equilibrium between the three phases that exists at the triple point to be disrupted. This would result in at least one of the phases undergoing a phase transition resulting in a maximum of only two phases existing at the new temperature and/or pressure.

7.6

- The liquidus is the line in a binary phase diagram that defines the temperature boundary above which there is a single liquid phase.
- The solidus is the line in a binary phase diagram that defines the temperature boundary below which there is a single solid phase.

7.7

- This region contains both solid and liquid phases.

7.8

- The eutectic point is the lowest melting point for a binary system. Mixtures with this composition are useful in pharmaceutical formulations because of their improved melting and dissolution behaviour.

7.9 At the point 2, the phase diagram shows that the phases present are liquid and solid B. The liquid has a composition of 82% (w/w) B and the solid has a composition 100% (w/w) B.

The lever rule gives the proportion of each phase:

%Soild=YZ/YB×100=(100–93)/(100–82)×100=39%.

%Liquid=ZB/YB×100=(93–82)/(100–82)×100=61%.

7.10 State the composition of the mixtures represented by points 2, 3 and 4 in Figure 7.16.

Point 2: 70% (w/w) A, 20% (w/w) B, 10% (w/w) C.

Point 3: 40% (w/w) A, 30% (w/w) B, 30% (w/w) C.

Point 4: 0% (w/w) A, 80% (w/w) B, 20% (w/w) C.

Chapter 8

8.1 Water molecules structure themselves around suspended globules in order to preserve local hydrogen bonding, and this arrangement has correspondingly low entropy. Coalescence reduces the interfacial area of the globules, liberating water molecules. Liberated water molecules in the bulk solvent have greater freedom and higher entropy. Coalescence therefore has a positive entropy change.

8.2

$$P = C_o/C_w = 66/21 = 3.14$$

$$\log P = 0.50$$

8.3 The log P is zero so caffeine is neither hydrophobic nor hydrophilic, relative to this octanol-water system.

8.4 D will increase. Increasing pH lowers the concentration of H^+. According to Le Chatelier's principle, the base ionization equilibrium will shift to the left, favouring the formation of B over BH^+. B is unionized and is able to enter the organic phase, causing D to increase.

8.5

$$P = 1/\text{intercept} = 1.0 \times 10^2$$

$$K_a = \text{gradient/intercept} = 1 \times 10^{-3}\ \text{M}$$

8.6 The chemical potential of the solute in the two phases is not the same so this system is not at equilibrium and it will spontaneously change over time. The chemical potentials of the solute in the aqueous and organic phases need to decrease and increase, respectively, if they are to become equal. As chemical potential depends on mole fraction, this can be achieved if there is a net movement of solute from the aqueous to organic phase.

8.7 1.27. The experimental value of log P is always preferred over the calculated value. The latter is only generally used when the former is not available. For compounds that have been studied extensively, log P and Clog P are often very similar. For new classes of compounds with little existing experimental data, log P and Clog P may be different.

8.8 Less than 0.32. A hypodiscriminating solvent is less able to discriminate between structurally similar solutes when compared to octanol.

8.9 An API dissolving in aqueous physiological fluids is the first stage of drug delivery. An API with a log P greater than 5 is highly hydrophobic and would be expected to have limited aqueous solubility. Moreover, once absorbed by a lipophilic cell membrane, an hydrophobic API is unlikely to partition back out and reach its intended target.

8.10 The free base form of fentanyl is unionized and is sufficiently lipophilic to partition into the hydrophobic barrier presented by the skin. The citrate salt of fentanyl is highly water-soluble and will readily dissolve in aqueous physiological fluids, being the first step before absorption can occur.

Chapter 9

9.1 Surface free energy is the energy required to increase the surface area of the boundary layer by one metre squared. It arises because the formation of a surface always requires that work is done ($\Delta G > 0$).

9.2 Surface tension arises because molecules at the boundary do not have like molecules on all sides of them. Consequently, they form stronger attractive cohesive forces with molecules below and adjacent to them. This enhancement of attractive forces at the surface is termed surface tension.

9.3 Interfacial tension is similar to surface tension, but exists at the boundary between two immiscible liquids to resist mixing.

9.4 C. A material with good wettability should have a small contact angle with water as the interfacial tension at the solid-liquid interface is then decreased so that wetting of the hydrophobic drug would be easier.

9.5 The spreading coefficient, S, must be equal to or greater than zero and is dependent on the surface tension of water being greater than the sum of the surface tension of the oleic acid and the interfacial tension between the two liquids.

9.6

$$S = \gamma_{SV} - \gamma_{LV} - \gamma_{SL}$$

Therefore

$$S = 72.8 - 28.9 - 35.0 = 8.9\ \text{dyn cm}^{-1}$$

Spreading will occur as $S > 0$.

9.7

$$S = \gamma_{SV} - \gamma_{LV} - \gamma_{SL}$$

$$S = 62.2 - 28.8 - 35.0 = -1.6\ \text{dyn cm}^{-1}$$

No further spreading occurs after equilibrium as $S < 0$.

9.8 **Adsorption** refers to the process of molecules binding to the surface of solids and liquids. **Absorption** refers to a molecule penetrating in to the bulk of the absorbing medium, such as water being absorbed by a sponge.

9.9 Physisorption is a reversible process utilizing weak van der Waals forces and can lead to multilayer adsorption. Chemisorption involves the formation of strong covalent or ionic bonds formed and only monolayer adsorption occurs.

9.10 The electric potential around a particles decreases with increasing distance from the surface. The electrical double layer surrounding a particle in a liquid is composed of two parts, a dense layer near the particle surface (Stern layer) and a diffuse layer away from it (Gouy–Chapman layer).

9.11 ΓMax is the maximum concentration of surfactants on the surface of a liquid while CMC is the critical concentration at which micelles begin to form. Upon increasing the concentration of surfactants in a liquid, they arrange themselves on the surface until it becomes saturated, at ΓMax, *before* the CMC is reached and they start forming micelles.

9.12 We must convert all units to SI before calculation.

Diameter of tube $= 0.2\ \text{mm} = 0.2 \times 10^{-3}\ \text{m}$

Therefore, $r = 0.1 \times 10^{-3}$ m.

$h = 3.42\ \text{cm} = 3.42 \times 10^{-2}$ m.

$\rho = 0.7914\ \text{g cm}^{-3} = 0.7914 \times 10^6\ \text{g m}^{-3} = 0.7914 \times 10^3\ \text{kg m}^{-3}$.

$$\gamma = \frac{\rho r h g}{2}$$

$\gamma = 0.7914 \times 10^3 \times 0.1 \times 10^{-3} \times 3.42 \times 10^{-2} \times 9.81/2.$

$\gamma = 13.3\ \text{mN m}^{-1}.$

9.13 Capillary action occurs when the adhesive forces between the liquid molecules and the walls of the tube are stronger than the cohesive forces between the liquid molecules. This leads to the liquid wetting the inside surface of the tube, spreading over it and causing the liquid to rise.

9.14 Mercury forms a convex meniscus in a glass capillary because the liquid does not wet the inside of the tube. The adhesive forces between liquid and the walls of the tube are weaker than the cohesive forces between the liquid molecules.

9.15 The correction factor is determined by analysing a sample with a known surface tension.

Chapter 10

10.1 (d) This is a polydisperse system as the particles range in size. It is a colloidal system because the particles size is in the range 1–1000 nm.

10.2 This is most likely a coarse dispersion as it has limited physical stability and can be separated by a filter.

10.3 If it existed, a gaseous coarse dispersion would consist of domains made up of one gaseous component, dispersed throughout another gaseous component. Intermolecular forces between gas particles are weak and would be unable to hold the domains together. This dispersion would spontaneously convert through diffusion into a homogenous gas solution of uniform concentration throughout. The driving force for this process would be the associated increase in entropy.

10.4 (a) emulsion, (b) microemulsion, (c) nanoemulsion.

10.5

$$r = 10\,\text{nm} = 10 \times 10^{-9}\ \text{m}$$

$$A_{\text{surface}} = 4\pi r^2 = 4 \times 3.14 \times (10 \times 10^{-9})^2 = 1.3 \times 10^{-15}\ \text{m}^2$$

$$V = 4/3\pi r^3 = 4.2 \times 10^{-24}\ \text{m}^3$$

10.6 Flocculation is where two or more domains cluster together without losing their individual identity. In coalescence, the domains join together so that their individual identity is lost.

10.7 Milk of magnesia is a suspension and is therefore not thermodynamically stable. Suspended particles may flocculate over time but this can be reversed by shaking, where work is done on the system, raising the free energy.

10.8 Benzocaine is the API and is a local anaesthetic. Pentane is a propellant and is a slower evaporating gas that will provide a cooling effect that would sooth burns.

10.9 Foams are more easily spread than creams. This is of considerable benefit when treating large areas of hairy and inflamed skin. Compared to a cream, there is reduced need to apply pressure or maintain prolonged contact.

10.10 DLVO theory predicts a secondary minimum. At this particle separation, dispersed domains may form stable associations and this is observed as flocculation. The attraction between domains at this interparticle separation is predicted to be weak and can be overcome by shaking.

Chapter 11

11.1 Lowering of vapour pressure, lowering of melting point, raising of boiling point, osmotic pressure.

11.2 Solvent molecules in a solution are more thermodynamically stable than those in the pure solvent as solutions have a higher entropy.

11.3 $i = 0.5$. A solution formed from two moles of the organic compound would contain one mole of dimer particles in solution. Thus, the van't Hoff factor is one divided by two.

11.4

$$\Pi = 1000i[\text{S}]RT = 1000 \times 2 \times 0.07 \times 8.314 \times 298 = 347\ \text{kPa}$$

NaOH has the same van't Hoff factor and is therefore predicted to have the same osmotic pressure at 298 K.

11.5 An isotonic solution is one that has an osmolarity that is the same as that of the cytosol under investigation. A hypertonic solution is one that has a greater osmolarity than the cytosol. A hypotonic solution is one having a lower osmolarity than the cytosol.

11.6 Standard saline is composed of both sodium and chloride ions in solution so the van't Hoff factor, $i = 2$. On this basis, the osmolarity of 0.15 M NaCl(aq) will be 0.3 osmol L^{-1}. This is isotonic with body fluids.

11.7

(a) Yes, if not imbibed in vast quantities.

(b) Yes, but normally only as a treatment for corneal edema.

(c) Yes, within limits and only if administered slowly.

(d) Yes, the skin can be safely exposed to both hypertonic (and hypertonic) solutions.

11.8 Glycerol will increase the viscosity of the eye drops and this may mean they are difficult to administer and uncomfortable to use.

11.9 In osmotic pump tablets, the API is release with zero-order kinetics (constant rate) for a greater proportion of tablet lifetime. The reliance on osmosis also minimizes patient-to-patient variability in the rate of delivery.

11.10 It ensures that the hypertonic solution within the engine is always saturated and, therefore, of constant concentration. This, in turn, ensures that the osmotic pressure on the piston and the rate of delivery of API is constant also.

11.11

$$\mu_{\text{H2O(l)}} - \mu^{\theta}_{\text{H2O(l)}} = -RTx_S$$

The left hand-side of this equation represents the drop in the chemical potential of water molecules on the formation, from pure water, of a solution with a mole fraction of solute, x_S.

11.12 The salt depresses the melting point of water. If this drops below the ambient temperature then the ice will melt, reducing the risk of accidents.

Chapter 12

12.1 (c) specific base catalysis.

The reaction rate depends on pH, not buffer concentration, so this is an example of specific catalysis. Rate increases as the buffers become more alkaline and this indicates base catalysis.

12.2 Hydrocortisone acetate is the API. Sodium metabisulphite is a reducing agent that inhibits oxidation and enhances stability of the formulation.

12.3 Acetone is involved in the rate determining step of this reaction that determines the overall rate. Iodine is not involved in the rate determining step.

12.4 Rate$=k[A]^2$ A linear plot of 1/[A] versus time is consistent with second-order kinetics. The rate law cannot be $v=k[A][B]$ as 1/[A] versus t would only give a straight line if the starting concentrations of A and B were the same.

12.5 Reactant particles must have the correct orientation upon collision and must meet the energy requirement (activation energy) for reaction to occur.

12.6 The production of gas helps to break up the tablet and increase the exposed surface area, increasing the rate of dissolution.

12.7 Catalase is an enzyme that catalyses the decomposition of hydrogen peroxide. The enzyme's catalytic activity relies on its structure. As temperature increases, the enzyme denatures meaning that key structural elements are lost.

12.8 The slope of an Arrhenius plot is proportional to $-E_a$, where E_a is the activation energy. As activation energies are always positive, it follows that Arrhenius plots will always have a negative slope.

Chapter 13

13.1 High-throughput screening is used to rapidly check large numbers of candidate compounds in order to identify the most suitable group of compounds to take into production.

13.2 A pharmacophore is the area of a drug's structure which is responsible for the molecule's biological activity.

13.3 QSAR stands for Quantitative Structure-Activity Relationships and log P is a physicochemical descriptor for lipophilicity.

13.4 The three components of a QSAR model are; (1) The data set for the biological activity, (2) Knowledge of the molecular structure and (3) A suitable statistical method. The quality of a QSAR model is limited by the quality and the amount of available experimental data.

13.5 Drug substance refers to the therapeutic candidate (active ingredient) and the finished dosage form (e.g. tablet, capsule, liquid) is the drug product.

13.6 The various studies carried out for drug profiling are solubility, pK_a, partition coefficient, stability and excipient compatibility. Analytical characterization involves assessing structure, purity and the development of assays for both qualitative and quantitative measurements.

13.7 Oral Liquid dosage forms are available in the form of Solutions, Suspensions and Emulsions. Oral solid dosage forms are available in the form of tablets and capsules.

13.8 (1) Oral, (2) Ocular, (3) Nasal, (4) Otic, (5) Vaginal, (6) Rectal, (7) Respiratory, (8) Topical, (9) Parenteral.

13.9 A suitable packaging form will;

- Protect the drug from damage as a result of mechanical stress such as during transport or if accidentally dropped.
- Prevent microbial infiltration of the product during transport and storage.
- Protect the product from physical factors such as light, moisture and oxygen to prevent the degradation of a formulation.
- Carry the relevant product information.

13.10 The general requirements for packaging of pharmaceutical products are listed in the pharmacopoeiae although the actual packaging requirements of each drug product will need thorough investigation.

13.11 Phase I pharmacological studies are aimed at providing the essential information on the tolerance, metabolism, interactions, pharmacokinetics and pharmacodynamics of a drug.

Phase II examines the effect of dosage and other therapeutic effect studies.

Phase III trials develop the safety profile for the drug at the same time as being used to reinforce the findings in the phase II trials.

Phase IV clinical trials investigate the effect of the drug over a range of patient segments as a means of identifying any unusual side effects which had not been previously seen in the trial process.

13.12 Single ascending dose studies (SAD), multiple ascending dose studies (MAD) and food effect studies are the three categories for phase I clinical trials.

SAD studies involve the administration of a single dose of the medication to a small subject group whom are then observed for their response over a period of time. So long as the group does not show signs of any side effects and also that the group responds to the medication in the expected manor as predicted by the pharmokinetic data, the dose is then increased and this higher dose is given to a separate group of subjects. This process is repeated until either the pre-determined safety level is reached or until side effects which are severe, this point is termed the MTD which is the maximum tolerated dose.

MAD studies are conducted to investigate the effect of multiple doses of the medication on subjects in order to further understand the pharmacokinetics and pharmacodynamics of the drug. To undertake the MAD studies, small groups of subjects are given multiple doses of the drug at a level which is known to be safe, they are then monitored in much the same way as for SAD studies and again if no side effects or changes in the pharmacokinetics and pharmacodynamics of the drug are seen then the dose is increased.

Food effect studies are usually quick and easy to perform but provide vital information on the effect of eating on the absorption of the drug into the body. The drug is given to subjects in a fasted state and the level of absorption is measured before the investigation is repeated again at a later date with the subjects having recently eaten. The results from the two are compared and recommendations such as 'take after eating' can be included in the administration instructions on the packaging.

Index

A

B

C

D

E

F

G

H

I

Q

R

S

T